# Racialized Health, COVID-19, and Religious Responses

W0113047

*Racialized Health, COVID-19, and Religious Responses: Black Atlantic Contexts and Perspectives* explores black religious responses to black health concerns amidst persistent race-based health disparities and healthcare inequities. This cutting-edge edited volume provides theoretically and descriptively rich analysis of cases and contexts where race factors strongly in black health outcomes and dynamics, viewing these matters from various disciplinary and national vantage points. The volume is divided into the following four parts:

- Systemic and Socio-Cultural Dimensions of Black Health
- Ecclesial Responses to Black Health Vulnerabilities
- Public Education and Policy Considerations
- Spirituality and the Wellness of Black Minds, Bodies, and Souls

Part I explores ways social and cultural factors such as racial bias, religious conviction, and resource capacity have influenced and delimited black health prospects. Part II looks historically and contemporarily at denominational and ecumenical responses to collective black health emergencies in places such as Nigeria, the UK, the US, and the Caribbean. Part III focuses on public advocacy, particularly collective black health, both in terms of policy and education. The final section deals with spiritual, psychological, and theological dimensions, understandings, and pursuits of black health and wholeness.

Collectively, the essays in the volume delineate analysis and action that wrestle with the multidimensional nature of black wellness and with ways broad public resources and black religious resources should be mobilized and leveraged to ensure collective black wellness.

**R. Drew Smith, PhD**, is a political scientist who serves as professor of Urban Ministry and director of the Metro-Urban Institute at the Pittsburgh Theological Seminary. He is a founding co-convener of the Transatlantic Roundtable on Religion and Race, a global network of scholars, religious leaders, and activists. His publications on religion and public life include more than eighty articles, chapters, and essays, nine edited books, and four themed academic journal issues. He also holds an appointment as Professor Extraordinarious at the Institute for Gender Studies at the University of South Africa.

**Stephanie C. Boddie, PhD**, is an assistant professor in the Diana R. Garland School of Social Work, the George W. Truett Theological Seminary, and the School of Education at Baylor University where she co-teaches Disrupting Racial Disparities in Health Care. She also is a co-convener of the Transatlantic Roundtable on Religion and Race, a professor extraordinarius in the Institute for Gender Studies at University of South Africa, a faculty associate at the Center for Social Development at Washington University and a fellow at the University of Pennsylvania's Program for Research on Religion and Urban Civil Society. She is coauthor of more than sixty journal articles, chapters, and reports, and of several books and short films.

**Bertis D. English, PhD**, is a professor of history at Alabama State University in Montgomery. He is owner of English Editing Services, LLC; author of the book *Civil Wars, Civil Beings in Civil Rights in Alabama's Black Belt: A History of Perry County*; and editor of the *International Journal of Africana Studies*. His scholarly writings appear in state, regional, national, and global publications.

# Racialized Health, COVID-19, and Religious Responses

Black Atlantic Contexts and Perspectives

Edited by
R. Drew Smith, Stephanie C. Boddie,
and Bertis D. English

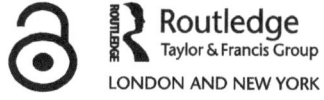

Routledge
Taylor & Francis Group

LONDON AND NEW YORK

First published 2022
by Routledge
2 Park Square, Milton Park, Abingdon, Oxon OX14 4RN

and by Routledge
605 Third Avenue, New York, NY 10158

*Routledge is an imprint of the Taylor & Francis Group,
an informa business*

© 2022 selection and editorial matter, R. Drew Smith, Stephanie C. Boddie, and Bertis D. English; individual chapters, the contributors

The right of R. Drew Smith, Stephanie C. Boddie, and Bertis D. English to be identified as the authors of the editorial material, and of the authors for their individual chapters, has been asserted in accordance with sections 77 and 78 of the Copyright, Designs and Patents Act 1988.

The Open Access version of this book, available at www.taylorfrancis. com, has been made available under a Creative Commons Attribution-Non Commercial-No Derivatives 4.0 license.

*Trademark notice*: Product or corporate names may be trademarks or registered trademarks, and are used only for identification and explanation without intent to infringe.

*British Library Cataloguing-in-Publication Data*
A catalogue record for this book is available from the British Library

*Library of Congress Cataloging-in-Publication Data*
A catalog record has been requested for this book

ISBN: 978-1-032-10223-8 (hbk)
ISBN: 978-1-032-10225-2 (pbk)
ISBN: 978-1-003-21428-1 (ebk)

DOI: 10.4324/9781003214281

Typeset in Times New Roman
by KnowledgeWorks Global Ltd.

# Contents

*List of tables*                                                             ix
*List of contributors*                                                        x

**Introduction: Black Health, Church Responsiveness,
and Transnational Metrics**                                                    1
R. DREW SMITH

**PART I
Systemic and Sociocultural Dimensions of Black Health**                       15

1  **Racializing Religious Institutions during the
   COVID-19 Pandemic**                                                        17
   STEPHANIE C. BODDIE AND JERRY Z. PARK

2  **Racialized Discourses on Disease at Intersections
   of Canadian and the Caribbean Contexts**                                   27
   GOSNELL L. YORKE

3  **Racialized Healthcare Inequities Dating to Slavery**                     35
   ERIC KYERE

4  **Cuban Public Healthcare, Economic Scarcity,
   and COVID-19 Management**                                                  43
   JUALYNNE E. DODSON

5  **Black Health, Ethics, and Global Ecology**                              51
   ERNST M. CONRADIE

6  Food Insecurity, Black Churches, and Black Household
   Vulnerabilities during COVID-19                                    58
   MARGARET LOMBE, VON NEBBITT, KHRISTIAN HOWARD,
   HEBER BROWN III, AND MANSOO YU

7  Setswana Medicinal Practices and Tensions with
   Western Healthcare Perspectives                                    67
   ITUMELENG DANIEL MOTHOAGAE

8  Racism and Clinical Trials of COVID-19, Tetanus,
   and Malaria Vaccines in Kenya                                      75
   ELIAS O. OPONGO


PART II
Ecclesial Responses to Black Health Vulnerabilities                   85

9  The African Methodist Episcopal Church
   and Its Reckonings with Deadly Plagues, 1793–2020                  87
   DENNIS C. DICKERSON

10 Pandemics, the Rev. Francis J. Grimké, and Life Lessons            99
   KATHRYN FREEMAN, ELISE M. EDWARDS, BERTIS ENGLISH,
   AND STEPHANIE C. BODDIE

11 Collins Chapel Hospital and the Christian Methodist
   Episcopal Church Responses to Healthcare Disparities
   in Memphis, Tennessee                                             110
   RAYMOND SOMMERVILLE AND GEORGE W. COLEMAN JR.

12 Black United Methodist Church Responses to COVID-19               120
   CYNTHIA MOORE-KOIKOI

13 The Redeemed Christian Church of God's Responses
   to Contemporary Health Urgencies in Nigeria                       126
   BABATUNDE ADEDIBU AND ADELEKE AWOJOBI

14 The Church of God in Christ, COVID-19,
   and Black Pentecostal Constructive Engagement                     134
   DAVID D. DANIELS III

15 Richard Allen, Black Aid Workers, and Civil Rights
Lessons of the First Great Epidemic in the United States 142
RICHARD NEWMAN

16 Caribbean Churches, Capacities, and Responses
to the COVID-19 Pandemic 148
RONALD A. NATHAN

17 Black Majority Church Responses to Black Health
Urgencies in the United Kingdom 158
NATASHA CALLENDER AND ALTON P. BELL

18 COVID-19, Cultural Competency, and Church
Responsiveness in Nigeria 165
JUSTINA OGODO, MARTHA FOLASHADE ATANDA, A. CHRISTSON ADEDOYIN,
SABRINA A. CARTER, AND JAMAR THRASHER

PART III
Public Education and Policy Considerations 175

19 The Black Church, Public Policy, and
the Challenge of Health Equity 177
QUARDRICOS DRISKELL

20 Black Mental Health Challenges and Responses
by Britain's Black Majority Churches 185
BABATUNDE ADEDIBU

21 Cultural and Religious Influences on Genetic Interventions
in Sub-Saharan Africa 192
MURUGI KAGOTHO AND NJERI KAGOTHO

22 Pastoral Care, the COVID-19 Pandemic, and
Oppression in Port-au-Prince, Haiti 202
B. DENISE HAWKINS AND ERVIN E. DYER

23 Black Women's Reproductive Health, Justice,
and COVID-19 Complications in the United States 208
BERNETTA D. WELCH

24  **Film as a Pedagogical Tool for Trauma- and
    Resiliency-Informed Theology and Liturgy**                           215
    PHIL ALLEN

25  **Shifting the Tide Toward Health Equity**                           225
    LYDELL LETTSOME


PART IV
**Spirituality and the Wellness of Black Minds,
Bodies, and Souls**                                                      235

26  **Nigerian Women, Mental and Physical Health, COVID-19,
    and Spirituality**                                                   237
    SAMUEL E. OLADIPO, A. CHRISTSON ADEDOYIN, JIMOH W. OWOYELE,
    AND HAMMED ADEOYE

27  **African American Palliative Care amid the COVID-19 Pandemic**      245
    JOHN C. WELCH

28  **Black Religion, Mental Health, and the Threat
    of Hopelessness during the COVID-19 Pandemic**                       252
    DANJUMA G. GIBSON


    *Index*                                                              257

# Tables

4.1   Cuba and the Region: Selected Indicators         45

16.1  COVID-19 in Selected Caribbean Countries, June 2020
        and September 2021         150

17.1  Percentage of Overweight or Obese Adults, 2019/2020      159

# List of Contributors

**Babatunde Adedibu, PhD**, is a professor of mission studies and African Christianity and provost of the Redeemed Christian Bible College, an affiliate of the University of Ibadan, Nigeria. He earned a doctorate in missiology at North West University, South Africa, and his research interests include new dynamics of religious experience and expression in Africa and throughout the African Diaspora, with a particular focus on non-Western Christianity.

**A. Christson Adedoyin, PhD**, is a professor of social work in the Department of Social Work, School of Public Health, Samford University, Homewood, Alabama. His research interests include program evaluation, social policy analysis, and faith-based interventions to address socioeconomic and health disparities among African Americans, African immigrants, and African refugees.

**Hammed Adeoye** is an associate professor of applied counselling psychology and educational evaluation sub-dean, College of Specialised and Professional Education, Tai Solarin University of Education, Ijebu-Ode, Nigeria. His research areas of interest include emotional intelligence, sexuality, and educational evaluation. He is a member of the International Society for the Study of Behavioural Development, the Society for Research on Adolescence, and the Counselling Association of Nigeria.

**Phil Allen Jr.** is a PhD degree candidate at Fuller Theological Seminary where he is a Pannell Center for Black Church Studies fellow. His research integrates Black Church theology and praxis, a theology of justice, theological insights for healing racial trauma, and fostering ethics of racial solidarity. He is the founder of the Racial Solidarity Project, a nonprofit, and author of *Open Wounds: A Story of Racial Tragedy, Trauma, and Redemption.*

**Martha Folashade Atanda, MSW**, is a missionary, attorney, and community-based social worker. Widely traveled across the African continent, she directs her energy toward establishing churches among unreached and unengaged groups. She also serves underresourced and underserved populations and is passionate about collaborations to identify and leverage the strengths and assets of individuals, families, and communities to help them flourish and achieve self-sufficiency.

**Stephanie C. Boddie, PhD**, is an assistant professor in the Diana R. Garland School of Social Work, the George W. Truett Theological Seminary, and the School of Education at Baylor University where she coteaches Disrupting Racial Disparities in Health Care. She also is a co-convener of the Transatlantic Roundtable on Religion and Race, a professor extraordinarius in the Institute for Gender Studies at University of South Africa, a faculty associate at the Center for Social Development at Washington University and a fellow at the University of Pennsylvania's Program for Research on Religion and Urban Civil Society. She is a coauthor of more than sixty journal articles, chapters, and reports, and of several books and short films.

**Heber Brown III, DMin**, is a pastor of the Pleasant Hope Baptist Church in Baltimore, Maryland. Reverend Brown also is founder of Black Church Food Security, a multistate alliance of congregations working together to inspire health, wealth, and power in black communities by organizing African American churches to establish gardens on church-owned land. Additionally, the alliance cultivates partnerships with African American farmers to create grassroots, community-led food systems.

**Sabrina A. Carter** is a graduate student in the Diana R. Garland School of Social Work at Baylor University. She also is president and cofounder of Black Leaders Moving Social Work, the first Black student organization of the Garland School. A United States Navy veteran, Carter is passionate about using her education to contribute to diverse, inclusive, and equitable practices for black communities.

**George W. Coleman Jr.** is a Christian Methodist Episcopal pastor and church archivist for the denomination. He also is the director of the First Episcopal District Technology Center.

**Ernst M. Conradie, PhD**, is a senior professor in the Department of Religion and Theology at the University of the Western Cape in South Africa. His work focuses on the intersection of Christian ecotheology, systematic theology, and ecumenical theology and is rooted in the Reformed tradition. He is the author of three books, lead or co-editor of two books, and was the international convener of the Christian Faith and the Earth project from 2007 to 2014.

**David D. Daniels III, PhD**, is the Henry Winters Luce Professor of World Christianity at McCormick Theological Seminary, having joined the faculty in 1987. Daniels earned a doctorate in church history from Union Theological Seminary, serves on the editorial board of the *Journal of*

*World Christianity*, and has authored more than sixty academic journal articles and book chapters. He specializes on the Black Church, world Christianity, and global Pentecostalism.

**Dennis C. Dickerson, PhD**, is the Reverend James Lawson Chair in History at Vanderbilt University. Previously, he was the Stanfield Professor of History at Williams College. He is author of *Out of the Crucible: Black Steel Workers in Pennsylvania, 1875–1980, Militant Mediator: Whitney M. Young, Jr., African American Preachers and Politics: The Careys of Chicago*, and *The African Methodist Episcopal Church*.

**Jualynne E. Dodson, PhD**, is a professor of sociology at Michigan State University. She earned a doctorate from the University of California, Berkeley, served as research director for Atlanta University School of Social Work, and dean of seminary life at the Union Theological Seminary in New York City. Dodson founded the African Atlantic Research Team at University of Colorado, Boulder from which MSU appointed her 'John Hannah Distinguished Professor' before recruiting her to join the faculty.

**Quardricos B. Driskell, MPS, MTS**, manages the legislative and political affairs department for the American Urological Association. He also is an adjunct professor of legislative politics at the George Washington University Graduate School of Political Management and serves as senior pastor of the Beulah Baptist Church in Alexandria, Virginia. His work appears in the *Hill*, the *New York Times*, Voice of America, NBC News, *Religion and Politics*, MSNBC, the Religion News Service, and the BBC.

**Ervin E. Dyer, PhD**, is a writer, editor, and sociologist based in Pittsburgh, Pennsylvania, where serves as adjunct professor in the University of Pittsburgh Africana Studies Department. A Pulitzer Center grant recipient, his research focuses on the African Diaspora.

**Elise M. Edwards, PhD**, is an assistant professor of Religion at Baylor University and a registered architect in Florida. Her research is interdisciplinary, drawing on theology, ethics, architectural theory, and religion. She develops Christian theological and ethical perspectives on civic engagement, cultural and artistic expressions of marginalized communities, and racial and gendered justice.

**Bertis D. English, PhD**, is a professor of history at Alabama State University in Montgomery. He is owner of English Editing Services, LLC; author of the book *Civil Wars, Civil Beings in Civil Rights in Alabama's Black Belt: A History of Perry County*; and editor of the *International Journal of Africana Studies*. His scholarly writings appear in state, regional, national, and global publications.

**Kathryn Freeman, JD, MDiv**, is a graduate of the University of Texas School of Law and the Baylor University George W. Truett Theological Seminary. She has ten years of experience in nonprofit advocacy and enjoys teaching faith leaders how to engage the political process for the common good and for God's glory. Freeman writes about the intersection of faith and pop culture and cohosts "Melanated Faith," a podcast that focuses on race, faith, and culture.

**Danjuma G. Gibson, PhD**, is the professor of pastoral care at Calvin Theological Seminary, and a licensed psychotherapist in Grand Rapids, Michigan. His book, *Frederick Douglass, A Psychobiography: Rethinking Subjectivity in the Western Experiment of Democracy*, investigates the formation of Douglass's psychological and religious identity in the context of trauma and American slavocracy.

**B. Denise Hawkins, MA**, is an award-winning journalist and communications consultant based in the Washington, DC, area. Before launching her consultancy, Orchard Hill Communications, LLC, she held senior-level positions at public relations firms and national media companies, focusing on higher education and science, technology, engineering, and mathematics. Her stories and photographs appear in the *Washington Post*, among other major news outlets.

**Khristian Howard, MSW**, is regional manager for SNAP Strategy at the Baylor Collaborative on Hunger and Poverty. Her research and service focuses on sustainable solutions to food insecurity, especially teenagers, coalition building, and participatory research methods. She earned an undergraduate degree from Georgia State University and completed graduate work at the Diana R. Garland School of Social Work at Baylor University.

**Murugi Kagotho, MSc**, is an education researcher based in Nairobi, Kenya, with an academic background in molecular genetics and educational neuroscience. Her interests and present work lie at the intersection of those subjects and environmental factors that contribute to learning attainment. She is the cofounder of Library-in-a-Box, a community initiative that promotes recreational reading by providing mobile libraries to underserved children in Nairobi and its environs.

**Njeri Kagotho, PhD**, is a social worker and associate professor in The Ohio State University College of Social Work. Her international practice influences her scholarly work, which spans multiple continents, applies a transformative lens, and centers community voices in furthering the pursuit of social justice. She often investigates influences of formal and informal institutions on economic and health behavior, concentrating on linkages between institutions, household wealth, and health outcomes.

**Eric Kyere, PhD**, is an assistant professor of social work and adjunct professor of Africana Studies at Indiana University–Purdue University Indianapolis. He theorizes racism, examining ways it denies African-descended people access to psychosocial, educational, and societal opportunities. Through his work, which also entails researching lasting effects of the transatlantic slave trade and colonialism, Kyere explores ways education can interrupt racism and advance social justice.

**Lydell C. Lettsome, MD, MDiv**, is a board-certified general surgeon who serves as clinical director for Quality Wound Care in Hawthorne, New Jersey. He earned degrees from Columbia University, Union Theological Seminary, and Jefferson Medical College. Lettsome studies Christian and medical ethics, and he authored the award-winning book, *Stolen Money, Stolen Health*.

**Margaret Lombe, PhD**, is an associate professor in the Boston University School of Social Work. She also is a faculty associate at the Center for Social Development at Washington University in St. Louis. She specializes in international social development, with an emphasis on global health equity, social inclusion/exclusion, and capacity building. She is author of more than thirty book chapters, reports, and peer-reviewed publications and is coeditor of *Children and AIDS: Sub-Saharan Africa*.

**Cynthia M. Moore-Koikoi, MDiv**, is a bishop of the United Methodist Church, a position she has held since 2017. She worked as a school psychologist for seven years before entering the ministry, whereupon she pastored a church in East Baltimore, Maryland, and served as associate pastor in Annapolis. Moore-Koikoi earned an undergraduate degree from Loyola College in Maryland and graduate degrees from the University of Maryland and Wesley Theological Seminary.

**Itumeleng Daniel Mothoagae, PhD**, is a lecturer of the New Testament and early Christian studies in the Department of Biblical and Ancient Studies at the University of South Africa. New Testament Ethics, cultural translation studies, post-colonial Bible translation, decoloniality, African biblical interpretation, and cultural studies are his specializations, though he also has interests in the Black Theology of liberation, African ethics, critical spatiality theory, space and literature, and identity studies.

**Ronald A. Nathan, MTh**, is an ordained elder with the AME Zion Church. He has been in Christian ministry for four decades, having served in Barbados, Kenya, Trinidad and Tobago, and the United Kingdom. He currently pastors the Hoggard AME Zion Church in Jackson, St. Michael, Barbados. Nathan has published scholarly articles on Africentricity, Pan-African theology, and the Black Church. He sits on several international boards, including the Transatlantic Roundtable on Religion and Race.

**Von Nebbitt, PhD**, is an associate professor in the Brown School at Washington University in St. Louis. His research assesses how exposure to community and household violence, peer networks, social cohesion, and belonging are related to the mental, behavioral, and physical health of adolescents. His book, *Adolescents in Public Housing: Addressing Psychological and Behavioral Health*, is a study of youth living in public housing facilities based upon data collected in multiple cities across the United States.

**Richard Newman, PhD**, is a professor of history at the Rochester Institute of Technology and author or editor of seven books on American and African American history, including *Freedom's Prophet: Bishop Richard Allen, the AME Church, and the Black Founding Fathers*. He also appeared as a commentator in the Public Broadcasting Service series, *The Black Church*, written, hosted, and directed by Harvard University professor Henry Louis Gates Jr.

**Justina A. Ogodo, PhD**, is an assistant professor in the Department of Curriculum and Instruction at the Baylor University School of Education. Her research centers on science curricula, teacher knowledge, and culturally relevant and responsive education in urban school settings, among other areas. She has published multiple peer-reviewed scholarly articles and book chapters.

**Samuel E. Oladipo, PhD**, is a professor of applied social psychology, dean of the College of Specialised and Professional Education, and director of the Directorate of Research and External Relations at Tai Solarin University of Education, Ogun State, Nigeria. A National Research Fund recipient, his research spans spirituality and health, educational research, human immunodeficiency virus, acquired immunodeficiency syndrome, gender-based violence, and child abuse.

**Adeleke Adeyemo Olujobi, PhD**, is a chaplain and acting academic dean at the Redeemed Christian Bible College, Nigeria, where he earned a doctorate in theology and a postgraduate diploma and master's degree. Olujobi also earned an undergraduate degree in agricultural economics and extension from the Ladoke Akinola University of Technology and an undergraduate degree in Christian Religious Studies from Ajayi Crowther University. Olujobi also has a postgraduate diploma from Redeemers University.

**Elias O. Opongo, PhD**, is a senior lecturer at Hekima Institute of Peace Studies and International Relations and director of the Centre for Research, Training and Publications at Hekima University College in Nairobi, Kenya. A Jesuit priest, Opongo earned a doctorate in peace studies from the University of Bradford in the United Kingdom and a master's degree in international peace studies from University of Notre Dame in the United Sates. His book publications include *African Theology in the 21st Century.*

**Jimoh Wale Owoyele, PhD,** is an associate professor of psychometrics and counselling psychology in the Department of Counselling Psychology and Educational Foundations, College of Specialized and Professional Education, Tai Solarin University of Education, Ijagun, Nigeria. He also is deputy director of the Directorate of Academic Planning and Quality Assurance at the university. Owoyele has published several articles and research papers in national and international academic journals.

**Jerry Z. Park, PhD,** is an associate professor of sociology at Baylor University. His research interests include the sociological study of religion, race, identity, culture, and civic participation. Recent publications focus on religion and inequality attitudes, religion and workplace attitudes, religious attitudes of academic scientists, and Asian American religiosity. He earned his bachelor's degree in psychology from the University of Virginia, and a master's and doctorate in sociology from University of Notre Dame.

**R. Drew Smith, PhD,** is a political scientist who serves as professor of Urban Ministry and director of the Metro-Urban Institute at the Pittsburgh Theological Seminary. He is a founding co-convener of the Transatlantic Roundtable on Religion and Race, a global network of scholars, religious leaders, and activists. His publications on religion and public life include more than eighty articles, chapters, and essays, nine edited books, and four themed academic journal issues.

**Raymond (Ron) Sommerville Jr., PhD,** is historian of the Christian Methodist Episcopal (CME) Church and Emeritus Professor of Church History at Christian Theological Seminary. A third-generation CME minister, he pastored churches in North Carolina and in Ohio. He earned an undergraduate degree from Miles College, a graduate degree from Duke Divinity School, and a doctorate from Vanderbilt University. His publications include *An Ex-Colored Church: Social Activism in the CME Church, 1870–1970.*

**Jamar Thrasher, MS,** is a press secretary at the Pennsylvania Department of Environmental Protection, owns the public relations firm Kennedy Blue Communications, which provides media relations, copywriting, and copyediting services to clients across the world. He earned an undergraduate degree in political science and communication from the University of Pittsburgh and a graduate degree in public policy and management from Carnegie Mellon University.

**Bernetta D. Welch, PhD,** is a senior pastor of the Bidwell Presbyterian Church. Her education includes a doctorate in healthcare ethics from Duquesne University, a Master of Divinity degree from Pittsburgh

Theological Seminary, a Bachelor of Science degree from Geneva College, and an associate degree from Robert Morris University. Reverend Welch has served as chaplain at the University of Pittsburgh Medical Center Western Psychiatric Hospital and spiritual care provider at the Family Hospice and Palliative Care.

**John C. Welch, PhD**, is a senior pastor of the Sixth Mount Zion Missionary Baptist Church in Pittsburgh, Pennsylvania. He served thirteen years as dean of students and vice president for Student Service and Community Engagement at the Pittsburgh Theological Seminary. Welch earned a bachelor's degree in chemical engineering and economics from Carnegie Mellon University, a master's degree in divinity from Pittsburgh Seminary, and a doctorate in healthcare ethics from Duquesne University.

**Gosnell L. Yorke, PhD**, is a senior lecturer in the Dag Hammarskjöld Institute for Peace and Conflict Studies at the Copperbelt University, Zambia. Born in the Caribbean, Yorke is a naturalized citizen of Canada and of South Africa. He is co-convener of the Transatlantic Roundtable on Religion and Race. Yorke has taught in Canada, Kenya, Nigeria, South Africa, the United States, and Zimbabwe. He has published on Pan-Africanism, biblical and translation studies, and on religion and human rights.

**Mansoo Yu, PhD**, is a professor in the University of Missouri-Columbia School of Health Professions with a joint appointment at the Missouri Department of Public Health. He is a fellow at the Society for Social Work Research and a member of the Delta Omega Public Health Honorary Society. His research and writing focus on health disparities and the interconnections of mental health, physical health, and health risk behavior.

# Introduction

## Black Health, Church Responsiveness, and Transnational Metrics

*R. Drew Smith*

This volume draws attention to multiple ways black health prospects and outcomes are configured by the actions, inactions, and cultural capital of social institutions and leaders, including within the governmental sector, the healthcare sector, and the religious sector. Facilitating and ensuring conditions conducive to public health, and capacities for provision of public healthcare, are macro tasks, requiring substantial institutional, financial, and technological resources. Government sectors and healthcare sectors around the globe are where this scale of resources are concentrated, though in varying degrees reflective of global wealth disparities. As these disparities and inequities have become increasingly evident, including as a result of the COVID-19 crisis, it has become more urgent to hold sectors charged with public health accountable in fulfilling their public charge.

Civil society leaders, including faith-sector leaders, have an important role to play in drawing attention to healthcare gaps and providing supplementary support and services in response to these gaps. Where gaps have existed in public health resources and commitments, faith sector leaders and institutions have sought oftentimes to leverage their institutional and moral resources as supplement and counterweight. This has been especially evident in black contexts, where an accumulation of social factors has unfavorably disposed their collective health prospects and their availability of systematic healthcare.

The urgencies are clear, given how much worse black populations across the transatlantic have fared than white and other ethnic population groups on important health indices as measured in life expectancy, frequencies of illnesses, access to professional healthcare, and (as seen during the COVID-19 emergency) vulnerability to major outbreaks of disease. Moreover, inequities in health profiles and prospects across global demographics and geographies have become more pronounced—with those inequities manifesting within countries as well as between countries. As reported by the World Health Organization's Commission on Social Determinants of Health in 2008: "In countries at all levels of income, health and illness follow a social gradient: the lower the socioeconomic situation, the worse the health."[1]

In addition to the level of resources channeled toward public health is the level of public will and commitment to a qualitative and quantitative maximizing of

DOI: 10.4324/9781003214281-1

public healthcare—and there have been vast differences and disparities on this matter as well from one social context to another. In all of these contexts, racial and ethnic disparities in health prospects have been undergirded by formalized social policies, institutional practices, and cultural rationales. Each of these factors affect social contexts and conditions in ways impacting health prospects, especially in regard to the relative healthiness or toxicity of the physical environment (e.g., air, water, soil, food sources) and of the social environment (e.g., inter- and intra-group relations, conceptions of personhood and peoplehood, collective discourses and conveyances more broadly), and as measured by access to resources bearing-upon wellness prospects (e.g., healthcare providers, health insurance, quality nutrition, and preventive care resources). Unfortunately, racial and ethnic biases and bigotries have skewed these factors in ways more fully facilitating the healthfulness of persons of means, especially whites, than of persons without means, especially blacks). The COVID pandemic has expanded public attention to these disparities and intensified their dire health consequences for black and brown populations.

The volume, focusing across the transatlantic, explores black religious responses to black health concerns amidst persistent race-based health disparities and healthcare inequities. In doing so, it provides theoretically and descriptively rich analysis of cases and contexts where race factors strongly in black health outcomes and dynamics, viewing these matters from various disciplinary and national vantage points. Collectively, the essays in the volume delineate analysis and action that wrestle with the multidimensional nature of black wellness and with ways broad public resources and black religious resources should be mobilized and leveraged to ensure collective black wellness.

The volume aligns theoretically with an increasing emphasis within public health research and analysis on nonmedical factors impacting health prospects and outcomes. Factors such as income, race/ethnicity, education, health beliefs, ideational contexts, and other factors framing physical and normative environments have been receiving at least as much attention as personal behavioral factors as determinants of public health.[2] Attention to systems and structures seems even more necessary given the growing occurrences of epidemics in recent decades—including major outbreaks of swine flu, cholera, measles, Ebola, and COVID-19 within the previous 20 years that resulted in thousands of deaths in each instance. Each essay in the volume opens out directly or indirectly on the COVID pandemic, especially the systems-level understandings and approaches out of which black faith-based actors have operated in their responses to the pandemic.

## Racially Disproportionate COVID-19 Infections and Mortalities

According to data on COVID deaths within the United States through August 2020, black deaths were almost four times the rate of white deaths, and Latino/ae deaths three times the rate of white deaths (with blacks at

118, Latino/ae at 99, and whites at 33 per 100,000 persons).[3] By March 2021, racial disparities had decreased somewhat although overall mortality rates had increased across the board, with US deaths per 100,000 for blacks at 178, for Latino/ae persons at 154, and for whites at 124.[4]

Canada also has evidenced racial disparities in rates of COVID infections. Data from October 2020 showed COVID mortality rates were 35 per 100,000 residents in Canadian neighborhoods where 25 percent or greater of the residents were "visible minorities," as compared to 17 per 100,000 in neighborhoods where less than 1 percent of residents were visible minorities and 13 per 100,000 where 1–10 percent of residents were visible minorities.[5] In February 2021, black Canadians constituted more than 20 percent of COVID infections even though they made up only 9 percent of the Canadian population.[6]

Race-specific data are less available on European contexts, but a July 2020 study showed that mortality rates in France for persons born in sub-Saharan Africa increased by 114 percent during March and April 2020 as compared to an increase of only 22 percent for persons born in France. An October 2020 report focusing on Britain indicated that "58,000 more people would have died in the first wave of the coronavirus in Britain if the white population had faced the same risk as Black communities."[7]

One can track COVID-19 infections and deaths across demographics and geographies in ways besides race—specifically, in regional difference between Global North and Global South countries.[8] In August 2020, for example, Africa had a far lower rate of COVID infections and deaths compared to several places in the Global North.[9] Africa had 1,037,135 persons infected and 22,916 deaths, whereas Europe had 3,061,264 people infected and 207,215 dead.[10] The US had 10,615,855 people infected and 389,793 deaths.[11] There were spikes in multiple sub-Saharan African countries from December through February 2021, especially in southern Africa and most noticeably in South Africa. Cases mostly subsided from March through May to pre-spike rates across most of southern Africa, but then escalated dramatically in June as part of a "third wave," propelled by COVID variants such as the Delta variant that has been traced to South Africa.[12]

The rate of new infections and deaths in South Africa increased dramatically during June and July 2021, with the country's COVID deaths rising to 42nd highest in the world at 1,098 per day, Namibia's rising to 54th in the world at 798 deaths per day, and Botswana's rising to 65th in the world at 522 deaths per day.[13] As of early July, South Africa reported 2.1 million cases of COVID infection and 63,000 deaths, far outpacing any other Sub-Saharan African country.[14]

In addition to the Global North–South social disparities South Africa embodies alongside other Global South countries, South Africa's legacy of separate development—apartheid—and its enduring manifestations of race-based inequalities, especially with respect to income, employment, housing, health conditions, and healthcare access, have contributed to greater

COVID vulnerabilities and frequencies of infection and death among black South Africans. As indicated in a January 2021 Oxfam International report, "it is black South Africans in rural, peri-urban, and informal settlements who are hit the hardest by the COVID-19 pandemic."[15]

Similarly, the COVID pandemic's impact within many Latin American nations also reflects the dual impact of Global North–South disparities and domestic racial disparities. For example, as July 12, 2021, Brazil has lost almost 531,000 persons to COVID, which was the second highest number of deaths per country in the world behind the United States.[16] Regionally, Brazil's COVID mortality numbers dwarfed those of other Latin American countries, with more than twice the number of Mexico's COVID deaths, almost three times the number in Peru, and roughly five times the number in Columbia and Argentina.[17] Other Latin American countries experienced fewer than 10 percent of Brazil's number of COVID deaths.[18]

Race has been a factor in frequencies of COVID infections and deaths in several Latin American countries. In Brazil, for example, COVID has dispro-portionately impacted its Afro-descendants (a contested demographic desig-nation but referring to the 83 million brown and 13 million black persons who constitute approximately half of Brazil's population).[19] In April 2020, Afro-descendants made up 35 percent of Brazil's COVID mortalities compared to 65 percent by non-Afrodescendants.[20] By June 2020, the numbers flipped with Afrodescendant persons constituting 60 percent of COVID mortalities and non-Afrodescendants constituting 40 percent.[21] Similarly, in Columbia, where up to 25 percent of persons have been reported to explicitly identify as Afro-Columbians, seven of the country's municipalities with the largest num-ber of Afrodescendant persons had the highest number of COVID cases and six of those municipalities had the highest number of COVID mortalities.[22]

The Caribbean region has fared much better than the rest of the Americas. While all North, Central, and South American countries except for Venezuela and Nicaragua were in the top 100 countries with respect to deaths per capita as of July 12, 2021, only Puerto Rico (55th), Trinidad and Tobago (61st), Jamaica (71st), and Dominican Republic (73rd) were among Caribbean countries ranked in the top 100 COVID-19 deaths per capita.[23] Because 7 Caribbean island nations had populations fewer than 100,000 people and only 8 had populations exceeding 500,000, the actual numbers of COVID deaths per country tended to be quite small compared to the world's more heavily populated countries.[24] The highest number of COVID deaths among Caribbean countries with fewer than 100,000 was Antigua and Barbuda's 42, while 5 of those countries had 1 or no death.[25]

## Structural and Systemic Influences on COVID Impact

There have been distinctive COVID vulnerabilities associated with par-ticular types of employment, especially related to food services, transpor-tation services, cleaning services, childcare services, agricultural work, manufacturing work, and other types of essential services in which black and brown populations are disproportionately involved. A December 2020 University of California-Merced study of COVID health impact on California workers showed a 30 percent increase since Mach in deaths among persons working in ten essential service industries—agriculture, bars, building services, food processing, grocery, landscaping, nursing care, restaurants/food service, warehousing, and wholesale trade—with 87 percent of deaths coming from low-wage workers.[26] The study also indicated that black people working in those industries had a 34 percent increased risk of death and that Latino/ae people had a 59 percent increased risk of death.[27] In Canada, meanwhile, almost two-thirds of black people reported commuting to work during the COVID crisis (with those persons twice as likely as other groups to use public transportation) and 50 percent more likely than non-black people to have sought medical treatment for COVID-related illnesses.[28]

A majority of the workforce in sub-Saharan Africa are involved in low-wage jobs requiring personal contact with other persons, leading to increased vulnerability to COVID exposure and infection. Reporting from South Africa has shown work of that sort, such as supermarket employment, have created COVID infection hotpots.[29] With respect to Latin America and the Caribbean, the Organisation for Economic Co-operation and Development points out 80 percent of the region's population lived in urban context, 21 percent live in slums, and 60 percent work in the informal sector—with all three factors contributing to increased vulnerability to COVID exposure and infection.[30]

Job loss is a secondary impact of the COVID crisis in black and brown communities (and at times has had major health implications). The US lost more than 20 million jobs in April 2020 alone as the pandemic forced businesses to suspend operation.[31] Nearly 4 million jobs were lost permanently, and roughly 100,000 businesses closed.[32] Black and brown workers were especially hard hit, given their concentration in leisure and hospitality, occupation in which the unemployment rate soared from roughly 5 percent in March to 40 percent in April.[33] Immediately north of the US, in Canada, 18 percent of black people who participated in an African-Canadian Civic Engagement Council and Innovative Research Group telephone survey reported being laid off from their jobs in June because of COVID, as compared with 13 percent of the national population in general.[34] Thirty-eight percent of black Canadians aged 45 or older experienced a significant negative impact on household finances from COVID, as compared with 22 percent of the national population in the same age group.[35]

In Africa, 45 percent of Nigerians had to stop work because of COVID by June 2020, as did 17 percent of Ugandans.[36] Here, again, increased COVID-period unemployment among African workers resulted in large part from concentrations of African workers in employment sectors particularly hard hit by the COVID shutdown, including the informal sector which comprises more than 50 percent of workers in Senegal and Namibia and 80 percent in Kenya.[37] With 60 percent of Caribbean and Latin American workers involved in the informal sector and with such a strong reliance in that region upon tourism industries, COVID restrictions have had detrimental impacts on the economic security and the overall well-being of people in general and low-wage laborers in particular.

Economic and employment insecurities are part of the poverty metrics that have made black and brown populations disproportionately vulnerable to the health perils of the COVID pandemic. Such insecurities translate into insufficient access to preventive and interventionary healthcare facilitated through employer health insurance benefits and through direct income they can apply toward healthcare services. Employment and income deficits, which worsened during the COVID shutdown, have compounded already fraught public health circumstances within low-income and racial/ethnic minority communities.

## Vaccination Disparities

In addition to the matters discussed above, scientists, medical researchers, and other observers have tied COVID vulnerabilities to whether people receive protections afforded by vaccinations. Racial/ethnic disparities have persisted in the United States, Canada, and European countries since vaccinations became available in December 2020.[38] Before the month ended, whites, Native Americans, Hispanics, and Asians in the United States were getting vaccinated at twice the rate of blacks.[39] By early February 2021, Native Americans (11 percent) were receiving vaccinations at four times the rate of blacks (2.5 percent), Asians and whites continued doing so at two times the rate of blacks, and Hispanics at about the same rate as blacks.[40] As of July 2021, 46 percent of Native Americans had received at least one dose of the vaccine, 37 percent of Asians, 34 percent of whites, and 33 percent of Hispanics but only 26 percent of blacks.[41]

In Canada, 68 percent of the population got at least one dose of vaccine by mid-July 2021 (compared to 48 percent of the US population), but willingness to become inoculated varied by race/ethnicity.[42] While 77 percent of nonvisible minority Canadians aged 12 or older indicated a willingness to receive the COVID vaccine (including 83 percent of the Asian Canadian population), only 66 percent of Latino/ae Canadians and 57 percent of black Canadians indicated a willingness to be vaccinated.[43] Among European countries, 68 percent of people in the United Kingdom had received at least on vaccination by mid-July, as had 60 percent of Italians, 59 percent of Germans, and 53 percent of French.[44] Once more, a pattern of lower racial/ethnic minority vaccination rates and willingness to receive vaccines was apparent. with mid-January 2021 data from Britain, for example, showing 21 percent of blacks over age 80 (as compared to 43 percent of whites) and

37 percent of black healthcare workers (as compared with 71 percent of white healthcare workers) being vaccinated.[45]

Vaccinations in Africa, Caribbean, and Latin America have trailed North America and Europe by a large margin. As of early July, dosages per 100 persons were 101 in North America, 71 in Europe, 42 in Latin America and the Caribbean, and 4 in Africa.[46] Vaccination rates were similarly wide in Caribbean nations. Trinidad and Tobago was on the low end of the spectrum: 4 percent of its population had gotten at least 1 dosage.[47] The island of Saba was at the high end, with 67 percent of its population receiving at least 1 dose.[48]

A lack of access to vaccines is one reason for low inoculation rates among Global South populations. A May 2021 report indicated distribution in the Caribbean was uneven.[49] Almost midway through the month, the Dominican Republic had forged agreements to receive enough vaccines from Western manufacturers to cover 132 percent of its population, while Jamaica had agreements sufficient to cover only 16 percent.[50] Similar disparities existed within Latin American countries. Chile had agreements to receive enough supply to cover 242 percent of its population, but Venezuela had agreements sufficient to cover less than 2 percent.[51] Despite large populations, African countries had less than 2 percent of the global supply in June.[52]

Low confidence levels in the safety or the effectiveness of vaccines is another cause of lagging vaccination rates among black and other ethnic minority groups, including those in the Global North. When governments worldwide began authorizing vaccines in December 2020, more than 50 percent of African Americans indicated they would take a "wait and see" approach to getting vaccinated.[53] Another 25 percent indicated taking a vaccine only if required.[54] By mid-June 2021 the percentage of African Americans who said they would wait and see had dropped to 15 percent, with another 15 percent saying only a mandate would cause them to become vaccinated.[55] Hispanic Americans were comparable to African Americans on those December 2020 and June 2021 data points.[56]

December 2020 polling in the UK showed 57 percent of black and ethnic minority people were willing to receive COVID vaccinations.[57] Among Caribbean countries, June 2021 findings from a survey conducted by the Caribbean Public Health Agency indicated 32 to 62 percent of the population was hesitant to become vaccinated.[58] Whatever the reason for low rates among black people, inequities and imbalances pose an ongoing threat to their health and, by extension, to global health.

## Placing Faith Sector Responses in Perspective

The religious sector often has served as a social as well as a spiritual resource for black communities in times of hardship and struggle. The importance of religion in those instances traces largely to its privileged position within black communities, both as a function of demand (i.e., high levels of religious commitment) and of default (e.g., abandonment of black people by other social support sectors). In the Americas, Europe, and Africa, there is substantial evidence of widespread black Christian adherence. According to data the Pew Research Center publicized in 2014, 79 percent of African Americans identified as Christian.[59] That percentage was 8 percent higher than Americans overall.[60]

By 2018, Africa had the largest number of Christians, 599 million, in the world (Latin America was second with 597 million), and scholars estimated the number of African Christians to increase to 1.25 billion by 2050 (Latin American Christians would increase to 700 million).[61] If realizes, Africa's share of world's Christians population would rise from 25 percent to 40 percent in that span of time.[62]

In Europe, African immigrants have been responsible in large part for new dimensions of church vitality and numerical growth within an otherwise declining European Christianity. That vibrancy has emanated mainly from Pentecostal expressions, particularly black Pentecostals, whose numerical expansion in the UK has been especially strong. Between 2005 and 2012 alone, 400 of 700 new Pentecostal congregations in London, the most populous city in the island nation, were black majority churches.[63]

Despite a prevalence of black Christian identification and involvement sufficient to generate characterizations of African American Christianity as "the cultural womb of the black community" and of African Christianity as a "new center of gravity in the Christian world," people worldwide have vigorously debated the social strengths of black Christianity from one place and time to another.[64] Analyses of African American Christianity through the mid-twentieth century often characterized that brand of Christendom as more of a refuge from hostile society than a resource for social empowerment.[65] For centuries, however, resourceful African American churches had engaged in institution-building and in delivering social services that incessant racism necessitated.[66] During the mid-twentieth century, moreover, African American churchgoers helped lead fights for racial justice and additional freedoms, including women's rights.[67] Future churchgoers have been active in movements to not only preserve but also expand the gains those earlier generations fought and won to advance human and civil rights.[68]

Black Christianity in Canada has run parallel to black Christianity in the United States in certain key respects. According to scholar Carol B. Duncan, black Canadian Christianity represents a "cross-border social, cultural, and religious experience ... directly tied to expressions of freedom and autonomy [and] resistance and adaptations to the exigencies of life under legalized chattel slavery and the legacy of racism."[69] Black Canadian Christianity, Duncan expounds, draws richly on black religious in-migrations from the United States, the Caribbean, Africa, and Europe, with all the "competing loyalties and hybrid identities" that might be expected from that social, geographical, and theological array.[70] In those ways, Afro-Canada symbolizes black Atlantic intersections in important ways that have translated into a plurality of understandings and expressions of the social role of black religion, especially within varying diasporic contexts in the Americas and Europe.

Actually, there has been a strong emphasis throughout black diasporic and continental Africa on a Christian focus on, in descending order of importance, spiritual fortification, religious discipleship, group connectivity, societal integration, and (to a lesser degree) political activism. The more social aspects frequently have operated in an active tension with aspects bearing more explicitly on religiosity. Scholar Paul Gifford argues that African Christianity too often has been more politically passive and socially conformist institution than transformational, far too willing to embrace rather than challenge unjust and nondemocratic practices within its African contexts.[71] Many other scholars, however, have criticizes the analytical frameworks out of which such assessments often operate as imposing flat liberationist measurements that insufficiently understand African churches' vitality and impact.[72] Scholars across the Black Atlantic have held similar debates about tensions and tradeoffs about black Christianity's social and spiritual contributions.[73]

Although not an area in which black churches have specialized, black health has been an area of interest, nonetheless, in the black religious sector. Black churchgoers have supported health education, advocated fair health policy, and championed equitable healthcare provisions. Black churchgoers also have established and helped operate clinics, created midwife networks and, more frequently, developed spiritual healing and therapy practices. Moreover, the black religious sector has engaged black health concerns through its broader responsiveness to, as well as critiques of, conditions influencing black health prospects, including legislative conversations about such matters.[74]

## Volume Structure

The essays in this volume examine myriad dimensions of Black Church engagement, but emphasize the impact of the COVID-19 pandemic. Section 1 explores ways social and cultural factors such as racial bias, religious conviction, and resource capacity have influenced and delimited black health prospects. Section 2 looks historically and contemporarily at denominational and ecumenical responses to collective black health emergencies in places such as Nigeria, the UK, the US, and the Caribbean. Section 3 focuses on public advocacy, particularly collective black health, both in terms of policy and education. The final section deals with spiritual, psychological, and theological dimensions, understandings, and pursuits of black health and wholeness.

## Notes

1  World Health Organization Commission on Social Determinants of Heath, *Closing the Gap in a Generation: Health Equity Through Action on the Social Determinants of Health* (Geneva: World Health Organization, 2008), ii.

2  Susan E. Short and Stefanie Mollborn, "Social Determinants and Health Behaviors: Conceptual Frames and Empirical Advances," *Current Opinion Psychology* 5 (October 2015): 78.

3  Wei Li, "Racial Disparities in COVID 19," *Harvard University Graduate School of Arts and Sciences Science in the News*, October 24, 2020, https://sitn.hms.harvard.edu/flash/2020/racial-disparities-in-covid-19/.

4  "COVID-19 Is Affecting Black, Indigenous, Latinx, and Other People of Color the Most," *COVID Tracking Project*, September 15, 2020, https://covidtracking.com/race.

5  Rajendra Subedi, Lawson Greenberg, and Martin Turcotte, "COVID-19 Mortality Rates in Canada's Ethno-Cultural Neighbourhoods," *Statistics Canada*, October 28, 2020, https://www150.statcan.gc.ca/n1/pub/45-28-0001/2020001/article/00079-eng.htm. According to the Employment Equity Act, visible minorities are defined as "persons, other than Aboriginal peoples, who are non-Caucasian in race or non-white in colour." *Statistics Canada*, March 25, 2021, https://www23.statcan.gc.ca/imdb/p3Var.pl?Function=DEC&Id=45152.

6  "Understanding the Impact of COVID-19 on Black Canadians: Q and A with Dr. Upton Allen," *Genome Canada*, February 26, 2021, https://www.genome-canada.ca/en/news/blog/understanding-impact-covid-19-black-canadians.

7  Victoria Waldersee, "COVID Toll Turns Spotlight on Europe's Taboo of Data by Race," *Reuters,* November 19, 2020, https://www.reuters.com/article/health-coronavirus-europe-data-insight/covid-toll-turns-spotlight-on-europes-taboo-of-data-by-race-idUSKBN27Z0M3.

8  Global South and Global North are contested terms, referring possibly to geography or to economics. The South (e.g., Africa, Asia, Latin America, Oceania) is less developed than the North (e.g., Australia, Canada, Europe, Israel, Japan, New Zealand, Russia, Singapore, South Korea, the United States). For representative scholarly discussions about such matters, see Nour Dados and Raewyn Connell, "The Global South," *Contexts* 11 (winter 2012): 12–3; and Jean-Philippe Thérien, "Beyond the North–South divide: The Two Tales of World Poverty," *Third World Journal* 20 (August 1999): 723–42.

9  Itai Chitungo et al., "COVID-19: Unpacking the Low Number of Cases in Africa," *Public Health in Practice* 1 (November 2020): 1, https://doi.org/10.1016/j.puhip.2020.100038.

10  Itai Chitungo et al., "COVID-19," 1.

11  Itai Chitungo et al., "COVID-19," 1.

12  "Africa's Third Wave is Killing Thousands and the World is not Paying Attention," *PATH*, July 1, 2020, https://www.path.org/articles/africas-third-wave-is-killing-thousands-and-the-world-is-not-paying-attention/; United Nations, "COVID-19: Africa 'Third Wave' not yet Over, while Vaccine Inequity Threatens All," July 22, 2021, https://news.un.org/en/story/2021/07/1096252 (hereafter cited as UN).

13  "Coronavirus (COVID-19) Deaths Worldwide per One Million Population" *Statista*, July 12, 2021, https://www.statista.com/statistics/1104709/coronavirus-deaths-worldwide-per-million-inhabitants/.

14  David McKenzie, "Southern Africa Hoped It was through the Worst of COVID-19. Then the Delta Variant Arrived," *CNN*, July 9, 2021, https://www.cnn.com/2021/07/09/africa/southern-africa-covid-delta-intl-cmd/index.html; UN "COVID-19."

15 Vuyokazi Futshane, "COVID-19 in South Africa: The Intersections of Race and Inequality," *Oxfam International*, March 16, 2021, https://oxfam.medium. com/covid-19-in-south-africa-the-intersections-of-race-and-inequality-e71696bd839c.

16 "Number of Novel Coronavirus (COVID-19) Deaths Worldwide... by Country," *Statista*, July 12, 2021, https://www.statista.com/statistics/1093256/novel-coronavirus-2019ncov-deaths-worldwide-by-country/.

17 "Number of Deaths Due to the Novel Coronavirus (COVID-19) in Latin America and the Caribbean... by Country," *Statista*, July 12, 2021, https://www. statista.com/statistics/1103965/latin-america-caribbean-coronavirus-deaths/.

18 World Population Review, "Brazil Population 2021 (Live)," https://worldpopulationreview.com/countries/brazil-population (the datum reflected death rates on July 12) (hereafter cited as WPR).

19 WPR, "Brazil Population [July 12,] 2021 (Live), https://worldpopulationreview.com/countries/brazil-population.

20 WPR, "Brazil Population [July 12,] 2021 (Live)."

21 United Nations Economic Commission for Latin America and the Caribbean, *People of African Descent and COVID-19: Unveiling Structural Inequalities in Latin America* ([Puerto España, Trinidad y Tobago]: United Nations, 2021), 5 (hereafter cited as UNECLAC).

22 UNECLAC, *People of African descent and COVID-19*, 6. See also Rebecca Bratspies, "'Territory is Everything': Afro-Colombian Communities, Human Rights and Illegal Land Grabs," *Human Rights Law Review Online*, May 27, 2020, 299, http://blogs.law.columbia.edu/hrlr/files/2020/05/12-Bratspies_Final.pdf.

23 "Coronavirus (COVID-19) Deaths Worldwide per One Million Population."

24 Caribbean Network of Researchers on Sickle Cell Disease and Thalassemia, "COVID-19 in the Caribbean," *Carest*, May 21, 2021, https://carest-network. org/?p=4197&lang=en (hereafter cited as CAREST).

25 CAREST, "COVID-19 in the Caribbean."

26 Matthew Nuttle, "Essential Workers Accounted for 87% of Additional COVID-19 Deaths in California, Data Shows," *ABC News*, April 30, 2021, https://www.abc10.com/article/news/health/coronavirus/essential-workers-covid-deaths-california-data-uc-merced/103-f0717263-7e33-497d-b1e4-b01ab-fc95a3f. (reporting the ten industries that researchers analyzed, "in descending order from the highest percentage increase in additional deaths, included warehousing, agriculture, bars, food processing, wholesale trade, restaurants/food service, nursing care, landscaping, grocery, and building services").

27 Advisory Board, "The Jobs Most At-Risk of COVID-19 Death, Charted," February 10, 2021, https://www.advisory.com/en/daily-briefing/2021/02/10/covid-jobs; Nuttle, "Essential Workers."

28 African-Canadian Civic Engagement Council and Innovative Research Group, *Impact of COVID-19: Black Canadian Perspectives* ([N.P.]: African-Canadian Civil Engagement Council and Innovative Research Group, 2020), 3, 8, 10, 12–13 (hereafter cited as ACCEC/IRC).

29 Futshane, "COVID-19 in South Africa" (providing data for 2020).

30 Organisation for Economic Co-operation and Development, "COVID-19 in Latin America and the Caribbean: An Overview of Government Responses to the Crisis," November 11, 2020, https://www.oecd.org/coronavirus/policy-responses/covid-19-in-latin-america-and-the-caribbean-an-overview-of-government-responses-to-the-crisis-0a2dee41/.

31 Jeff Cox, "US Private Payrolls Drop by 20.2 Million in April, the Worst Job Loss in the History of ADP Report," *CNBC*, May 6, 2020, https://www.cnbc. com/2020/05/06/adp-private-payrolls-april-2020-drop-by-record-20point2-million.html.

32　Heather Long, "Small Business Used to Define America's Economy. The Pandemic Could Change that Forever," *Washington Post*, May 12, 2020, https://www.washingtonpost.com/business/2020/05/12/small-business-used-define-americas-economy-pandemic-could-end-that-forever/; RTT News, "U.S. Private Sector Employment Plunges by More than 20 Million Jobs in April," *Nasdaq*, May 6, 2020, https://www.washingtonpost.com/business/2020/05/12/small-business-used-define-americas-economy-pandemic-could-end-that-forever/.

33　Congressional Research Service, *Unemployment Rates During the COVID-19 Pandemic: In Brief (Updated January 12, 2021)* (Washington: Congressional Research Service, 2021), 6.

34　ACCEC/IRC, *Impact of COVID-19*, 21.

35　ACCEC/IRC, *Impact of COVID-19*, 23.

36　Michael Weber, Amparo Palacios-Lopez, and Ivette Maria Contreras-González, "Labor Market Impacts of COVID-19 in Four African Countries," *World Bank Blogs*, November 18, 2020, https://blogs.worldbank.org/opendata/labor-market-impacts-covid-19-four-african-countries.

37　Weber, Palacios-Lopez, and Contreras-González, "Labor Market Impacts."

38　European Centre for Disease Prevention and Control, "First COVID-19 Vaccine Authorised for Use in the European Union," December 21, 2010, https://www.ecdc.europa.eu/en/news-events/first-covid-19-vaccine-authorised-use-european-union; Government of Canada, "Health Canada Authorizes First COVID-19 Vaccine," December 9, 2020, https://www.canada.ca/en/health-canada/news/2020/12/health-canada-authorizes-first-covid-19-vaccine0.html; United States Food and Drug Administration, "FDA Takes Key Action in Fight Against COVID-19 By Issuing Emergency Use Authorization for First COVID-19 Vaccine," December 11, 2020, https://www.fda.gov/news-events/press-announcements/fda-takes-key-action-fight-against-covid-19-issuing-emergency-use-authorization-first-covid-19.

39　Centers for Disease Control and Prevention, "Percent of People Receiving COVID-19 Vaccine by Race/Ethnicity and Date Reported to CDC, United States," July 12, 2021, https://covid.cdc.gov/covid-data-tracker/#vaccination-demographics-trends (hereafter cited as CDC).

40　CDC, "Percent of People Receiving COVID-19 Vaccine by Race/Ethnicity."

41　CDC, "Percent of People Receiving COVID-19 Vaccine by Race/Ethnicity."

42　Katie Adams, "States Ranked by Percentage of Population Fully Vaccinated: July 14," *Becker's Hospital Review,* July 14, 2021, https://www.beckershospitalreview.com/public-health/states-ranked-by-percentage-of-population-vaccinated-march-15.html; Government of Canada, "COVID-19 Vaccination in Canada," July 12, 2021, https://health-infobase.canada.ca/covid-19/vaccination-coverage/.

43　Statistics Canada, "COVID-19 Vaccine Willingness among Canadian Population Groups," March 26, 2021, https://www150.statcan.gc.ca/n1/pub/45-28-0001/2021001/article/00011-eng.htm.

44　Hannah Ritchie et al., "Coronavirus (COVID-19) Vaccinations," *Our World in Data*, July 15, 2021, https://ourworldindata.org/covid-vaccinations.

45　Mohammad S. Razai, "COVID-19 Vaccine Hesitancy among Ethnic Minority Groups: Tackling the Reasons for Hesitancy Requires Engagement, Understanding, and Trust," *BMJ* 372 (February 26, 2021): 1–2, https://www.bmj.com/content/372/bmj.n513.

46　McKenzie, "Southern Africa Hoped It was Through the Worst of COVID-19."

47　CAREST, "COVID-19 in the Caribbean."

48　CAREST, "COVID-19 in the Caribbean."

49  Jason Marczak, Pepe Zhang, and Cristina Guevara, "COVID-19 Vaccine Tracker: Latin America and the Caribbean," *Atlantic Council,* May 12, 2021, https://www.atlanticcouncil.org/in-depth-research-reports/covid-19-vaccine-tracker-latin-america-and-the-caribbean/.
50  Marczak, Zhang, and Guevara, "COVID-19 Vaccine Tracker."
51  Marczak, Zhang, and Guevara, "COVID-19 Vaccine Tracker."
52  Rich Mendez, "Africa Sees 44% Spike in New COVID Infections, 20% Increase in Deaths," *CNBC,* June 16, 2021, https://www.cnbc.com/2021/06/16/africa-sees-44percent-spike-in-new-covid-infections-20percent-increase-in-deaths-.html.
53  Kaiser Family Foundation, "KFF COVID-19 Vaccine Monitor," July 15–27, 2021, https://www.kff.org/coronavirus-covid-19/dashboard/kff-covid-19-vaccine-monitor-dashboard/?gclid=EAIaIQobChMInuv-n5rm8QIVhpyzCh3K-dgxDEAAYASAAEgJkYPD_BwE (hereafter cited as KFF).
54  KFF, "KFF COVID-19 Vaccine Monitor."
55  KFF, "KFF COVID-19 Vaccine Monitor."
56  KFF, "KFF COVID-19 Vaccine Monitor."
57  Royal Society for Public Health, "New Poll Finds Ethnic Minority Groups Less Likely to Want COVID Vaccine," December 16, 2020, https://www.rsph.org.uk/about-us/news/new-poll-finds-bame-groups-less-likely-to-want-covid-vaccine.html.
58  Janine Mendes-Franco, "Vaccine Hesitancy in Smaller Caribbean Islands Benefits Larger Neighbours with High COVID-19 Rates," *Global Voices,* June 10 2021, https://globalvoices.org/2021/06/10/vaccine-hesitancy-in-smaller-caribbean-islands-benefits-larger-neighbours-with-high-covid-19-rates/.
59  David Masci, Besheer Mohamed, and Gregory A. Smith, "Black Americans Are More Likely than Overall Public to be Christian, Protestant," *Pew Research Center,* April 23, 2018, https://www.pewresearch.org/fact-tank/2018/04/23/black-americans-are-more-likely-than-overall-public-to-be-christian-protestant/, citing Pew Research Center, "Religious Landscape Study," 2014, https://www.pewforum.org/religious-landscape-study/ (hereafter cited as PRC).
60  Masci, Mohamed, and Smith, "Black Americans"; PRC, "Religious Landscape Study."
61  Todd M. Johnson et al., "Christianity 2018: More African Christians and Counting Martyrs," *International Bulletin of Mission Research* 42 (January 2018): 20–28; David McClendon, "Sub-Saharan Africa Will Be Home to Growing Shares of the World's Christians and Muslims," *Pew Research Center,* April 19, 2017, https://www.pewresearch.org/fact-tank/2017/04/19/sub-saharan-africa-will-be-home-to-growing-shares-of-the-worlds-christians-and-muslims/.
62  Johnson et al., "Christianity 2018."
63  Ruth Gledhill, "Church Attendance has been Propped Up by Immigrants, Says Study," *Guardian,* June 3, 2014, https://www.theguardian.com/world/2014/jun/03/church-attendance-propped-immigrants-study.
64  C. Eric Lincoln and Lawrence H. Mamiya, *The Black Church in the African American Experience* (Durham, NC: Duke University Press, 1990), 8 (first quotation); Philip Jenkins, *The Next Christendom: The Coming of Global Christianity* (New York, NY: Oxford University Press, 2011), 1 (second quotation).
65  See, for example, E. Franklin Frazier, *The Negro Church in America* (New York, NY: Schocken Books, 1964), 50–51.
66  Lincoln and Mamiya, *Black Church*; Albert J. Raboteau, *Slave Religion: The "Invisible Institution" in the Antebellum South,* updated ed. (New York, NY: Oxford University Press, 2004).

67  See, for example, Vincent Harding, *There Is a River: The Black Freedom Struggle in America* (New York, NY: Harcourt, Brace and Company, 1981).

68  R. Drew Smith, ed., *New Day Begun: African American Churches and Civic Culture in Post–Civil Rights America* (Durham, NC: Duke University Press, 2003).

69  Carol B. Duncan, "Historical and Contemporary Perspectives on Multiculturalism and Black Christianities in Canada," chap. 2 in R. Drew Smith, William Ackah, and Anthony G. Reddie, eds., *Churches, Blackness, and Contested Multiculturalism: Europe, Africa, and North America*, 31–46 (quotation on 34) (New York, NY: Palgrave Macmillan, 2014).

70  Duncan, "Historical and Contemporary Perspectives," 42.

71  Paul Gifford, *African Christianity: Its Public Role* (Bloomington: Indiana University Press, 1998).

72  See Paul Gundani, review of *African Christianity: Its Public Role*, by Paul Gifford, *Zambezia: The Journal of Humanities of the University of Zimbabwe* 25, no. 2 (1998): 243–246, esp. 243–44; J.N.K. Mugambi, *Christianity and African Culture* (Nairobi: Acton, 2002).

73  See Kortright Davis, *Emancipation Still Comin': Explorations in Caribbean Emancipatory Theology* (Eugene, OR: Wipf and Stock, 2008); Noel Leo Erskine, *Decolonizing Theology: A Caribbean Perspective* (1981; repr., Trenton, NJ: Africa World Press, 1998); Gerrie ter Haar, "Enchantment and Identity: African Christians in Europe," *Archives de Sciences Sociales des Religions* 143 (July–September 2008): 31–48; and Michael N. Jagessar and Anthony G. Reddie, *Black Theology in Britain: A Reader* (2007; repr., London: Routledge, 2017).

74  See David McBride, *Caring for Equality: A History of African American Health and Healthcare* (Lanham, MD: Rowman and Littlefield, 2018), 55; and Larry G. Murphy, "African American Churches, Health Care, and the Health Reform Debate," chap. 10 in *From Every Mountainside: Black Churches and the Broad Terrain of Civil Rights*, ed., R. Drew Smith, 203–20 (New York, NY: State University of New York Press, 2013).

Part I

# Systemic and Sociocultural Dimensions of Black Health

# 1 Racializing Religious Institutions during the COVID-19 Pandemic

*Stephanie C. Boddie and Jerry Z. Park*

## Introduction

Since March 11, 2020, when the World Health Organization declared COVID-19 a pandemic, researchers, journalists, and other observers have drawn attention to the racially/ethnically disproportionate impact of COVID on healthcare.[1] As of August 8, 2021, rates of infection and death continued to increase in some parts of the United States (US) but were declining in most states after the Centers for Disease Control and Prevention, familiarly the CDC, announced a record-setting number surpassing 300,000 daily coronavirus cases on January 8, 2021 (about the same population as St. Louis or Pittsburgh).[2] According to a July 5, 2020 article in the *New York Times* newspaper, the CDC had not made COVID racial/ethnic impact data available for analysis until the *Times* filed a Freedom of Information Act lawsuit to obtain the data.[3] The *Times* found evidence of racialized patterns of infection and death, with black and Latino Americans being three times as likely to contract COVID and nearly twice as likely to die from it than white Americans.[4]

While biochemical causes for the abovementioned differences remain unapparent, socio-environmental factors aggravate the spread of COVID-19, affecting consequences of the disease. The risk of exposing and infecting other people is one consequence. Health officials have called for decreasing public exposure by reducing the size and the frequency of gatherings, whether work, worship, or leisure. A second consequence arises from inadequate testing and treatment. Neither consequence is novel; high risks of exposure to disease and limited access to care are longstanding factors in racialized social systems.

In this essay, we propose expanding research into essential dimensions of social life that bear considerably on racial/ethnic patterns of the COVID-19 pandemic. Religion is foremost. Concentrating on the US and using recent discernments about the complex relationship between religious affiliation and intersecting social identities—namely sex, race, gender, ethnicity, and class—we contend that understanding the impact of racial/ethnic and related inequities of the pandemic requires considering religious beliefs,

DOI: 10.4324/9781003214281-3

participation, and collective resources (e.g., funds, facilities, and networks). In our judgment, religion offered communities a salve for various vulnerabilities but also has increased the spread of COVID because of insufficient access to care among social minorities such as African and Latino Americans.

## Intersecting Race and Religion

Race and religion have a complex relationship.[5] As scholar Vincent Lloyd noted in 2013, "Racial categories are supported by institutions [such as religion and] applied to bodies, marking them, through the explicit and implicit effects of power."[6] According to Lloyd, such ideas had produced provocative scholarship, including studies that demonstrated "how the racializing logic that produced Jews as a race depended on Christian theological ideas that also produced blacks and Native Americans as races in different contexts."[7] Fellow scholars Grace Yukich and Penny Edgell elaborated this in 2020.[8] "Religion is raced," they declared.[9] That is to say, the racialized character of social life in the US has shaped religious identity and beliefs as well as religious interactions and structures.[10] For example, much of the sociology of Christianity (e.g., normative assumptions, definitions and constitution of religious beliefs, behaviors, and identity) has centered on white Protestant experiences while marginalizing or omitting the experiences of other ethnicities.[11]

Many scholars of historically black Protestantism have noted the above-mentioned scholarly bias, which exists in part because white academics have written the majority of studies about Christianity in the US. By interrogating the assumptions of white Christian norms, a more diverse pool of scholars can develop and expand the literature by examining the intersection of race/ethnicity and religion by focusing on social minorities who share religious affiliation. Few studies explore this intersection, but the COVID-19 pandemic has created an opportunity to resolve this issue. Investigating racial inequities the pandemic has highlighted will increase understanding of religion and health among Black Church members, clearing a pathway to explore health disparities throughout the country.[12]

This essay presents African American Christians and their churches as primary examples of racializing religion. We concentrate on the Black Church because of its unique history. Although some Africans practiced Christianity before the explosion of international slavery from the late 1400s and into the 1500s, numerous white slave traders, slave owners, and slaveless commoners who supported slavery used force to convert Africans from indigenous African belief systems to Christianity. While some white people indoctrinated black people to quell the possibility of rebellion instead of viewing them as real brothers and sisters in Christ, many black people nevertheless synthesized native African religious expressions with the theology their white oppressors foisted upon them.

In the European colonies of North America and later in the US, black Christians created one of the most significant and lasting cultural institutions in continental history.[13]

Organized churches in the present-day US have been community hubs for people of African descent since the colonial period. Enslaved Baptists were pioneers. In 1750, a visionary group in South Carolina raised a church on the Southwestern bank of the Savannah River close to Augusta, Georgia.[14] Eight years later, a comparably minded set of enslaved black Christians in Virginia raised a church on a plantation of the late author, planter, and statesman William Byrd II, founder of Richmond.[15] Decades later in Philadelphia, Pennsylvania, black Methodists Richard Allen and Absalom Jones led a revolutionary 1787 walkout to protest racially segregated worship at St. George's Methodist Church.[16] Demonstrating an emerging sense of black consciousness and self-determination, Allen and Jones started the independent Black Church movement.[17] Jones founded the African Church of Philadelphia under the governance of the Protestant Episcopal Church of North America in 1794.[18] The same year, Allen established an autonomous church known as Mother Bethel, and he oversaw formation of the African Methodist Episcopal Church denomination in 1816.[19]

Black churches grew in number during the antebellum period, but four years of civil war from 1861 to 1865 halted much church building among black subjects and citizens. When the war ended officially and federal officials wrote the Thirteenth Amendment abolishing the legalized racial/ethnic slavery in the US Constitution in 1865, shared faiths between black and white Christians could have presented an opportunity for religious integration.[20] However, the same racism that necessitated the creation of black "invisible institutions" (e.g., hush harbors, clandestine services) and independent black denominations such as the African Methodist Episcopal Church, the African Methodist Episcopal Zion Church, and The Church of God in Christ persisted in predominately white denominations.[21] Ultimately, African American renderings of Christian collective expression became institutionalized in the most enduring sector of the African American community, the Black Church.[22]

## Racialized Religion and the COVID-19 Pandemic: Exposure Risks

As racism was partly responsible for the creation of black churches in the US, racism is responsible for black people being at greater risks of exposure to COVID-19 than white people. Because of persistent patterns of residential segregation, black people are more likely than whites to live or work in adverse conditions and to have limited access to healthcare, healthy foods, and reliable public transportation. In general, predominantly black neighborhoods also have greater housing densities and higher crime rates than white neighborhoods.[23]

Based on Bureau of Labor Statistics data from 2019, 30 percent of white Americans and 37 percent of Asian Americans could have worked from home in 2017 or in 2018 compared with 19.7 percent of black Americans and 16.2 percent Latin Americans.[24] By 2020, according to social epidemiologists David R. Williams and Lisa A. Cooper, racial/ethnic minorities tended to work in restaurants, grocery stores, healthcare settings, and other essential services, where there was great risk of exposure to COVID-19.[25] These minorities also were most likely to have not much if any sick leave, to live from paycheck to paycheck, to be underinsured or uninsured, to commute to work by public transportation, and to live in close quarters.[26] Each one of these circumstances made physical, or social, distancing challenging.

The situations above help explain why in 2020 the infection rate of COVID-19 in predominately black counties in the US was more than threefold the rate in predominately white counties.[27] The rate of death from COVID complications in counties where black people comprise the majority was twice that number in 2020.[28] Those disparities, which had not shrunk by mid-2021, continued to highlight "the compounding, elevated risks from our systems of housing, the labor force, healthcare system and policy responses" that have resulted from systemic racism, particularly residential segregation.[29] Such clustering of disadvantages results in stigma and a vicious cycle of economic, psychological, and physical distress.[30]

As journalists and other media personalities noted, religious facilities were virus hotspots. Despite the good that physical fellowshipping provided, the "most segregated hour of the week," as the Rev. Martin Luther King Jr. characterized each Sunday morning from 11 a.m. to 12 p.m., in-person worship services during COVID-19 pandemic have a real potential for harm.[31] In addition to the racial/ethnic segregation King referenced, many religious leadership and laity do not abide by CDC, local, or state guidelines to distance physically; consequently, instead of praise houses and buffers for discrimination, among other upliftingly safe places, churches expose congregants to COVID.[32]

Black churches are social hubs and public resources that provide positive energy through collective effervescence and offer emotional and psychological benefits.[33] While congregations face many social pressures for minimizing group gatherings during the COVID-19 pandemic, empathy lies at the heart of most religious practices in the US and elsewhere in the world. For example, as the number of black deaths rose in the US in 2020, millions of surviving black churchgoers who once supported in-person services began to question meeting in person; instead, they voiced concern for public health, promoted civic responsibility, and held virtual services.[34] Meanwhile, numerous white churchgoers, emphasizing constitutional liberty and freedom to worship as an important First Amendment right, continued to worship in person.[35]

As many church leaders and ordinary parishioners across the US considered such matters, some debated religious institutions receiving funds via the Coronavirus Aid, Relief, and Economic Security Act the federal government put into effect on March 27,[36] sixteen days after the World Health Organization affirmed COVID-19 was a pandemic.[37] Though eligible, many black congregations who requested loans through the paycheck protection programs and related means never received the public assistance they sought. Most bank officials were white men, and they routinely prioritized existing clients. Those acts disadvantaged churches with large numbers of ethnic/racial minorities. Much federal aid went to churches, but distribution was inequitable.[38]

While COVID-19 has resulted in great peril, it also has created new opportunities for individuals and communities to design innovative solutions to myriad problems.[39] To avoid some of the in-person infection risks we discussed above, innumerable church leaders began livestreaming religious worship services online. Other leaders recorded sermons and other activities, which they broadcasted later. The internet allowed churchgoers to approximate religious gatherings without being in the same physical spaces. One megachurch pastor, John K. Jenkins Sr. of the First Baptist Church of Glenarden, Maryland, organized an entire team to simulate call-and-response worship rhythms while livestreaming.[40]

## Racialized Religion and the COVID Pandemic: Access to Care

In light of racial/ethnic disparities in relation to COVID-19 exposure risks, that similar disparities exist regarding access to healthcare is no surprise to us. We therefore provide a rationale for more research about the role of religion as a corrective tool. In particular, we believe religious institutions can facilitate access to mental and physical healthcare, food collection and distribution, and related assistance. As stated earlier in this essay, black Americans are more likely than white Americans to have inadequate or no health insurance. Consequently, such black people often do not seek professional medical treatment until ailments are in advanced stages. In addition to that occurrence, a history of medical mistrust causes some contemporary black Americans to place more confidence in their pastors than in healthcare providers.[41]

Beyond mistrust, black congregations in the US typically provide more general health and substance abuse assistance to persons who need it than white, Asian, or Hispanic congregations.[42] Multiple black congregations also led the charge to provide specialized assistance, to include free COVID-19 testing. While many religious centers were ill-equipped or unwilling to test people until late 2020, the Friendship-West Baptist Church in Dallas, Texas, was testing by midyear.[43] Later, as congregations of every racial/ethnic demographic joined Friendship-West Baptist as testing centers, the Catalyst Church in Philadelphia, Pennsylvania, recognized the toll the COVID pandemic was having on the mental health of local citizens and began to offer crisis management sessions online.[44]

Despite attempts to curtail COVID-19, death is often inevitable. As rates increased in 2020 and into 2021, black people experienced an uptick in funerals.[45] Traditional home-going services are hours long if not all-day events when one considers viewing bodies, celebrating decedents' lives, internments, and fellowship meals.[46] Such rituals, which are powerful communal means of remembering and mourning in black communities, are hard to replicate using internet and related technologies. Nevertheless, millions of black funeralgoers have adapted because further misery is a feasible outcome if they hold customary in-person services.

## Future Research

We think it is important to explore the ways black congregations adapt to navigate the COVID-19 environment, particularly as they provide new forms of worship, inreach, and outreach services. Many congregants who employed technology to hold religious events, carry out social programs, and perform similar duties had done so before the COVID-19 pandemic. In numerous instances, instead of letting their unfamiliarity with various technologies defeat them, congregants expanded their use to provide new services, to include student laptop loans, grocery deliveries, carry-out soup kitchens, drive-through food pantries, and pop-up vaccine distribution sites.[47]

In our judgment, future research should examine, among other occurrences, how black congregations have maintained traditions while adapting to the challenges of the COVID-19 pandemic?[48] How well have churchgoers improvised? Where are they innovating and leading change? How, too, have they been able to continue providing adequate financial resources (e.g., benevolent offerings) to people in need during the pandemic, especially considering black congregations tend to have fewer monetary resources than white congregants?[49]

For generations, when black Americans have exhausted monetary resources, religion has been a vital source of emotional and psychological as well as spiritual assistance for people in need.[50] Numerous scholarly studies demonstrate that religious coping can be invaluable during trying times.[51] Limited financial or physical resources notwithstanding, black congregants historically have reached deep into their humanitarian reservoirs to serve vulnerable people in their midst.[52] How, then, have congregations continued to provide services during the COVID-19 pandemic? Are congregants moving beyond racial/ethnic boundaries to work with white congregants? In sum, how are black congregants living out their raced religion?

## Conclusion

Scholars David Williams and Lisa Cooper deem COVID-19 "a magnifying glass that has highlighted the larger pandemic of racial/ethnic disparities in health."[53] Indeed, such disparities were present in the US long before the

COVID-19 pandemic, but the disparities have intensified during the pandemic. Black, Latino, Asian, and other generally underserved people of color have been hit particularly hard. We, however, believe religious institutions can perform not only spirit-lifting but also potentially life-saving functions.

## Notes

© 2021 by the authors. Licensee MDPI, Basel, Switzerland. This essay is adapted from an open access article distributed under the terms and conditions of the Creative Commons Attribution (CC BY) license (https://creativecommons.org/licenses/by/4.0/).

1 "WHO Director-General's Opening Remarks at the Media Briefing on COVID-19," *World Health Organization*, March 11, 2020, https://www.who.int/director-general/speeches/detail/who-director-general-s-opening-remarks-at-the-media-briefing-on-covid-19.

2 Centers for Disease Control and Prevention, "COVID Data Tracker," https://covid.cdc.gov/covid-data-tracker/#trends_dailytrendscases (source of the 312,488 datum and hereafter cited as CDC); Johns Hopkins University and Medicine Coronavirus Resource Center, "America Is Re-Opening. But Have We Flattened the Curve?," May 9, 2021, https://coronavirus.jhu.edu/data/new-cases-50-states; Paulina Villegas et al., "U.S. Surpasses 300,000 Daily Coronavirus Cases, the Second Alarming Record this Week," The Washington Post, January 8, 2021, https://www.washingtonpost.com/nation/2021/01/08/coronavirus-covid-live-updates-us/.

3 Richard A. Oppel Jr. et al., "The Fullest Look Yet at the Racial Inequity of Coronavirus," *New York Times*, July 5, 2021, https://www.nytimes.com/interactive/2020/07/05/us/coronavirus-latinos-african-americans-cdc-data.html?action=click&module=Top%20Stories&pgtype=Homepage&ncid=newsltushpmgnews.

4 Oppel Jr. et al., "Fullest Look."

5 Melissa J. Wilde, "Complex Religion: Intersections of Religion and Inequality," *Social Inclusion* 6 (May 2018): 82.

6 Vincent Lloyd, "Race and Religion Contribution to Symposium on Critical Approaches to the Study of Religion," *Critical Research on Religion* 1 (April 2013): 80–86.

7 Lloyd, "Race and Religion Contribution."

8 Grace Yukich and P. Edgell, eds., *Religion Is Raced: Understanding American Religion in the Twenty-First Century* (New York: New York University Press, 2020).

9 Yukich and Edgell, *Religion Is Raced*.

10 Yukich, and Edgell, "Introduction: Recognizing Raced Religion," in *Religion Is Raced*, 1–16.

11 Courtney Bender et al., "Introduction: Religion on the Edge—De-Centering and Re-Centering," in Bender et al., eds., *Religion on the Edge: De-Centering and Re-Centering the Sociology of Religion* (New York: Oxford University Press, 2013), 1–22.

12 Regarding the dearth of scholarly studies about the intersections of race/ethnicity and religion, see Jerry Z. Park, Joyce C. Chang, and James C. Davidson, "Equal Opportunity Beliefs beyond Black and White American Christianity," *Religions* 11 (July 2020): 348.

13  Albert J. Raboteau, *Slave Religion: The "Invisible Institution" in the Antebellum South* (New York: Oxford University Press, 2004).

14  C. Eric Lincoln and Lawrence H. Mamiya, *The Black Church in the African American Experience* (Durham, NC: Duke University Press, 1990), 23.

15  Lincoln and Mamiya, *Black Church*, 23.

16  Richard S. Newman, *Freedom's Prophet: Bishop Richard Allen, the AME Church and the Black Founding Fathers* (New York: New York University Press, 2008), esp. 63–68.

17  Gary B. Nash, *Forging Freedom: The Formation of Philadelphia's Black Community 1720-1840* (Cambridge, MA: Harvard University Press, 1988), 132–33.

18  Nash, *Forging Freedom,* 125–33. The African Church of Philadelphia was later renamed the African Episcopal Church of St. Thomas.

19  Dennis C. Dickerson's *The African Methodist Episcopal Church: A History* (New York: Cambridge University Press, 2020) is one of the most recent published scholarly books about the formation of the denomination.

20  Laurie F. Maffly-Kipp, "The Burden of Church History," *Church History* 82 (June 2013): 353–67.

21  Raboteau, *Slave Religion* (the term *invisible institution* is in the subtitle).

22  Sandra L. Barnes, "Enter into His Gates: An Analysis of Black Church Participation Patterns," *Sociological Spectrum* 29 (March–April 2009): 173–200; W. E. Burghardt Du Bois, "The Organized Life of Negroes," chap. 12 in *The Philadelphia Negro: A Social Study* (Philadelphia: University of Pennsylvania, 1899), 197–221; Henry Louis Gates, Jr., *The Black Church: This Is Our Story, This Is Our Song* (New York: Penguin Press, 2021); and Kelly McCarthy, "How the Black Church Has Been a Rock Community and a Catalyst for Change," *ABC News*, June 19, 2020, https://abcnews.go.com/US/black-church-rock-community-catalyst-change/story?id=71344308.

23  CDC, "COVID-19 in Racial and Ethnic Minority Groups," April 22, 2020, https://www.hsdl.org/?view&did=837299.

24  Bureau of Labor Statistics, "Table 1: Workers Who Could Work at Home, Did Work at Home, and were Paid for Work at Home, by Selected Characteristics, Averages for the Period 2017–2018," *Economic News Release*, September 24, 2019, https://www.bls.gov/news.release/flex2.t01.htm.

25  David R. Williams and Lisa A. Cooper, "COVID-19 and Health Equity—A New Kind of 'Herd Immunity,'" *JAMA: Journal of the American Medical Association* 323 (June 2020): 2478–80.

26  Don Bambino Geno Tai et al., "The Disproportionate Impact of Covid-19 on Racial and Ethnic Minorities in the United States," *Clinical Infectious Diseases* 72 (February 15, 2021): 703–6.

27  Clyde W. Yancy, "COVID-19 and African Americans," *JAMA: Journal of the American Medical Association* 323 (May 19, 2020): 1891–92.

28  Yancy, "COVID-19 and African Americans."

29  Stephanie C. Boddie and Jerry Z. Park, "Racializing the Religious during the COVID-19 Pandemic," *Religions* 12 (May 2021): 341, https://doi.org/10.3390/rel12050341.

30  Sanni Yaya et al., "Ethnic and Racial Disparities in COVID-19-Related Deaths: Counting the Trees, Hiding the Forest," *BMJ Global Health* 5 (June 2020): 1–5, http://dx.doi.org/10.1136/bmjgh-2020-002913.

31  "Meet the Press," *NBC*, March 28, 1965, https://m.youtube.com/watch?v=fAtsAwGreyE.

32  Christina Carrega and Lakeia Brown, "'Sorrowful': Black Clergy Members and Churches Reeling from COVID-19 Losses," *ABC News*, May 21, 2020, abcnews.go.com/US/sorrowful-black-clergy-members-churches-reeling-covid-19/story?id=70434181; Claire Gecewicz, "Amid Pandemic, Black

and Hispanic Worshippers More Concerned about Safety of In-Person Religious Services," *Pew Research Center*, August 7, 2020, https://www. pewresearch.org/fact-tank/2020/08/07/amid-pandemic-black-and-hispanic-worshippers-more-concerned-about-safety-of-in-person-religious-services/; Aneri Pattini, "Amid COVID and Racial Unrest, Black Churches Put Faith in Mental Health Care," *Philadelphia Tribune*, December 9, 2020, https://www.phillytrib.com/news/health/amid-covid-and-racial-unrest-black-churches-put-faith-in-mental-health-care/article_58182f7c-0aa4-5d8e-bf48-e33768e6fb6a.html.

33  Randall Collins, *Interaction Ritual Chains* (2004; repr., Princeton, NJ: Princeton University Press, 2004); Émile Durkheim, *The Elementary Forms of the Religious Life: A Study in Religious Sociology*, trans. Joseph Ward Swain (New York: Macmillan Company, 1915).

34  Carrega and Brown, "Sorrowful"; Gecewicz, "Amid Pandemic, Black and Hispanic Worshippers More Concerned about Safety."

35  Keely Arthur and Maggie Chatter, "Christian Leaders Rally in Raleigh Demanding Reopening of Churches," *WRAL.com*, May 15, 2020, https://www.wral.com/coronavirus/christian-leaders-rally-in-raleigh-demanding-re-opening-of-churches/19097741/.

36  Pub. L. 116–136, March 27, 2020.

37  "WHO Director-General's Opening Remarks."

38  Tom Gjelten, "Black Pastors Say They Have Trouble Accessing SBA Loan Program," *NPR*, April 25, 2020, https://www.npr.org/2020/04/25/844802957/black-pastors-say-they-have-trouble-accessing-sba-loan-program.

39  L. Gregory Jones, *Christian Social Innovation: Renewing Wesleyan Witness* (Nashville, TN: Abingdon Press, 2016).

40  John K. Jenkins Sr., "God is Doing a New Thing," part 3, *First Baptist Church of Glenarden [Maryland]*, January 25, 2021, https://www.youtube.com/watch?v=VXhpnVRmXeY&feature=youtu.be.

41  Jane Caffrey, "Pastor Says Medical Mistrust Is an Obstacle to Vaccination," *WBDJ7*, February 17, 2021, https://www.wdbj7.com/2021/02/17/pastor-says-medical-mistrust-is-an-obstacle-to-vaccination/.

42  R. Khari Brown and Amy Adamczyk, "Racial/Ethnic Differences in the Provision of Health-Related Programs among American Religious Congregations," *Journal of Sociology and Social Welfare* 36 (June 2009): 105–23.

43  "To Combat Disparities, Black Churches in Dallas Offer Coronavirus Testing," *NPR*, June 13, 2020, www.npr.org/sections/health-shots/2020/06/13/874950245/to-combat-disparities-black-churches-in-dallas-offer-coronavirus-testing-Black.

44  Pattini, "Amid COVID and Racial Unrest, Black Churches Put Faith in Mental Health Care."

45  James Peterson, "The Color of Coronavirus: Our Mournful Undertaking," *Philadelphia Citizen*, June 18, 2020, https://thephiladelphiacitizen.org/black-mourning-during-covid/.

46  J. Lee Hill Jr, "Opinion: The Pandemic has Forced Black Churches to Rethink the Funeral Traditions We Hold Sacred," *San Diego Union-Tribune*, March 5, 2021, https://www.sandiegouniontribune.com/opinion/commentary/story/2021-03-05/opinion-black-families-church-homegoing-covid-19.

47  Stephen M. Modell and Sharon L. R. Kardia, "Religion as a Health Promoter during the 2019/2020 COVID Outbreak: View from Detroit," *Journal of Religion and Health* 59 (October 2020): 2243–55; Sarah Rigg, "Ypsi-Area Churches Respond to COVID-19 with Virtual Worship and Expanded Community Outreach," *Concentrate*, April 7, 2020, www.secondwavemedia.com/concentrate/features/covidypsichurches0544.aspx.

48  L. Gregory Jones, *Christian Social Innovation: Renewing Weslyan Witness* (Nashville: Abingdon Press, 2016). Churches bring the traditions of the past forward to find new ways to fulfill church traditions.

49  Lluis Oviedo and Sara Lumbreras, "What Will Happen to Religion After Covid Pandemic?," *SocArXiv*, November 26, 2020, https://doi.org/10.31235/osf. io/chktm.

50  Modell and Kardia, "Religion as a Health Promoter."

51  Jeremy P. Cummings and Kenneth I. Pargament, "Medicine for the Spirit: Religious Coping in Individuals with Medical Conditions," *Religions* 1 (December 2010): 28–53; Byron R. Johnson, and Thomas S. Kidd, "Responding to COVID-19 Would Be a Lot Harder without Churches and Christian Groups," *Dallas News*, March 25, 2020, www.dallasnews.com/opinion/commentary/2020/03/29/responding-to-covid-19-would-be-a-lot-harder-without-churches-and-christian-groups/.

52  Ram A. Cnaan et al., *The Invisible Caring Hand: American Congregations and the Provision of Welfare* (New York: New York University Press, 2002); Cnaan et al., *The Other Philadelphia Story: How Local Congregations Support Quality of Life in Urban America* (Philadelphia: University of Pennsylvania Press, 2006).

53  Williams and Cooper, "COVID-19 and Health Equity," 2478.

# 2 Racialized Discourses on Disease at Intersections of Canadian and the Caribbean Contexts

*Gosnell L. Yorke*

## Introduction

This essay compares human immunodeficiency virus/acquired immuno-deficiency syndrome (HIV/AIDS) and COVID-19, focusing on the African Diaspora in general and the AfriCanadian community in particular. In doing so, the essay addresses adverse human rights impacts that both pandemics have had on the AfriCanadian community. As regard HIV/AIDS, such impacts include the racially driven scapegoating of Africana people. For COVID-19, the number of African-descended people who have suffered with or succumbed to the disease is a major impact. Their infection and death rates are disproportionately high when compared with their European-descended contemporaries in Canada.[1]

I am a naturalized Canadian citizen born in the English-speaking Caribbean, and the story I tell is part of a larger narrative concerning the spread, prevention, and treatment of disease as well as various means to control those who are infected or have substantial risk factors for becoming infected. My essay fleshes out the existing narrative by exploring certain underemphasized social determinants of disease or conditions precedent to disease that often render masses of marginalized people—in this instance, AfriCanadians—susceptible to infection, which in turn affects their autonomy.[2]

## Disputed Linkages between Haiti and Canada on Infectious Diseases

In the summer of 2006, after serving as a church worker in multiple parts of Africa for fifteen years, I journeyed to Canada. While in Montreal, Quebec, I visited the bookstore of McGill University, my alma mater. Curious about what faculty members were teaching medical students about the etiology and the spread of HIV/AIDS, I decided to take a look at the assigned textbook in microbiology. The text contained an explicit statement about the origin of the disease being an unsettled matter.[3] That idea appeared in print even though the European-descended authors of the text acknowledged

DOI: 10.4324/9781003214281-4

the scientific consensus was HIV/AIDS originated in Africa and made its way to North America via the Caribbean—for example, Haiti.

In 2006, during the early period of the HIV/AIDS pandemic, as some people debated its genesis and others tried to determine if HIV/AIDS was a pandemic,[4] countless white Canadians scapegoated Haiti, the first republic in the Northern or Western hemisphere established by Africana people who liberated themselves from European colonial rule.[5] Those who believed Haiti was the birthplace of HIV/AIDS, anthropologist Susan S. Hunter noted, hurriedly inducted natives of the island country into a "'4-H Club': homosexuals, heroin users, Haitians, and hemophiliacs."[6] Criticism was as widespread among white people in the US as it was in Canada. As Hunter's fellow anthropologist, Julian C.H. Lee, would affirm in 2011: "Haiti was one of the first countries in which AIDS was recognized and thus Haitians came to be blamed for the AIDS [virus'] spread to the US."[7]

The ideas Hunter and Lee presented were not novel. In 2000, two nurses, educators, and authors, Marie-Anne Santana and Barbara L. Dancy, affirmed that calling Haitians principal "AIDS carriers" was simply a means of compounding existing stereotypes.[8] Already, Santana and Dancy recollected, ignorant, or informed but biased people had an extensive list of negative sobriquets for Haitians. "Boat people," "voodoo worshippers," and "illiterate" were common derisions.[9] Some European American parents in Haiti went further than pejorative language: They withdraw their children from schools with Haitian students.[10]

Such disease-based and racialized scapegoating of Haitians did not go unchallenged. In 2004, approximately two years before some news outlets began calling HIV/AIDS a pandemic,[11] medical anthropologist Paul Farmer questioned the notion of the HIV/AIDS coming to North America by way of Haiti.[12] In his judgment, Haiti was more a victim than a vector of the disease.[13] Given the country's history of prolonged colonial exploitation and modern citizens' determined desire to improve their financial conditions through tourism, on which Haiti and most of the Caribbean was and remains dependent, Farmer reasoned there was a connection between HIV/AIDS sufferers in Haiti and North American tourists: "The Haitian men who had been the partners of North Americans were by and large poor men; they were trading sex for money. The Haitians in turn transmitted HIV to their wives and girlfriends. Through affective and economic connections, HIV rapidly became entrenched in Haiti's urban slums and then spread to smaller cities, towns, and, finally, villages."[14]

This scapegoating of Haitians and Haiti, an important country in African diasporic history, amounts to racialized discourse that targets mainly non-European immigrants who have settled throughout the Global North. In that region, whose exact geography scholars have debated for decades, countless people of European descent have used sexually transmitted diseases and other infections to stigmatize other ancestry groups for centuries.

Present-day Canada is a fitting example. European-descended people routinely claim that, among non-European immigrants, African-descended people are the primary carriers of disease. As with other localities worldwide, in framing such racialized discourse, Canadian media personalities have not been immune to spreading false narratives.[15]

To me, numberless white people's general tendency to scapegoat or to stigmatize people of color, especially those with African ancestry, when discussing the origin or circulating of disease is no surprise. Countless modern white people have viewed virtually everything and everyone associated with the African Diaspora through an Enlightenment, Darwinian, or Spencerian lens that privileges Europeanism. As regard contemporary Africa, for instance, a large number of white people around the world still perceive the continent as a monolith whose governing structures, political practices, economic arrangements, indigenous knowledge systems, and other societal phenomena as primitively ineffective. Consider health and healing. Colonial era practitioners of Western medicine helped create an image of Africa as a continent fraught with death, disease, and degeneration.[16] According to Sarah Hunter, a woman with European ancestry who has resided in Africa for decades, "European medical science used Africa as a 'diseased environment' ripe for research. Africa was a laboratory to test the new bacteriology, a place where scientific reputations could be made. One-fifth of all newly trained medical graduates left Britain for practice in tropical and subtropical climates after six months of training to investigate insect-borne and other exotic diseases."[17]

In Canada, people of Haitian descent and other dark-skinned people of the African Diaspora have borne the brunt of white people's scapegoating when it comes to HIV/AIDS. For me, that occurrence is explicable, in that ambivalence has characterized the historical relationships between Haitians and Canadians of European descent, especially in Quebec—despite linguistic affinities between Haitians and Francophone Canada.

As residents of a predominantly, and justifiably, proud French-speaking province with the motto *"Je me souviens"* ("I remember"), white people in Quebec have sought stubbornly to keep alive their French heritage. Their determination is in spite, or perhaps because, of the official formation of a predominantly English-speaking Canada via the 1867 British North America Act, or Constitution, which united Canada, New Brunswick, and Nova Scotia "into one Dominion, under the name of Canada."[18] As of 2021, Quebec still boasted the largest French-speaking community outside France, and Haiti was the oldest independent French-speaking republic in the Western hemisphere. Quebec had a strong Roman Catholic tradition, extending to early periods of the locality when French missionaries saw Haiti as a natural target for their evangelistic, educational, charitable, and health-related work.[19]

The missionary view of Haiti explains much of the intense ambivalence I referenced above. In the early 1600s, when Catholics began missionizing in Quebec, many people of European descent were socialized in and conditioned by white supremacy. Hence, they considered people of African descent as inferior. That African-descended people comprised the numerical majority in Quebec and usually spoke the French language, though maybe with a unique dialect, was immaterial to the Catholic missionaries. To the typical European, a Haitian was a backward at best and a repugnant at worse creature in need of a civilizing.[20]

## HIV/AIDS and Racialized Discourse in the Twenty-First Century

During the 1960s, as Africana people staged revolutions across the world, white officials in Canada were easing immigration policies in the country.[21] Many native Haitians, concerned that increasingly inhospitable political and economic environments in their homeland would not cease anytime soon and seeking better educational and employment, among other opportunities, opted to resettle in Quebec. As with many people who relocate from primarily agricultural settings, whether such people are asylum seekers, refugee claimants, or economic migrants, large numbers of Haitians who made Quebec their new homes during the 1960s chose urban areas. Montreal, a cosmopolitan city, was a preferred destination. They settled mainly in the eastern quadrant of Montreal, while predominantly English-speaking immigrants chose the Western section.[22] Later emigrations resulted in movements from Montreal to places such as Toronto. The Quebec government's insistence that local residents respect the French heritage was mainly responsible for those demographic shifts. As AfriCanadians relocated from one place to another, their white contemporaries engaged in racialized discourse about disease, claiming nonwhite people were principal carriers and spreaders. Most often, people of African descent bore the brunt of such unwarranted criticism.[23]

As late as 2021, many Haitians still felt marginalized in Quebec society even though a few people of Haitian origin had become influential decision makers in preceding decades.[24] In 2002, for example, Quebec high officials appointed Daniel Dortélus to a judgeship.[25] A woman of Haitian origin, Michaëlle Jean, held even higher positions than Dortélus: she served as governor general of Canada from 2005 to 2010 and secretary-general of the International Organization of the Francophonie from 2015 to 2019.[26]

Not long after Jean began her tenure as governor general in 2005, the HIV/AIDS pandemic made its way into Canada. Even though the first known case in the country dated to 1979, according to a timeline the Canadian AIDS society posted online in 2021, white citizens routinely scapegoated AfriCanadians, especially Haitian immigrants, for being the primary carriers of the disease while Jean was in office from 2005 to 2010.[27] Whites continued to stigmatize blacks when Jean left office, and research by scholars such as Viviane K. Namaste indicates that Montreal, the site of the 1979 HIV/AIDS case, was a center of bigotry and meanness.[28]

Toronto was another place where disease-based discrimination was prevalent during the 2010s. Fortunately for some AfriCanadians whom biased white people targeted for abuse, decent individuals and respectable organizations such as the Canadian Council of Churches and the Canadian AIDS Society remained vigilante in their efforts to stem the tide of inequity. As early as winter-spring 2006, months before information sources like the *Boston Globe* newspaper in the US began reporting HIV/AIDS had risen from an epidemic to a pandemic,[29] the Canadian Council of Churches cosponsored a pre-ecumenical conference in advance of a summer international HIV/AIDS conference to be held in Toronto.[30] At the conference, held in mid-August and cohosted by the Canadian AIDS Society,[31] popular US actor and activist Richard Gere declared he and other celebrities along with the media were "key to reducing [the] stigma of disease," the *Ottawa Citizen* newspaper announced.[32]

## COVID-19

Whereas much of the story about the HIV/AIDS pandemic in Canada has to do with the racialized defaming of African-descended people, a large section of the COVID-19 tale deals with disproportionate rates of infection and death compared with European-descended people. Numerous scholarly and popular studies have shown that institutional racism and ethnic bias are principal causes of disproportionality. In 2020, the African-Canadian Civic Engagement Council and the Innovative Research Group conducted a study in Toronto that found 21 percent of AfriCanadians know someone who died because of a COVID-related condition.[33] At the time of the study, AfriCanadians made up 9 percent of the population, which was one percentage point more than white Canadians who knew someone who succumbed to COVID.[34]

## Conclusion

The lopsided statistics I cite above are not unique to Toronto. Credible groups have reported similar data from elsewhere in Canada. Beyond misfortune, AfriCanadians and other vulnerable Canadian citizens, including destitute white people, face a number of social determinants of health that racial/ethnic bias and economic classism influence. As discussed previously in this essay, those determinants include unemployment to working as frontline laborers. Substandard education, inadequate housing, and residential segregation are three additional factors that increase the likelihood of not having nutritious foodstuffs, quality medical facilities, and other resources essential for healthy living. Consequently, rates of obesity, diabetes, and related underlying conditions increase, thereby heightening vulnerabilities to potentially fatal diseases such as COVID-19. Those realties, together with the persistent scapegoating of AfriCanadians for being primary disease carriers in Canada, have contributed to an environment where countless white people continue to believe "immigrants can be deadly" simply because they are immigrants.[35]

## Notes

1 Emily Chung, Vik Adhopia, and Melanie Glanz, "Black Canadians Get Sick More from COVID-19, Scientists Aim to Find Out Why," *CBC News*, September 25, 2020, https://www.cbc.ca/news/health/black-covid-antibody-study-1.5737452; Nadine Spencer and Mohamed Elmi, "Ep.40: Realities for Black Canadians in COVID-Times," *Public Policy Forum*, February 25, 2021, https://ppforum.ca/policy-speaking/ep-40-covid-19-impacts-on-black-communities/; "Understanding the Impact of COVID-19 on Black Canadians: Q and A with Dr. Upton Allen," *Genome Canada*, February 26, 2021, https://www.genomecanada.ca/en/news/blog/understanding-impact-covid-19-black-canadians.

2 Susan S. Hunter, *Who Cares? AIDS in Africa* (New York: Palgrave Macmillan, 2003), 144.

3 See, for example, Mirko D. Grmek, *History of AIDS: Emergence and Origin of a Modern Pandemic*, Russell C. Maultz and Jacalyn Duffin, trans. (Princeton, NJ: Princeton University Press, 1990).

4 John Donnelly, "Ten Steps Africans Can Take to Curb AIDS Epidemic," *Boston Globe*, June 5, 2006, C5 (calling southern Africa the epicenter of a pandemic and not simply an epidemic).

5 The years 1791 to 1804 are the traditional dates of the Haitian Revolution, which ended French domination in its colony known as Saint-Domingue, whose spelling varies.

6 Hunter, *Who Cares?*, 41.

7 Julian C. H. Lee, *Policing Sexuality: Sex, Society, and State* (London: Zed Books, 2011), 94.

8 Marie-Anne Santana and Barbara L. Dancy, "The Stigma of Being Named 'AIDS Carriers' on Haitian American Women," *Health Care for Women International* 21 (April/May 2000): 161–71.

9 Santana and Dancy, "Stigma," 162.

10 Lee, *Policing Sexuality*, 94.

11 Donnelly, "Ten Steps."

12 Paul Farmer, "An Anthropology of Structural Violence," *Current Anthropology* 45 (June 2004): 305–25.

13 Farmer, "Anthropology of Structural Violence."

14 Farmer, "Anthropology of Structural Violence," 316. The United States, South Korea, Singapore, Russia, New Zealand, Japan, Israel, Europe, Canada, and Australia are places that many scholars include when referring to the geographical Global North. Other scholars prefer economic characterized of the Glob South, which they agree is developed economically. Regarding some of those matters and the COVID-19 pandemic, see Udo Schuklenk, "The Ethical Challenges of the SARS-CoV-2 Pandemic in the Global South and the Global North—Same and Different," *Developing World Bioethics* 20 (June 2020): 62–63.

15 Sylvia Reitmanova et al., "'Immigrants Can Be Deadly': Critical Discourse Analysis of Racialization of Immigrant Health in Canadian Press and Public Health Policies," *Canadian Journal of Communication* 40 (2015): 471–87.

16 See Megan Vaughn, "Syphilis in East and Central Africa: The Social Construction of an Epidemic," in *Epidemics and Ideas: Essays on the Historical Perception of Pestilence*, Terence Ranger and Paul Slack, eds., 269–302 (1992; repr., New York, NY: Cambridge University Press, 1999).

17 Hunter, *Who Cares?*, 142–43. See also Pamela A. Andanda, *The Law and Regulation of Clinical Research: Interplay with Public Policy and Bioethics* (Nairobi: English Press, 2006), 18, 261.

18 "By the Queen. A Proclamation for Uniting the Provinces of Canada, Nova Scotia, and New Brunswick, into One Dominion, Under the Name of Canada," June 5, 1867, in, among other works, *Journal of the House of Assembly of the Province of New Brunswick, From the 11th of May to the 17th of June 1867; Being the Second of the Twenty-First General Assembly* (Fredericton: G. E. Fenety, 1867), 151–52.

19 Laënnec Hurbon, "Haiti," in *The Encyclopedia of Caribbean Religions*, vol. 1: *A–L*, Patrick Taylor and Frederick I. Case, ed., 313–15 (Urbana, IL: Illinois University Press, 2013).

20 Hurbon, "Haiti."

21 See, for example, "'Haiti Then and Now' Interviews Professor Ron Charles," Haiti Then and Now, July 1, 2020, haitithenandnow.wordpress.com/2020/07/01/haiti-then-and-now-interviews-professor-ronald-charles/. I am grateful to Charles, an influential Haitian-born AfriCanadian who directed me to some of the main Canadian sources I used to draft this essay.

22 Sarah-Jane Mathiew, *North of the Color Line: Migration and Black Resistance in Canada, 1870–1955* (Chapel Hill, NC: University of North Carolina Press, 2010).

23 See Robyn Maynard, *Policing Black Lives: State Violence in Canada from Slavery to the Present* (Nova Scotia: Fernwood Publishing, 2017); and Mills, *Place in the Sun*.

24 Frances Henry et al., *The Equity Myth: Racialization and Indigeneity at Canadian Universities* (Vancouver: University of British Columbia Press, 2017); Maryse Potvin "Second-Generation Haitian Youth in Quebec. Between the 'Real' Community and the 'Represented' Community," *Canadian Ethnic Studies Journal* 31 (1999): 43–72; Gosnell L. Yorke, "Visible but Voiceless Minorities No More: New Readings of the Bible in Canada," in Néstor Medina, Alison Hari-Singh, and HyeRan Kim-Cragg, eds., *Reading In-Between: How Minoritized Cultural Communities Interpret the Bible in Canada*, 112–14 (Eugene, OR: Pickwick Publications, 2019).

25 Rhéal Séguin, "Quebec Appoints First Haitian Judge," *Globe and Mail*, May 18, 2002, https://www.theglobeandmail.com/news/national/quebec-appoints-first-haitian-judge/article4135466/.

26 Michaëlle Jean, *La Drancophonie des Exigences au Service des Peuples et au Coeur des Urgences du Monde: Plaidoyer: Discours et Interventions (2015–2018)* (Bruxelles: Bruylant, 2019).

27 Canadian AIDS Society, "History of Canadian AIDS Society," https://www.cdnaids.ca/about-us/history/.

28 Viviane Namaste, "AIDS Histories: The Case of Haitians in Montreal," in *AIDS and the Distribution of Crises*, Jih-Fei Cheng et al., eds., 131–47 (Durham, NC: Duke University Press, 2020); Namaste, *Savoirs Créoles: Leçons du Sida pour l'Histoire de Montréal* (Montreal: Mémoire d'Encrier, 2019).

29 Donnelly, "Ten Steps."

30 Canadian Council of Churches, "HIV and AIDS," n.d., https://www.councilofchurches.ca/social-justice/hiv-and-aids/.

31 Canadian AIDS Society, "History."

32  "Icons, Media Key to Reducing Stigma of Disease, Gere Says," *Ottawa Citizen*, August 15, 2006, A5.
33  African-Canadian Civic Engagement Council and Innovative Research Group, *Impact of COVID-19: Black Canadian Perspectives* ([N.P.]: African-Canadian Civil Engagement Council and Innovative Research Group, 2020), 3, 11 (hereafter cited as ACCEC/IRC).
34  ACCEC/IRC, *Impact of COVID-19*, 3, 11.
35  Reitmanova et al., "Immigrants Can Be Deadly."

# 3 Racialized Healthcare Inequities Dating to Slavery

*Eric Kyere*

## Introduction

The Black Lives Matter movement makes the case that black lives have not always mattered in the United States. Viewed in historical perspective, it seems clear that countless black lives—specifically, the lives of enslaved people—did not matter at all. Foremost among the unrelenting cruelties that masters, overseers, and other white people heaped upon those individuals was a lack of healthcare.[1] Infants and children fared especially poorly. After childbirth, mothers were forced to return to the fields as soon as possible, often having to leave their infants without care or food. One contemporary scholar estimates that, at one time before emancipation, the infant mortality rate was as high as 50 percent.[2] As for adult people who were enslaved, they often were beaten for showing signs of exhaustion or depression.[3]

Healthcare inequities remain evident in the US. In the early part of 2020, as the COVID-19 pandemic developed, its global nature conveyed the message that everyone was equally impacted by this global health epidemic but not equally resourced in the fight against the disease. When preliminary data and research related to the morbidity and mortality rates emerged, and when measures to contain the pandemic (e.g., physical distancing, stay-at-home orders) were implemented, the international community witnessed differential impacts on its citizens.

The US Centers for Disease Control and Prevention (CDC) found that, compared with whites and Hispanics, blacks in fourteen states were disproportionately hospitalized in the early stages of the pandemic.[4] While the total population of blacks living in the selected states was 18 percent on average, they comprised 33 percent of the infection and hospitalization rates compared to whites, who were 45 percent of the population and 8 percent of the hospitalizations.[5] Hispanics also had disproportionately high hospitalization rates, constituting 59 percent of hospitalizations though only 14 percent of the total population in the fourteen states the CDC surveilled.[6] In examining fatalities, data from New York showed COVID-related deaths per 100,000 population at 92.3 for blacks, 74.3 for Hispanic/Latinx people, 45.2 for whites, and 34.5 for Asians.[7]

DOI: 10.4324/9781003214281-5

Additional research and data showed African Americans and other racial minorities registering disproportionate COVID-19 morbidity and mortality rates.[8] For example, using July 2020 data from the Epic health record system for 7 million black patients and 34.1 million white patients, a group of research scholars estimated hospitalization and death rates per 10,000 patients.[9] According to their research, black people had 24.6 hospitalizations and 5.6 deaths, and white people had 7.4 hospitalizations and 2.3 deaths.[10] Those scholars and others have identified racial segregation as a key driver of the disproportionate impact of COVID-19 on African Americans and other persons of color.[11] African Americans are more likely to live in multigenerational households, live in crowded conditions, and have jobs such as nursing aids, transit workers, and grocery store clerks that are difficult to perform remotely. In addition to those factors, many people in predominantly black communities do not own vehicles and therefore are likely to use public transportation.[12] Moreover, high-risk individuals to COVID-19 tend to have at least one chronic condition (e.g., diabetes, hypertension, obesity, cardiovascular disease).[13]

Racism experienced by African Americans is linked to several chronic illnesses.[14] The COVID-19 pandemic has cast a light on the reality of many African Americans, one that has been long denied or ignored by many scholars: medical racism exists.[15] A review of the history illustrates that pathways of racism situate black people in socially murderous conditions that reproduce or perpetuate adverse health consequences. Most important, a critical historical review can help discover potential resources that African Americans have used to endure, resist, and thrive despite racism's unrelentingly pernicious effects on black communities. This essay documents the Black Church as a spiritual and healing resource dating from slavery.

## History of Racial Health Inequalities

Racialized ideologies and practices, including those in medicine that undermine health and lead to avoidable deaths in black communities, date back to the slave era in the US. Such practices have produced unequal access to healthcare in ways that disproportionately affect African Americans. Scholarship on the evolution of racism and medical history in the US documents white people's reliance on the racist ideas of black people's animal-like inferiority to justify the dehumanization and exploitation of black people for capital accumulation. Medical science, which evolved slowly in colonial North America compared with Europe, assumed biological differences between black and white people to justify the racist idea of black inferiority and the control over black people through oppressive practices.

Colonial racism also justified the precarious living and working conditions, and even rationed medical care, by white slave owners to enslaved black people. Oftentimes, enslaved people were isolated geographically into environments where they were overworked, fed poorly, and housed in overcrowded conditions. Those circumstances promoted the transmission of germs, thereby increasing vulnerability to disease. Moreover, because enslaved people received no pay, they equally as often lacked proper resources to maintain good personal hygiene. They lived with unwashed clothes, infrequent baths, limited dental care, and unclean beds. These living conditions, coupled with sexual, physical, psychological, and spiritual abuses, not only facilitated adverse conditions such as body lice, ringworm of the skin and scalp, and bedbugs[16] but also perpetuated the "assumption of poor health as 'normal' for Blacks."[17]

The oppressive practices and dehumanizing treatments mentioned above began at slave dungeons in forts established by Europeans on the coastal shores of Africa, where they captured and kept Africans before shipping them.[18] In Ghana, for example, such dungeons had very limited ventilation. Captives could not shower for months. Dungeons were where they ate, urinated, defecated, and did everything else. Archeological evidence indicates that, because of deadly conditions, even cleaning dungeons was a feared operation for white people: they were likely to contract smallpox, an intestinal infection, or some other condition.[19]

Numerous white slave traders and physicians across the globe justified the horrendous treatment of enslaved people on partial readings of both the Old and New Testaments.[20] For example, an 1833 report indicated the Harmony Presbytery of South Carolina passed a resolution noting that human bondage had "existed from the days of those good old slave-holders and patriarchs Abraham, Isaac and Jacob (who are now in the kingdom of heaven), to the time when the Apostle Paul sent a runaway home to his master, Philemon."[21] Therefore, the report concluded, "the existence of slavery itself is not opposed to the will of God."[22]

The generally terrible conditions that enslaved people endured in the US and elsewhere in the world led to their tending to have a higher prevalence of disease than free people.[23] Common health problems among those who were enslaved in the US included typhus, measles, mumps, chickenpox, typhoid, and other respiratory or intestinal diseases.[24] Because an enslaved labor force was essential to the wealth of free people, some masters showed interest in the health of their human chattel. Such masters relied on three primary sources to provide care: the enslaver himself or herself, someone enslaved (e.g., older woman, granny doctor), or, frequently of last resort, a white physician.[25]

In numberless instances, white slave masters called for white physicians to treat enslaved black people only when illnesses were severe or when normal procedures became complicated; difficult pregnancies were exemplars.[26] Slave masters typically summoned white physicians to provide services to certify enslaved people were fit to work,[27] and patients, as chattel, often had no say in their plans of care.[28] The possibility that white people would use sick black bodies for experimentation generated substantive fear and mistrust in the healthcare that white physicians provided to enslaved black people in an already class and caste stratified, ethically/racially segregated health system.[29] As a result of the aforementioned tendencies, the best healthcare an enslaved person could expect was combined treatment from a fellow enslaved person, a master, and a physician.[30]

African health practices became part of cooperative exchanges within an emerging Black Church.[31] Overall, the history of health and status of blacks in colonial America presents a nuanced and complicated picture of religion, racism, and health before the creation of the US. When black bodies were certified fit to work, they provided free labor and benefited whites financially. When black people became sick or died, their bodies were integral to establishing medical institutions, training white medical professionals, and achieving medical breakthroughs.[32]

White scientists inflicted tremendous pain on pregnant enslaved women, resulting at times in infant deaths. Nevertheless, many white physicians and medical institutions gained considerable wealth or fame. James M. Sims, a physician and a practicing Christian known today as the "father of American gynecology," treated black women in his care as commodities.[33] One enslaved woman, Lucy, was the subject of thirty gynecological surgeries that Sims performed without anesthesia to perfect his medical procedure before using it on white women he anesthetized.[34] Sims's brand of Christianity aligned with biased concepts, so he accepted a false belief regarding the divine order of slavery and there being both spiritual and physical differences between white and nonwhite people.[35]

Today, racism remains embedded in American society and culture. In many places, racism sustains individual and collective structures that concentrate black people in segregated spaces characterized by under resourced schools, limited employment prospects, food insecurity, a lack of access to healthcare, and higher mortality rates.[36] In a 2020 survey exploring black adult perceptions of racism during the COVID-19 pandemic, 73 percent identify individual acts of racism while 79 percent named structural or systemic racism as obstacles to achieving equal outcomes with white people.[37] In the same survey, the majority of blacks—65 percent of whom were men, and 59 percent were women—indicated that it was a bad time to be living as a black person in the US.[38] Their experiences were continuums of a long history of racism that continues to breed mistrust in black communities. Widespread black concern about COVID-19 vaccinations reflect that stained legacy.[39]

Historical and contemporary evidence suggests that residential segregation is another critical pathway through which racism operates to adversely affect the health of African Americans. Although the court-ordered desegregation of public places like hospitals has existed for generations, high levels of residential segregation have persisted for many more generations. Even churches have been affected. Most blacks and whites still worship separately, so Sunday from 11 a.m. to 12 p.m. remains "the most segregated hour of the week," to quote a 1965 statement by the Rev. Martin Luther King Jr.[40]

Continued residential segregation affects the health and other elements of African Americans' well-being in multiple ways, including access to quality healthcare services, food, housing, schooling, and employment. High poverty and violence rates in many neighborhoods hurt economic status. The concentration of individuals and families into different neighborhoods by race/ethnicity exacerbates matters. A racial empathy gap exists between racial/ethnic groups rather than members within homogenous groups, according to scholars David Williams and Lisa Cooper.[41] The gap, moreover, is longstanding. Because slave owners, including so-called Christian slave owners, dehumanized their human property, enslaved blacks people often fended for themselves. Today, the involvement of black communities in their healthcare needs are rooted in the historical legacies of white exploitation and racial/ethnic bias.

## How Have Black Communities Responded?
## The Black Church as a Case in Point

In the same way that racism has been unrelenting in undermining African Americans' health, black communities have been actively resisting racism's effect on their health.[42] Spirituality, as expressed through black churchgoing, has been a central mechanism by which African Americans from slavery forward have had at their disposal for promoting health and coping with sickness.[43] Spirituality provides comfort and strength to cope with health and has been shown to have a positive effect on the progression of disease and, in some cases, mortality.[44]

Historically, the Black Church has been the cornerstone of black communities, providing the context for developing substantial economic, political, and social capital. It remains a viable institution to confront racism and negative health consequences in black communities.[45] Beyond direct advocacy, black churches engage in several approaches to good healthcare (e.g., education, food pantries, counseling, prayer, collaboration with professionals).[46] Black churches also collaborate with independent researchers as well as colleges and university departments to deliver healthcare services.[47] In addition to those endeavors, black churchgoers provide emotional support to suffers and encourage a range of other health-related activities, to include physical exercise and nutritional guidance, to help others promote wellness.[48]

According to social and behavioral scientist Marino Bruce, faith within black communities represents assets and competencies that address acute health crisis like COVID-19 and sequelae; hence, people should support black churches and engage in the fight against the racial health inequities the COVID pandemic has amplified.[49] Indeed, the pandemic has cast a spotlight on the pre-COVID injustice contexts: many advances in biomedical research did not address health inequity among racial/ethnic groups before COVID; therefore, concerned individuals must understand that advances in medicine alone likely will not address post-COVID challenges in black communities.

The Black Church has been a safe haven for black communities. They have received spiritually affirming messages and social supports that have bolstered their coping capacities in racialized healthcare contexts. The role of black churches in deconstructing racial mistrust and increasing African Americans' access to quality healthcare services in culturally responsive ways is key to achieving equitable healthcare services and better health outcomes.

The COVID-19 pandemic has cast a spotlight on the everyday reality of many individuals within black communities. This reality is likely attributable to both historical and contemporary forms of racism. Moving forward, efforts to care for the health needs of African Americans and to acknowledge the consequences of racial health inequities must also recognize the indispensable role of black churches in promoting health and connecting communities to healthcare practitioners and other healthcare resources.

## Notes

1 Patricia M. Lambert, "Infectious Disease among Enslaved African Americans at Eaton's Estate, Warren County, North Carolina, ca. 1830–1850," *Memórias do Instituto Oswaldo Cruz* 101, supplement 2 (2006): 107–17.
2 Deirdre Cooper Owens and Sharla M. Fett, "Black Maternal and Infant Health: Historical Legacies of Slavery," *American Journal of Public Health* 109 (October 2019): 1342–45.
3 Uchenna Umeh, "Mental Illness in Black Community, 1700–2019: A Short History," *BlackPast*, March 11, 2019, https://www.blackpast.org/african-american-history/mental-illness-in-black-community-1700-2019-a-short-history/.
4 Shikha Garg et al., "Hospitalization Rates and Characteristics of Patients Hospitalized with Laboratory-Confirmed Coronavirus Disease 2019—COVID-NET, 14 States, March 1–30, 2020," *Morbidity and Mortality Weekly Report* 69 (April 17, 2020): 458–64.
5 Garg et al., "Hospitalization Rates and Characteristics."
6 Garg et al., "Hospitalization Rates and Characteristics."
7 Centers for Disease and Control and Prevention, "COVID-19 in Racial and Ethnic Minority Groups," *Homeland Security Digital Library*, April 22, 2020, https://www.hsdl.org/?abstract&did=837299.
8 Baligh R. Yehia, Angela Winegar, and Richard Fogel, "Association of Race with Mortality among Patients Hospitalized with Coronavirus Disease 2019 (COVID-19) at 92 US Hospitals," *JAMA Network Open* 3 (August 2020): 1–9.
9 Leo Lopez III, Louis H. Hart III, and Mitchell H. Katz, "Racial and Ethnic Health Disparities Related to COVID-19," *JAMA: Journal of the American Medical Association* 325 (February 23, 2021): 719–20.
10 Lopez, Hart, and Katz, "Racial and Ethnic Health Disparities."
11 Lopez, Hart, and Katz, "Racial and Ethnic Health Disparities."
12 Lopez, Hart, and Katz, "Racial and Ethnic Health Disparities."
13 Cindy Ogolla Jean-Baptiste and Tyeastia Green, "Commentary on COVID-19 and African Americans. The Numbers Are Just a Tip of a Bigger Iceberg," *Social Sciences and Humanities Open* 2 (2020): 1–3.

14 David R. Williams, Jourdyn A. Lawrence, and Brigette A. Davis, "Racism and Health: Evidence and Needed Research," *Annual Review of Public Health* 40 (2019): 105–25.

15 Jean-Baptiste and Green, "Commentary on COVID-19 and African Americans."

16 Todd L. Savitt, "Black Health on the Plantation: Owners, the Enslaved, and Physicians," *Organization of American Historians Magazine of History* 19 (September 2005): 14–16.

17 W. Michael Byrd and Linda A. Clayton, *The American Health Dilemma*, vol. 2: *Race, Medicine, and Health Care in the United States 1900–2000* (New York, NY: Routledge, 2002), 13.

18 Wazi Apoh, James Anquandah, and Seyram Amenyo-Xa, "Shit, Blood, Artifacts, and Tears: Interrogating Visitor Perceptions and Archaeological Residues at Ghana's Cape Coast Castle Slave Dungeon," *Journal of African Diaspora Archaeology and Heritage* 7 (July 2018): 105–30.

19 Apoh, Anquandah, and Amenyo-Xa, "Shit, Blood, Artifacts, and Tears."

20 Kirk A. Johnson, *Medical Stigmata: Race, Medicine, and the Pursuit of Theological Liberation* (New York, NY: Palgrave Macmillan, 2019); and Ibram X. Kendi, *Stamped from the Beginning: The Definitive History of Racist Ideas in America* (New York, NY: Nation Books, 2016).

21 *Analysis of the Report of a Committee of the House of Commons on the Extinction of Slavery. With Notes by the Editor* (1814; repr., London: Society for the Abolition of Slavery throughout the British Dominions, 1833), 30.

22 *Analysis of the Report of a Committee of the House of Commons on the Extinction of Slavery*, 30.

23 Jennifer Bronson and Tariqah Nuriddin, "'I Don't Believe in Doctors Much': The Social Control of Health Care, Mistrust, and Folk Remedies in the African American Slave Narrative," *Journal of Alternative Perspectives in the Social Sciences* 5 (May 2014): 706–32.

24 Savitt, "Black Health on the Plantation."

25 Bronson and Nuriddin, "I Don't Believe in Doctors Much."

26 Savitt, "Black Health on the Plantation."

27 Harriet A. Washington, *Medical Apartheid: The Dark History of Medical Experimentation on Black Americans from Colonial Times to the Present* (New York, NY: Harlem Moon, 2006).

28 Savitt, "Black Health on the Plantation."

29 Owens and Fett, "Black Maternal and Infant Health."

30 Bronson and Nuriddin, "I Don't Believe in Doctors Much."

31 Albert J. Raboteau, *Slave Religion: The "Invisible Institution" in the Antebellum South*, updated ed. (New York, NY: Oxford University Press, 2004).

32 Owens and Fett, "Black Maternal and Infant Health."

33 Washington, *Medical Apartheid*, 66.

34 Washington, *Medical Apartheid*.

35 J. Marion Sims, *The Story of My Life*, ed. H. Marion-Sims (New York, NY: D. Appleton and Company, 1888).

36 Williams, Lawrence, and Davis, "Racism and Health"; and David R. Williams and Lisa A. Cooper, "COVID-19 and Health Equity—A New Kind of 'Herd Immunity,'" *JAMA: Journal of the American Medical Association* 323 (June 2020): 2478–80.

37. Liz Hamel et al., "KFF/The Undefeated Survey on Race and Health," *Kaiser Family Foundation*, October 13, 2020, https://www.kff.org/racial-equity-and-health-policy/report/kff-the-undefeated-survey-on-race-and-health/.

38   Liz Hamel et al., "KFF/The Undefeated Survey on Race and Health."

39   Lonnae O'Neal, "Half of Black Adults Say They Won't Take a Coronavirus Vaccine," *Undefeated*, October 14, 2020, https://theundefeated.com/features/half-of-black-adults-say-they-wont-take-a-coronavirus-vaccine/. Concern—or outright mistrust—keeps many black people from accessing other health resources that are essential for achieving and maintaining quality health outcomes. In the process, gaps in life outcome expectancies between black people and other ethnic groups grow.

40   "Meet the Press," *NBC*, March 28, 1965, https://m.youtube.com/watch?v=fAtsAwGreyE (quotation); Michael Lipka, "Many U.S. Congregations Are Still Racially Segregated, but Things are Changing," *Pew Research Center*, December 8, 2014, https://www.pewresearch.org/fact-tank/2014/12/08/many-u-s-congregations-are-still-racially-segregated-but-things-are-changing-2/.

41   Williams and Cooper, "COVID-19 and Health Equity."

42   "Amplifying Black Perspectives in Pursuit of Improved Health Outcomes," *Keystone Policy Center*, December 18, 2020, https://www.keystone.org/amplifying-black-perspectives-in-pursuit-of-improved-health-outcomes/.

43   Thabiti M. Anyabwile, *The Decline of African American Theology: From Biblical Faith to Cultural Captivity* (Downers Grove, IL: InterVarsity Press, 2007); and Marino A. Bruce, "COVID-19 and African American Religious Institutions," *Ethnicity and Disease* 30 (summer 2020): 425–28.

44   Anyabwile, *Decline of African American Theology*; Bruce, "COVID-19 and African American Religious Institutions."

45   Anyabwile, *Decline of African American Theology*; Bruce, "COVID-19 and African American Religious Institutions"; "Fighting COVID-19 Vaccine Mistrust in The Black Community," *NPR*, December 19, 2020, https://www.npr.org/2020/12/19/948316306/fighting-covid-19-vaccine-mistrust-in-the-black-community.

46   Lydia R. Figueroa et al., "The Influence of Spirituality on Health Care-Seeking Behaviors among African Americans," *ABNF Journal* 17 (spring 2006): 82–88; and Keith Dempsey, S. Kent Butler, and LaTrece Gaither, "Black Churches and Mental Health Professionals: Can This Collaboration Work?," *Journal of Black Studies* 47 (January 2016): 73–87.

47   Figueroa et al., "Influence of Spirituality on Health Care-Seeking Behaviors"; Dempsey, Butler, and Gaither, "Black Churches and Mental Health Professionals."

48   Tyra Toston Gross et al., "'As a Community, We Need to Be More Health Conscious': Pastors' Perceptions on the Health Status of the Black Church and African-American Communities," *Journal of Racial and Ethnic Health Disparities* 5 (June 2018): 570–79.

49   Bruce, "COVID-19 and African American Religious Institutions."

# 4 Cuban Public Healthcare, Economic Scarcity, and COVID-19 Management

*Jualynne E. Dodson*

## Introduction

On the weekend of July 11, 2021, thousands of Cuban citizens born after the fall of the Soviet Union joined protests for governmental changes. They were tired and frustrated with frightful economic conditions and surges in COVID-19 cases. Electrical blackouts; shortages in available food, medicines, and other basic necessities; inflated prices; long lines for purchases; and deteriorating infrastructures were some of the major problems they faced on a daily basis. For days after July 11, Cubans expressed their desire for sought governmental adjustments and corrections through demonstrations spanning an estimated sixty cities and towns.[1]

Despite the protests and an eightfold surge in COVID infections from July through August, Cuba's healthcare system has been one of the largest successes the nation has produced in the years since achieving political independence in 1959. Nevertheless, the strengths of Cuba's healthcare system have proven insufficient in the face of the evolving coronavirus and shortages of supplies, including medical supplies, and embargoes the United States helped impose and have led for decades.[2]

This essay examines healthcare delivery in multiracial Cuba, focusing both on formal and informal systems that have mobilized around various collective health imperatives. In highlighting achievements, I draw on information acquired through directed and informal interviews I conducted with Cubans—particularly, Afro-Cubans/Blacks/*Afrodescendientes*—and through focus group conversations and systematic observations from 1992 through 2010.

## Cuba and Independence

The Caribbean region has thirteen sovereign island nations and twelve dependent territories. Cuba is the largest of six islands known as the Greater Antilles and has a population of approximately 11.5 million citizens whose ethnic and cultural heritages are mainly indigenous Taíno, African, Chinese, Spanish, and other Western European nationalities.[3] Apart from Chinese Cubans, whose foreparents mostly were brought during the

DOI: 10.4324/9781003214281-6

nineteenth century, descendants of these other population groups have been on the island in before, during, and since Spanish colonization.[4] Members of Cuban racial/ethnic groups struggled together in each military war for national independence and self-determination.

Producing a racially inclusive society was one goal of Cuba's independence struggles, but it took two nineteenth-century campaigns and a 1950s revolution to begin constructing a sovereign order to help accomplish the goal.[5] An 1868 military campaign against Spanish colonialism was unsuccessful, and although the 1895 to 1898 War of Independence succeeded, Cuban efforts were usurped by US intervention that resulted in Spain surrendering control of Guam, Puerto Rico, the Philippines, and Cuba to their Northern neighbors. The US government subsequently installed a military protectorate over Cuba and directed many economic, political, and social affairs on the island.

Cuban challenges to external influences and US dependency, including the presence of organized crime by the mafia, continued until 1953.[6] On July 26 of that year, Fidel Ruiz Castro, Afro-Cuban Juan Almeida Bosque, and other rebels attacked the Moncada military barracks of Santiago de Cuba. In 1959, the Cuban Revolution triumphed, and leaders began organizing new governing structures with the intent of implementing social inclusivity of all Cubans.[7] Implementation was made difficult by hardships from the US economic trade embargo, centuries of social presumptions about African descendants' inherent inferiority, if not subhuman nature, and light-skinned Cubans' control of leadership and resource distribution infrastructures.[8] Much of the population enthusiastically supported the new government, with Fidel Ruiz Castro becoming President, and the inclusionary changes.

As new social structures were evolving, economic and material resources were so scarce that most Cubans' daily life did not improve immediately. Six years of devastating war left horrific economic and agricultural conditions made tolerable by revolutionary promotion and practice aimed at dissolving social class divisions between citizens. The nationwide distribution of healthcare and education, especially in rural areas, demonstrated the real possibility of a new order.

### Healthcare Accomplishments

Although Cuban medical personnel sometimes use colloquial vocabularies about racial/ethnic attributes of their patients, I found no race or ethnic demographics in Cuban healthcare data or in healthcare training or reporting. Without official records that include racial/ethnic categories, I cannot conclude that Cuba has persistent disparities racially/ethnically even though black Cubans/Afro-Cubans/*Afrodescendientes* complained regularly with me about problems. Their grievances centered on the absence of medicines and supplies to care adequately for their conditions and not racial/ethnic discrimination.

Cuba's healthcare sector functions without the amount or the caliber of material resources that many countries consider standard for delivering services. The system also has garnered consistent international recognitions and accolades, to include:

*   a 2015 certificate from the World Health Organization for the elimination of mother-to-child transmission of syphilis and HIV;
*   full vaccination of the population against diphtheria, tetanus, and whooping cough;
*   the elimination of polio and endemic malaria;
*   legislative revisions regarding maternal leave, including time off for prenatal medical care, a six-week leave of absence before birth and three-month leave of absence after birth, time off for pediatrician appointments, and other benefits; and
*   successful handlings of dengue fever during the 1980s and the 2000s.[9]

There are additional data that compare healthcare performance on select indicators, and Table 4.1 presents some hemispheric comparisons. The table demonstrates that, despite an exceptional scarcity of resources, Cuba has delivered strong healthcare services on the selected indicators and compares well with the US, which bears responsibility for trade embargoes and sanctions against Cuba that hinder additional achievements.

Cuba's medical scientific sector has conducted research on issues linked to the population for decades. As the country expanded use of apartment propane gas burners during the 1990s, the devices burned many Cubans. Ana Quirot, an Afro-Cuban track and field middle-distance runner and Olympic medalist from the Oriente region, is the most well-known case. In 1993, a fire caused second- and third-degree burns to more than 30 percent of her body. Medical personnel were able to use an assortment of recently developed treatments to heal Quirot, enabling her to compete and win again.[10] During each one of my stays in Oriente thereafter (Santiago, Guantánamo, Bayamo), I spoke with community members about the innovative treatment. Each person referred to laboratories in Havana developing a specialized cream for burns used successfully on Quirot.[11] Some stories were exaggerated, but I verified basic truths.

The Latin American School of Medicine (ELAM) is a star in the healthcare system. Founded in 1999 in Havana, ELAM admits low-income medical

*Table 4.1* Cuba and the Region: Selected Indicators

| Region | Infant Mortality Per 1,000 Live Births | Under 5 Mortality Per 1,000 Live Births | Life Expectancy: Male | Life Expectancy: Female | Life Expectancy: Overall |
|---|---|---|---|---|---|
| Caribbean | 22 | 33.4 | 66.9 | 71.7 | 69.3 |
| Latin America | 22 | 27.7 | 70.3 | 76.4 | 73.3 |
| United States | 7 | 8 | 75 | 80.4 | 77.7 |
| Cuba | 5.3 | 8 | 75.8 | 79.5 | 77.6 |

students from such global locations as Africa, Asia, and the Americas and women comprise half of the Cuban student population. Medical students of color from the US who study at ELAM often return home to pass board examinations at high levels. Moreover, the Cuban government covers many of the fees that ELAM charges to train international students. While some buildings are not as pleasing aesthetically as structures in wealthier countries, but ELAM facility is clean and healthy.[12]

While attending professional meetings with academics and church laypeople from Ghana, Trinidad, Costa Rica, Kenya, Dominican Republic, and other nations of the Global South (Africa, Asia, Latin America, Oceania), colleagues heard of my Cuban research, as well as my training students, and were eager to share their experiences with Cuban medical personnel.[13] Professional colleagues were unanimous in their view that Cuban doctors in their countries were some of the world's best and with a strong sense of obligation to serving the people.

An important component of the national healthcare system revolves around delivering services through large hospital facilities. The number of hospitals per city within Cuba include four in Havana and in Holguín; three in Matanzas; two each in Cienfuegos, Villa Clara, Ciego de Avila, Camagüey, and Santiago; and one in Pinar del Rio and in Guantanamo. There are also military hospitals.[14]

Although hospitals deliver important health services, neighborhood *policlínicos* carry the larger load of healthcare delivery to the Cuban population. *Policlínicos* are foundational to Cuba's healthcare system. Many facilities are two-story houses painted in distinct colors centrally located in rural and city neighborhoods that serve as community offices for family nurses and doctors. Each *policlínico* provides medical care to neighbors in its catchment area and is responsible for maintaining patients' health records. Personnel deliver recurring care for common illnesses, conduct regular eye examinations, administer vaccinations for common diseases, monitor blood pressure and other vital signs, perform early maternity examinations, conduct dermatological screenings, monitor individuals with diabetes, cardiac conditions, and weight concerns, among other activities. *Policlínicos* usually are located within transportation distance of residents, but doctors and nurses make home visits to those who cannot travel easily.

Community-based centers also function as accredited locations for research and for teaching medical, nursing, and other students in the health sciences.[15] Richard S. Cooper, Joan F. Kennelly, and Pedro Orguñez-Garcia have shown that many highly developed nations' "unwillingness to take account of the Cuban experience … represents an important oversight… . In virtually every critical area of public health and medicine facing poor countries Cuba has achieved undeniable success."[16] My work is an attempt to substantiate data gathered and collected through Cuba's healthcare system. *Policlínicos* treated me successfully, and I had several conversations with their personnel.

Emergency centers constitute the next level in the Cuban healthcare system. In Havana, Holguín, Guantánamo, and Santiago, emergency centers are situated strategically near tourist hotels and *casas particulares* (guest housing facilities equivalent to bed-and-breakfast establishments in the US). There is no charge to non-Cubans who receive care although medicine and injections must be purchased in hard currency instead of by credit cards, among other means. Hospitals are not designated emergency centers but do dispense emergency care.[17]

Cuba maintains residential birthing houses for women in the last stages of pregnancy. Called aptly mothers' houses, the facilities are not used as emergency centers but are specifically for women about to deliver. The birthing houses are located throughout the island and contribute to its reputation as having one of the lowest infant mortality rates, better than several more resourced nations. In 2001, I visited a mother's house in the small Eastern town of Baracoa. In 2003, I lived in a Santiago *casa particular* with a woman who gave birth during my visit. She spoke regularly about preparing to go to the mother's house. After attendants deemed her baby healthy, she returned home. I have read personal accounts of mothers' houses rife with "absurd mechanisms" and other negative experiences, but my encounters while visiting such houses were different.[18]

No health facility I observed was dilapidated. Chairs, desks, lights, benches, curtains, beds, gurneys, blood pressure monitors, thermometers, and other tools were not the most contemporary but appeared exceptionally clean. Hospitals seemed to be constructed during the 1960s, but physical appearances are not as significant as treatment waiting times. When I have gone to a hospital to receive medical examinations, laboratory procedures, diagnostic assessments, or other courses of conventional treatment, I did not receive special or quick attention but, like Cubans there, entered the emergency area, signed-in, took a seat, and waited for staff to take passport information. I described physical symptoms to a nurse, was examined by a doctor, received laboratory tests and results, discussed diagnoses and treatments, was given prescriptions and/or medicine, and left the hospital in just over two hours. My experiences at public hospital emergency rooms in the US, particularly regarding the speed of care before the advent of urgent care facilities countrywide, was much different than my experiences in Cuba. Although healthcare received in Oriente was a bit better than in other regions, the quality of care throughout the island was above average.

My experiences in the Cuba support the idea that its healthcare system can be a bedrock of citizen commitment to the national government. One Afro-Cuban woman asked me, "Why should I go to the US? They don't like black people there and won't protect my baby boy! Here the government cares about all babies, and we get health care."[19]

Coupled with statistical data, such remarks bespeak an Afro-Cuban community whose members believe the state can handle any medical crisis that arises. That health professionals display less racial or ethnic bias than certain professionals in occupations doubtless engenders deep trust and willing support. Accordingly, Afro-Cubans tend to offer their assistance enthusiastically when crises do occur.

## COVID-19 in Cuba

The COVID-19 pandemic has loomed heavy across the globe. In March 2020, a British cruise ship called *MS Braemar* arrived near Havana, Cuba. There were 682 passengers, and several had COVID. The ship's captain wanted to dock and arrange for their transfer to London. Officials in the US and in several Caribbean countries had refused his request, and he was searching desperately for a country whose officials would allow him berth and help in managing the medical emergency. Despite the real danger of COVID, Cuban officials, "out of 'humanitarian concerns,'" journalist Christina Zdanowicz reported, allowed the ship to dock because they comprehended "the difficult situation these passengers find themselves in."[20] It is not clear if the ship brought COVID to Cuba, but the officials' allowance reflects the general spirit of humanitarianism on the island.

In March 2021, a year after the *MS Braemar* incident, the Center for Democracy in the Americas publicized COVID data for Cuba.[21] Among the island's almost 11.5 million residents,[22] there had been 3,318 active cases and 413 deaths since March 2020.[23] In terms of percentages, by my calculations, 0.00028 of the national population had active COVID cases, and 0.00004 died during a year's time.[24]

Comparing phenomena in large and developed countries to small and economically restricted countries can be confusing and misleading; nevertheless, as of April 2021, there were 6,879,670 million active COVID-19 cases in the US (the country had 328.2 million residents at the time), and 573,988 people had died from the disease.[25] In terms of percentages, 0.09667 of the US population had contracted COVID, and 0.00174 had died from it.[26] Such numbers pointed to differences in how the US government managed COVID compared with other governments, such as Cuba. Trade sanctions, however, made managing COVID in Cuba more difficult than in the US. For example, although vaccines were plentiful in the international economic market, there was no guarantee Cuban officials could purchase enough doses to treat all people on the island given existing sanctions.

## Conclusion

During the sixty plus years, Cuba has been sanctioned/embargoed/block-aded, the island government and its people have become exceptionally self-reliant. The March 2021 statement by the Center for Democracy in the Americas also reported Cuban "authorities could seek emergency use authorization in June for the island's Soberana 02 and Abdala vaccines, both of which are currently in the final stage of clinical trials."[27] There also were three vaccines that already had "progressed through various stages of clinical trials: the Soberana 01, Soberana 01A, and Mambisa vaccines."[28]

Despite Cuba's ability to keep COVID infections relatively low more than a year into the pandemic, by mid-2021 the delta variant of the virus was breaking through its firewalls. Consequently, COVID infections and deaths surged. By mid-August 2021, 20 percent (four times the world average) of the Cuban population was testing positive for the virus, and COVID-related deaths were at 52 per million inhabitants (six times the world average).[29] Viewed in terms of actual numbers of cases, COVID infections in Cuba increased from 2,340 to 689,674 between June 2020 and September 2021, and the numbers of COVID deaths increased from 86 to 5,703.[30]

I cannot predict how long Cuba can hold up under its many external and internal pressures. Countless people have questioned its survival since the revolution from 1953 to 1959. Nevertheless, the island country's healthcare system continues to function effectively compared with many other countries. Despite the 2021 protest, Cubans are managing the COVID pandemic in a manner worthy of consideration. They know well the physical consequences of hunger produced by internal shortages from external economic restrictions; nonetheless, Cubans are working effectively to mitigate the impact of COVID.

## Notes

1 Jon Lee Anderson, "Is Cuba's Communist Party Finally Losing Its Hold on the Country?," *New Yorker*, July 22, 2021, https://www.newyorker.com/news/daily-comment/is-cubas-communist-party-finally-losing-its-hold-on-the-country; Beth Daley, "Cuba's Mass Protests Are Driven by the Misery of COVID and Economic Sanctions," *Conversation*, July 16, 2021, https://the-conversation.com/cubas-mass-protests-are-driven-by-the-misery-of-covid-and-economic-sanctions-164505.

2 On the summer 2021 COVID-19 surge in Cuba, see Sarah Marsh, "Coronavirus Surge Pushes Cuba's Healthcare System to Brink," *Reuters*, August 11, 2021, https://www.reuters.com/world/americas/coronavirus-surge-pushes-cubas-healthcare-system-brink-2021-08-11/.

3 United States Central Intelligence Agency. "Cuba," *World Factbook*, June 13, 2006, http://www.umsl.edu/services/govdocs/wofact2006/geos/cu.html.

4 Evelyn Hu-Dehart, "Chinese Coolie Labor in Cuba in the Nineteenth Century: Free Labor or Neoslavery?" *Slavery and Abolition* 14 (April 1993): 67–86.

5 Alejandro de la Fuente, *A Nation for All: Race, Inequality, and Politics in Twentieth-Century Cuba* (Chapel Hill, NC: University of North Carolina Press, 2001).

6 "The Mafia in Cuba," *Cubamafia.com*, n.d., https://www.cubamafia.com/history-of-mafia-in-cuba.html.

7 See Jane Franklin, Cuba and the U.S. Empire: A Chronological History (New York, NY: Monthly Review Press, 2016), 8–12; and "History as Prologue," 7–9.

8 As Philip S. Foner noted in 1977, biased presumptions about the inherent inferiority of Afro-Cubans persisted into the mid-twentieth century despite the fact that Afro-Cubans such as General Antonio Maceo led independence struggles in 1868 and 1895. Foner, *Antonio Maceo: The "Bronze Titan" of Cuba's Struggle for Independence* (1977; repr., New York, NY: Monthly Review Press, 1989).

9 "Dengue Fever Infects Cuba," *Infection Control Today*, February 4, 2002, https://www.infectioncontroltoday.com/view/dengue-fever-infects-cuba. More than 1,600 inhabitants of Cuba were infected with dengue fever between November 2001 and February 2020. Many inhabitants believed the fever's resurgence on the island (following successful handling during the 1980s) was deliberate.

10  "Quirot Gives Birth," *New York Times*, January 26, 1993, B12.

11  Nuria Barbosa León, "Heberprot-P: A Revolutionary Treatment Brings Hope," *Granma*, March 29, 2018, http://en.granma.cu/cuba/2018-03-29/heberprot-p-a-revolutionary-treatment-brings-hope.

12  For information about Medical Education Cooperation with Cuba, visit https://medicc.org/ns/.

13  Regarding traditional geographical localities of the Global South, see, for example, Nour Dados and Raewyn Connell, "The Global South," *Contexts* 11 (winter 2012): 12–13.

14  United States Embassy in Cuba, "Hospitals and Physicians," n.d., https://cu.usembassy.gov/u-s-citizen-services/local-resources-of-u-s-citizens/doctors/medical-information/.

15  Gail Reed, "Cuba's Primary Health Care Revolution: 30 Years On," *Bulletin of the World Health Organisation*, 86 (May 2008): 327–29.

16  Richard S. Cooper, Joan F. Kennelly, and Pedro Orguñez-Garcia, "Health in Cuba," *International Journal of Epidemiology* 35 (August 2006): 817–18.

17  I visited centers for allergy medication, antibiotic injections, and other medicines. Cuban nurses and/or doctors administered the procedures. My charges never exceeded $25 in US currency.

18  Isbel Diaz Torres, "Giving Birth in Cuba," *Havana Times*, September 1, 2010, https://havanatimes.org/diaries/isbel-diaz/giving-birth-in-cuba/.

19  I quote the woman from memory.

20  Christina Zdanowicz, "Multiple Cruise Ships Are Left Stranded as Coronavirus Cases Increase," *CNN*, March 17, 2020, https://www.cnn.com/travel/article/cruise-ships-stranded-coronavirus-trnd/index.html.

21  The data I cite comes from a statement the Center for Democracy in the Americas made on March 26, 2021, https://www.democracyinamericas.org/us-cuba-news-brief/2021-03-26-cuban-migrant-smuggling-ring-busted (hereafter cited as CDA Statement).

22  "Cuba Country Profile," *BBC News*, May 1, 2018, https://www.bbc.com/news/world-latin-america-19583447.

23  CDA Statement.

24  "Total Coronavirus Cases in Cuba," *Worldometer.com*, https://www.worldometers.info/coronavirus/country/cuba.

25  "COVID-19 Update," *DocWireNews*.Com, April 9, 2021, https://www.docwirenews.com/docwire-pick/covid-19-update-eu-regulator-investigating-links-between-j-and-more/.

26  Dillard, "COVID-19 Update."

27  CDA Statement.

28  CDA Statement. The vaccine Mambisa, similar to many other Cuban names, is from African descended soldiers who experienced enslavement but who chose to fight in the 1868 war for Cuban independence.

29  Marsh, "Coronavirus Surge."

30  World Health Organization, "Coronavirus Disease (COVID-19) Situation Report—162," June 3, 2021, https://www.who.int/docs/default-source/coronaviruse/20200630-covid-19-sitrep-162.pdf?sfvrsn=e00a5466_2; Reuters, "COVID-19 Tracker: Latin America and the Caribbean," September 7, 2021, https://graphics.reuters.com/world-coronavirus-tracker-and-maps/regions/latin-america-and-the-caribbean/.

# 5 Black Health, Ethics, and Global Ecology

*Ernst M. Conradie*

## Introduction

The reflections offered here come from someone the South African government classified as white or as European under apartheid, who continues to be classified in that manner under affirmative action, and who has worked at a historically black university, the University of the Western Cape, since 1993. I teach systematic theology and ethics in a religion and theology department, and I focus on Christian ecotheology. I welcome theologian Jürgen Moltmann's reversal of interlocutors in calling for Latin American liberation theology for the First World, black theology for white people, and feminist theology for men. Consistent with backgrounds and beliefs, I treasure finding ways to reflect about common challenges with colleagues and students, both locally and internationally, in ways that are not limited to one set of interlocutors but remain ecumenical in both vision and scope.[1]

Two contrasting observations within global public discourse on the COVID-19 pandemic offer me a point of departure for reflection on black health. First, the pandemic has exposed grave social and economic inequalities (e.g., infections, associated disease burden, housing conditions, access to water and sanitation for personal hygiene, access to healthcare and to healthcare funding). Racial, gender, geographic location, and age reinforce economic inequalities of class. Public health statistics on infections and deaths only partially capture such inequalities. For example, where, how, and who tests for COVID-19, as well as the costs of testing, can influence data. In many instances, I propose, those who do not count to the powers-that-be are not counted. Inversely, what public officials and health experts cannot count—and, for me, human dignity comes to mind—does not really count within this public calculus.

The second observation is a truism: the pandemic has infected, and hence affected, all human societies, cultures, racial-ethnic groups, and tribes. While the virus possibly is the result of illegal global trade in animal products, and was first spread by travelling classes, it is not merely a white affluent disease. The novel coronavirus has reached every nook and cranny of the world, so complete isolation is impossible. This current outbreak has

DOI: 10.4324/9781003214281-7

reinforced, in theory at least, the equal vulnerability of the human body to viruses such as COVID-19. In practice, the same virus affects people in different ways depending on age, immune system, and underlying comorbidity. The resulting disease cannot be addressed selectively from one demographic to another, for example addressed among privileged groups but not among less privileged groups. If inadequate sanitizing due to lack of access or instruction leads to the spread of virus among less affluent populations, it has negative impacts on higher classes. The weakest link matters. This essay situates the current COVID outbreak within an analysis of broader human and environmental ecologies in which it operates.

## Perspectives on Ecologies and Systems

In understanding the human and environmental ecologies in which we operate, there are creative tensions between the global and the local, the public and the private, the similar and the dissimilar, the universal and the particular. It is a focus upon the particular that allows for a discovery of what may be universal, or upon the private (e.g., patriarchy in the household) that allows for understanding of what is manifest in public. But a recognition of what is universal reinforces the significance of the particular.

The implication of my general observations is this: one has to understand black health in a planetary perspective and understand the health of the blue planet from a black perspective (i.e., from the perspective of how planetary health is manifested in black health). I argue that the one cannot be addressed adequately without the other. One needs to zoom out to see the bigger picture of the blue planet, but this is only possible from outer space and with sophisticated levels of technology, which necessarily skews the picture. Therefore, it also is necessary to zoom in on individual cases of health that result in black pain. There is a white fallacy that seeing the blue planet is best done from a white perspective because of white masculine, muscular science. Another part of the fallacy is that science is indeed a white prerogative and domain, which is clearly not the case. Instead, what is needed are perspectives on these urgencies from a broad range of intellectual vantage points, including nature conservation, social justice, and socio-structural analytical frameworks, and that incorporate ethical and experiential concerns identified by persons across spectrums of race, ethnicity, gender, geography, sexual orientation, and faith.[2]

Discourse on environmental racism across the Atlantic, from the United States to South Africa, has rightly focused on issues of toxic waste. It is not possible to remain healthy in a toxic environment. This applies especially to the water we drink, the air we breathe, and the food we eat.[3] The energy we use is a source of many of these toxins so that all four the primal elements (earth, fire, water, air) are involved. However, the main point is that it is not possible to speak of a collective "we" here: the sources of pollution are not equally distributed amongst the population, while the victims are predominantly those already marginalized—again along differences of race, gender, age, and especially class and caste. The sickness may be systemic but the symptoms are particular.

This argument is typically derived from experiences and observations at a local level, in local neighborhoods, based on local testimonies. However, there is a growing recognition that the same problem applies as one zooms out. The underlying systemic disease is not only applicable to ecosystems at a micro or even a macro level but also to whole bioregions and indeed to earth systems.[4]

The terms *earth system* and *earth system science* refer to the way planetary systems interact. These dimensions include the biosphere (living organisms), the atmosphere (various gases in different layers), the hydrosphere (oceans, fresh water, ice), and the lithosphere (solid earth). Each of these can be further subdivided and all are influenced by fluctuations in the earth's axis, the earth's orbit around the sun, solar radiation, the moon, and other forces in the solar system. One would also need to add the influence of the noosphere (the human mind) and its outcomes in terms of technology, culture, and (contested) notions of civilization.

Earth system science (in the singular) emerged over the past two decades to study the interaction between these sub-systems. The landmark "2001 Amsterdam Declaration on Earth System Science," which the International Geosphere-Biosphere Programme issued, reported that the relative stability that characterized the Holocene (roughly the 12,000 years since the last ice age) and also the Pleistocene (roughly the last 2.5 million years characterized by intermittent ice ages) had become disturbed.[5] The report observed that "The interactions and feedbacks between the component parts are complex and exhibit multi-scale temporal and spatial variability" and added the following:

> Human activities are significantly influencing Earth's environment in many ways in addition to greenhouse gas emissions and climate change. Anthropogenic changes to Earth's land surface, oceans, coasts and atmosphere and to biological diversity, the water cycle and biogeochemical cycles are clearly identifiable beyond natural variability. They are equal to some of the great forces of nature in their extent and impact. Many are accelerating. Global change is real and is happening now.... . Earth System dynamics are characterised by critical thresholds and abrupt changes. Human activities could inadvertently trigger such changes with severe consequences for Earth's environment and inhabitants. The Earth System has operated in different states over the last half million years, with abrupt transitions (a decade or less) sometimes occurring between them. Human activities have the potential to switch the Earth System to alternative modes of operation that may prove irreversible and less hospitable to humans and other life. The probability of a human-driven abrupt change in Earth's environment has yet to be

quantified but is not negligible... . In terms of some key environmental parameters, the Earth System has moved well outside the range of the natural variability exhibited over the last half million years at least. The nature of changes now occurring simultaneously in the Earth System, their magnitudes and rates of change, are unprecedented. The Earth is currently operating in a no-analogue state.[6]

Scholars have conducted ongoing research in the field of earth system science since 2001. Some have monitored changes in biogeochemical cycles regarding the nine planetary boundaries that define "a safe operating space for humanity based on the intrinsic biophysical processes that regulate the stability of the Earth system."[7] The nine boundaries focus on climate change, biosphere integrity, or the rate of biodiversity loss, stratospheric ozone depletion, ocean acidification, biogeochemical flows, especially phosphorous and nitrogen, land-system change, freshwater use, atmospheric aerosol loading, and the introduction of novel entities such as chemical pollution. The assumption is that these boundaries describe a state of the earth system that does not risk destabilizing the Holocene epoch within which human civilizations emerged.[8] Humanity has faced environmental constraints throughout its history at local and regional levels, but one today should recognize constraints at the planetary level; furthermore, the magnitude of challenges now is vastly different than past generations.[9]

With regard to black health and environmental racism, as mentioned above, one of the planetary boundaries is the introduction of novel entities in the form of chemical pollution. Chemicals form part of nature, but their concentration is the result of human industries and power relations involved. More than 100,000 chemicals are used industrially, and it is well-nigh impossible to monitor the health impact of those chemicals in great detail; hence, black health in highly industrialized societies is important— for the sake of the victims of forces well beyond their control but also for all other people who perhaps are less exposed but still vulnerable to chemical use. Put bluntly, black health should be a concern for affluent whites as well as for black people.[10]

From the perspective of earth system science, people predicted pandemics such as COVID-19 before the World Health Organization labelled COVID a pandemic in 2020.[11] I think the pandemic will last longer than some persons expect; moreover, international citizens should anticipate further outbreaks involving different viruses and not simply mutations of existing viruses.[12] My predictions are sobering to me, given past and present impacts of COVID on human health and the global economy (e.g., unemployment, poverty, hunger).

Yet again, from the perspective of earth system science, I do not think the COVID pandemic is the worst challenge humanity will face during the twenty-first century. A 2009 report, updated in 2015, described the interaction between the nine planetary boundaries. The climate and the biosphere are core because the climate system is a manifestation of the amount, distribution, and net balance of energy at Earth's surface, while the biosphere regulates material and energy flows in the earth system and determines its resilience to abrupt and gradual change.[13] Both the climate and the biosphere have the potential to drive the Earth system into a new state should the two items be transgressed substantially and persistently. As the International Geosphere-Biosphere Programme suggested in 2015, "transgressing one or more planetary boundaries may be deleterious or even catastrophic due to the risk of crossing thresholds that will trigger non-linear, abrupt environmental change within continental to planetary-scale systems."[14]

The programme sought to quantify such boundaries to circumscribe what a safe operating space might be. On that basis, the programme could define a zone of uncertainty, with increasing levels of risk beyond such a boundary. The programme's findings suggest that nitrogen and phosphorous flows, together with genetic diversity loss, already pose high risks and that indicators for climate change and land-system change are in a zone of uncertainty with increasing levels of risk.[15] During the same year, 2015, chemist Will Steffen and his research colleagues spelled out the implications of a failure to heed planetary boundaries:

> Incremental linear changes to the present socioeconomic system are not enough to stabilize the Earth System. Widespread, rapid, and fundamental transformations will likely be required to reduce the risk of crossing the threshold and locking in the Hothouse Earth pathway; these include changes in behavior, technology and innovation, governance, and values.... The Stabilized Earth trajectory requires deliberate management of humanity's relationship with the rest of the Earth System if the world is to avoid crossing a planetary threshold. We suggest that a deep transformation based on a fundamental reorientation of human values, equity, behavior, institutions, economies, and technologies is required.[16]

Such notions of planetary boundaries have inspired a so-called lifebelt, or doughnut, economics that suggests a safe operating space for the economy between outer planetary boundaries and inner social boundaries vis-à-vis minimum requirements for decent living in terms of water, nutrition, healthcare, education, and equity—those boundaries appear as a lifebelt with a hole in the middle, hence the name. My sense is that two implications follow from such observations. On the one hand, people worldwide should expect inequalities to become aggravated as present challenges deepen and worsen. Climate change will affect all human beings, indeed all forms of life on this planet, but not equally. This occurrence translates into moral and ethical principles of common but differentiated responsibilities: countries with historically high carbon emissions should aid countries with historically low carbon emissions, particularly in terms of mitigation and adaptation efforts, technological transfer, and financial support.

## Conclusion

I think it is important to recognize inequality as at least one of the underlying causes of instability among earth systems. One needs to look no further than socioeconomic and other inequalities (e.g., sex, race, gender, ethnicity, class, caste) to understand this truism. In 2009, the South African Council of Churches asserted inequality was the reason many people worldwide thwarted efforts to address climate change.[17] Consider carbon emissions. Consumer culture and significant acceleration in human activity across many metrics since 1945 have correlated directly with and manifested clearly in rising emissions. In highly unequal societies, such phenomena have had a double effect: lower and middle classes have aspired to emulate the lifestyles of affluent classes, only for those with affluence to thwart their dreams.

It comes as no surprise to me that consumerism, supported by the so-called gospel of prosperity, has spread rapidly from the North Atlantic to Asia, Latin America, Eastern Europe, and Africa. To maintain their position amidst the instabilities associated with stark inequalities, affluent people have sought to protect their privilege. For that reason, it is exceptionally hard to move the global economy toward sustainable alternatives or to advance collective thinking beyond hope in technological miracles to address what is at heart a cultural, moral, and spiritual problem.[18]

## Notes

1 Jürgen Moltmann, *Experiences in Theology: Ways and Forms of Christian Theology* (Minneapolis, MN: Fortress, 2000).
2 In South Africa, the tension between green (nature conservation) and brown (social justice) agendas is a familiar topic of conversation. Red infers socialist movements; pink lesbian, gay, bisexual, transgender, queer or questioning, intersex, and asexual or allied; and purple faith-based organizations. See James Cone, "Whose Earth Is It Anyway?," in Dieter T. Hessel and Larry Rasmussen, eds., *Earth Habitat: Eco-Injustices and the Church's Response* (Minneapolis, MN: Fortress Press, 2000), 23–32; and Steve de Gruchy, *Keeping Body and Soul Together: Reflections by Steve de Gruchy on Theology and Development* (Pietermaritzburg, South Africa: Cluster Publications, 2015).
3 See Ernst M. Conradie and David N. Field *A Rainbow Over the Land: Equipping Christians to Be Earthkeepers* (Wellington, South Africa: Bible Media, 2016).
4 Ernst M. Conradie, *Secular Discourse on Sin in the Anthropocene: What's Wrong with the World?* (Langham, MD: Lexington Books, 2020).
5 See Berrien Moore III et al., "2001 Amsterdam Declaration on Earth System Science," *International Geosphere-Biosphere Programme*, July 13, 2001, http://www.igbp.net/about/history/2001amsterdamdeclarationonearthsystemscience.4.1b8ae20512db692f2a680001312.html.
6 Moore et al., "2001 Amsterdam Declaration."

7 Will Steffen et al., "Planetary Boundaries: Guiding Human Development on a Changing Planet," *Science* 347 (January 2015): 737.
8 Will Steffen et al., "Planetary Boundaries," 747.
9 Steffen et al., "Planetary Boundaries," 737.
10 Tyrone B. Hayes and Martin Hansen extend concerns about environmental racism to concerns for frogs, the proverbial canaries in the mine that serve as warnings that things have gone wrong. Hayes and Hansen, "From Silent Spring to Silent Night: Agrochemicals and the Anthropocene," *Elementa Science of Anthropocene* 5 (September 2017), https://www.elementascience.org/articles/10.1525/elementa.246/.
11 "WHO Director-General's Opening Remarks at the Media Briefing on COVID-19," *World Health Organization*, March 11, 2020, https://www.who.int/director-general/speeches/detail/who-director-general-s-opening-remarks-at-the-media-briefing-on-covid-19. March 11, 2020.
12 See, for example, James Gorman, "Potential for New Coronaviruses May Be Greater than Known," *New York Times*, February 16, 2021.
13 See Steffen et al., "Planetary Boundaries," 737.
14 Rockström et al., "Planetary Boundaries."
15 See Steffen et al., "Planetary Boundaries."
16 Will Steffen et al, "Trajectories of the Earth System in the Anthropocene," *Proceedings of the National Academy of Sciences of the United States of America* 115 (August 2018): 8257.
17 South African Council of Churches, *Climate Change: A Challenge to the Churches in South Africa* (Marshalltown, South Africa: South African Council of Churches, 2009).
18 For a set of recent reflections structured around global inequalities, see Ernst M. Conradie and Hilda P. Koster, eds., *The T&T Clark Handbook on Christian Theology and Climate Change* (New York, NY: Bloomsbury, 2019).

# 6   Food Insecurity, Black Churches, and Black Household Vulnerabilities during COVID-19

*Margaret Lombe, Von Nebbitt,*
*Khristian Howard, Heber Brown III,*
*and Mansoo Yu*

## Introduction

Before the COVID-19 pandemic devastated the globe, food insecurity presented a threat to health outcomes for communities of color. Research shows connections between food insecurity and health for children, adults, and senior citizens ranging from conditions like anemia and asthma in children, depression and suicide ideation in adults, and limitations to independence and daily functioning for senior citizens.[1] Experiences of food insecurity are rife with disparities for black and Hispanic/Latinx communities, reflecting the effects of socioeconomic inequities like poverty and unemployment.[2] With black and Hispanic/Latinx communities experiencing food insecurity at rates nearly double that of white communities, communities of color can experience more detrimental health outcomes and are less insulated against the effects of a global pandemic.[3]

The disproportional onslaught of COVID has exacerbated the food insecurity and health burden experienced by communities of color. The pandemic has revealed race-ingrained inequities exemplified in economic inequities like limited asset ownership, housing instability, and weak attachment to jobs that pay a decent wage. We contend food security should be regarded as a critical human rights and public health issue rather than a matter of charity.[4] The Center on Budget and Policy Priorities found that adults who reported their households had "not enough to eat" at some point in the last 12 months nearly tripled from 2019 (3.4 percent) to 2020 (9 percent). Although the impacts of the pandemic on food insecurity have been widespread, it is particularly prevalent among black and Hispanic/Latinx adults, and other people of color.[5]

In this essay, we use the layered vulnerabilities framework to better understand the factors that contribute to food insecurity and health outcomes in general, and the cumulative effects of COVID. We conclude by highlighting the roles of black churches as community resources that mitigate food insecurity and its effects.

DOI: 10.4324/9781003214281-8

## Layered Vulnerabilities, Black Communities, and Food Insecurities

Understanding experiences of food insecurity during the COVID pandemic in black communities through a lens of layered vulnerabilities enables one to identify and uncover myriad aspects of susceptibility.[6] Bioethicist Florencia Luna introduced the concept during the early twentieth century to highlight problems ranging from job insecurity to crowded housing.[7] She contends a vulnerability is not a permanent trait in a subpopulation; instead, a vulnerability can be contextual or transient. As this essays will show, her layered approach helps explain how the pandemic has affected the black community in the US by uncovering negative effects of concentrated poverty, job insecurity, and crowded housing.[8] For example, fast food restaurants and convenient stores, as opposed to places offering healthy menus, were abundant in many low-resourced communities of color before COVID decimated the communities.[9] The pandemic and attendant lacks of employment opportunities and healthcare facilities have constituted additional layers of vulnerability in those communities, and we believe Luna's concept can help guide public policy and practice to design successful interventions.

### *Extent of Food Security during COVID*

The United States Department of Agriculture (USDA) defines food insecurity as uncertainty about or inability to obtain enough food to feed everyone in a household at some point during the year.[10] The government measures food insecurity annually using an eighteen-item survey that contains ten adult and eight child items.[11] Prior to the pandemic, about 11 percent of households were food insecure, according to the USDA.[12] Data from the Urban Institute's Health Reform Monitoring Survey suggest that from March 25 to April 10, 2020, approximately 22 percent of households with nonelderly adults were insecure.[13] A January 2021 estimate indicated that such insecurity had risen to 38 percent of American households.[14]

Regarding adults solely, food insecurity rates declined to around 15.3 percent between April 2020 and April 2021. For households with children under age nineteen, the rate dropped from 23.8 percent in 2020 to 17.7 percent in 2021. However, for racial and ethnic minorities such as black and Latinx adults, food insecurity rates still are disproportionately high in 2021, at 19.6 percent and 25.7 percent, respectively. For white adults, in contrast, the April 2021 rate was 11.7 percent.[15]

The disparities in the preceding paragraph are consistent for households with young children as well as households that women head. According to a Feeding America report, two in five female-headed households with children under age twelve were food insecure in early 2021.[16] Compared with 2018, food insecurity in households with children has increased by about 130 percent; however, the most recent projections from Feeding America show slight improvement, estimating that around 13 million children, or one in six, will be food insecure in 2021, a change Feeding America attributes to improved unemployment rates and safety net responses.[17] Nonetheless, today's food insecurity rates still surpass those from before the pandemic.[18]

Experiences of food insecurity and COVID show variation across race and ethnic group, with people of color bearing the worst. Indeed, in 2018 only about 25 percent of black households with children were food insecure. Today, nearly four in ten black households with children struggle to feed their families. That surge in households experiencing food insecurity is higher than rates during the Great Recession of December 2007 to June 2009.[19]

A dramatic spike in food insecurity likely will exacerbate racial and ethnic inequities and potentially threaten the health of millions of young black Americans. Food insecurity often results in health problems such as obesity, diabetes, asthma, anemia, depression, and anxiety.[20] Pre-COVID health disparities existed for black and Latinx populations, who experienced higher rates of diabetes, obesity, hypertension, and HIV than white populations; compounded with food insecurity and the threat of COVID, those disparities can worsen.[21]

Food insecurity in the US is a social justice issue entrenched deeply in the country's history of slavery and persistent structural racism.[22] Food insecurity also is ingrained in residential segregation and other forms of inequality, to include concentrated poverty, weak affiliation to jobs that pay decent wages, and housing instability. Many African American households are more likely to report weak affiliation to the labor market and to be disproportionately affected by poverty, factors that make combatting hunger and food insecurity more difficult to defeat.

Coupled with the hardships mentioned above, black households face challenges related to housing affordability. Reliable scholarship demonstrates that many households in poverty often have to make hard choices between rent obligations and consumption needs—often sacrificing consumption.[23] Other tradeoffs include prioritizing medicine over food, consuming cheaper and shelf-stable foods, skipping meals, or engaging in transactional sex for meals.[24] The COVID-19 pandemic has impacted the food security of black families directly through illness-related income loss and indirectly through loss of productivity, weakened social networks, and compromised health.[25]

*Employment*

Households experiencing unemployment during the pandemic makeup about 25.3 percent of households experiencing food insecurity.[26] Because black and Latino workers tend to occupy low paying jobs, they have challenges accumulating the savings and other benefits that help cushion blows from challenging times such as the present economic rage caused or exacerbated by COVID. While unemployment has increased sharply among all groups of workers during the pandemic, the rate of unemployment among racial minorities has remained disproportionately high.[27]

From February to April 2020, unemployment skyrocketed, approximating 14.2 percent for white workers and 16.7 percent for black workers.[28] Using February 2020 as a baseline, we note the unemployment rate for black workers was 5.8 percent compared to 3.1 percent for white workers. The actual rate might have been higher, as certain sources classified people as employed despite their being absent from work.[29] In any event, unemployment rates declined after April 2020. In April 2021, the rate was 5.3 percent for white workers, 7.9 percent for Latinx workers, and 9.7 percent for black workers.[30] Even so, unemployment for black people almost doubled the unemployment of their white counterparts. Such statistics are noteworthy and suggest that black people bear the brunt of the pandemic-induced economic crisis.[31]

### Housing Instability

Data link housing instability, characterized by overcrowding and eviction, to food insecurity.[32] Pointing to a connection between housing stability and food security, many scholars agree that having stable and affordable housing enables families to dedicate leftover income to food and to other necessities—after paying rent, mortgage, or a related cost.[33] Housing vulnerabilities exemplified by unaffordability have been on the increase for years; however, COVID-19 pushed housing affordability and food security to the forefront of policy discussions. The pandemic has not only exacerbated housing challenges experienced by low-income households but also revealed racial inequalities in housing.

Data reveal a wide gap in white and black homeownership—a difference of 30 percentage points in 2017. This margin reflected the highest homeownership gap since the Great Recession, with white homeownership at 71.9 percent and black homeownership at 41.8 percent, surpassing the homeownership gap during times of legal housing discrimination.[34] Such data are important for two reasons: homeownership historically has been an important means for Americans to accumulate wealth, and black households are more likely than any other group to rent; therefore, black Americans tend to suffer most from any housing related phenomenon, including eviction.[35]

Current data suggest an increase in housing unaffordability before the pandemic. More than 40 percent of renters are cost-burdened, with one in four spending more than half their income on housing. In 2019, by contrast, households classified as cost burdened spend more than 30 percent their income on housing.[36] In 2019, only 21 percent of white renters were cost burdened.[37] Given that black households are more likely to rent, such households also are more likely to experience eviction related to loss of a job and other insecurities. Black women, often in households with children, bear the greatest risk.[38]

High rates of evictions connected to COVID-19 have hit low-income communities especially hard. Disruption in utility services and over-crowded housing (three to five people in a two-bedroom apartment), among other layers to the housing problem, make it difficult for people to social distance properly or to quarantine if needed. As the pandemic laid bare the layers of vulnerabilities experienced by black households and their communities, local organizations like black churches were organizing their assets.[39]

### The Role of Black Churches in Mitigating Food Insecurity

In communities of color, it is not unusual to encounter families experiencing employment or income losses due to the pandemic. As families strive to put food on the table, maintain housing, and keep utilities on, they sometimes turn to local churches for assistance. As in many other cases, black churches have risen to the challenge by addressing not only spiritual needs but also building relationships and attending to physical needs.[40] In fact, some black church ministries have started looking for ways to go beyond traditional soup kitchen models to address systemic food shortages.[41] Among other acts, ministries have called attention to food deserts and, moreover, to systemic injustices that create deserts and similar food problems.[42]

New faith-based models addressing food insecurity reflect communal and collectivist approaches of the first church in the Book of Acts and notable black faith leaders. A black initiative we describe below was inspired by the food sovereignty work of faith leaders such as Fannie Lou Hamer and the Revs. Vernon Johns, Major Jealous (Father) Divine, and Albert B. Cleage Jr.[43] They not only protested but also shifted paradigms and built institutions. In 1969, for example, Hamer established the 680-acre Freedom Farm Cooperative.[44] Owned by African American families, the co-op included a head start facility, a commercial kitchen, affordable housing, and other accommodations. Today, a new generation of leaders is extending that legacy in agriculture, food distribution, and lodging.

The Black Church Food Security Network, or simply the Network, a faith-based initiative based in Baltimore established in 2015, offers a sustainable solution to food injustice.[45] Responding to the rising number of diet-related illnesses among Pleasant Hope Baptist Church members, Rev. Dr. Heber Brown III engaged church elders to provide leadership and instruction for a micro farm.[46] Born in the South, the elders grew up on multigenerational farms before moving north as a part of the Great Migration of circa 1916 to 1970.[47] The Church harvests 1,200 pounds of produce each year on only 1,500 square feet of land.[48]

The Network focuses on both food access and food system agency. Discovering the benefit of gardening and distributing produce to church members, the Network developed several programs to replicate success at other black churches. For example, Operation Higher Ground works with black churches to establish gardens or other agricultural projects on church property to give people greater ownership of their food environments. Soil to Sanctuary Market, another Network program, organizes miniature farmers' markets inside churches on days of worship to give parishioners access to nutrient-rich food and to support black farmers and business owners.

In fall 2020, the Network launched a program called the Black Church Supported Agriculture (BCSA). Community-supported agriculture was its precedent. Noting how churches established food distribution sites during the COVID-19 pandemic, the Network created the BCSA to establish a pathway for black churches to buy products in bulk from black farmers to support their communities. The Network organized meetings between rural black farmers and urban black pastors to coordinate transportation, storage, and distribution of nutrient-rich produce and related goods.

Pastor Brown and other members of the Network are not simply organizing the resources of local black churches; Brown and his Network associates are weaving together member congregations across the country. They provide education about black food histories, train churches to obtain control of their food environments, and help establish collective health goals by leveraging existing relationships and assets. More than fifty congregations from across the country participated in 2020. The next year the Network formed partnership with The Balm in Gilead to expand its reach and the capacity to engage in health education.

## Conclusion

The long-term consequences of COVID-19 on food insecurity and the health of black communities is unknown. The pandemic, however, has made several ugly truths including systemic racism, deeply ingrained economic inequity, and the layered vulnerability of healthcare quite visible. Today, across the US, millions of people already susceptible to food insecurity continue to face unimaginable challenges as 40 percent (80 billion lbs.) of food ends up in landfills each day.[49]

We believe the intersectionality of race, place, housing, employment, food security, and health has become more visible than ever before. Given the layered character of societal vulnerabilities, addressing a singular need is not enough to create positive change. The challenges revealed by COVID call for a multidimensional response that starts with understanding long-term effects of systemic racism, related inequities, and connections between jobs, housing, food insecurity, and health. There is also a need for health promoting resources in communities of color, going beyond COVID to include surveillance of food insecurities and diseases that disproportionately affect low-income neighborhoods, especially communities of color whose members often struggle to attain sufficient housing and employment because of the sordid legacy of American injustice.

## Notes

1  Craig Gundersen and James P. Ziliak, "Food Insecurity and Health Outcomes," *Health Affairs* 34 (November 2015): 1830–39.
2  Angela M. Odoms-Young and Marino M. Bruce, "Examining the Impact of Structural Racism on Food Insecurity: Implications for Addressing Racial/ Ethnic Disparities," *Family and Community Health* 41, no. 2, supplement 2: Food Insecurity and Obesity (April–June 2018): S3–S6.
3  Elaine Waxman and Poonam Gupta, "Food Insecurity Fell Nearly 30 Percent between Spring 2020 and 2021," *Urban Institute*, May 26, 2021, https://www.urban. org/research/publication/food-insecurity-fell-nearly-30-percent-between-spring-2020-and-2021.
4  Mariana Chilton and Donald Rose, "A Rights-Based Approach to Food Insecurity in the United States," *American Journal of Public Health* 99 (July 2009): 1203–11; and Maritza Vasquez Reyes, "The Disproportional Impact of COVID-19 on African Americans," *Health and Human Rights Journal* 22 (December 2020): 299–307.
5  "Tracking the COVID-19 Recession's Effects on Food, Housing, and Employment Hardships," *Center on Budget and Policy Priorities*, August 9, 2021, https://www.cbpp.org/sites/default/files/8-13-20pov.pdf.
6  Florencia Luna, "Elucidating the Concept of Vulnerability: Layers Not Labels," *International Journal of Feminist Approaches to Bioethics* 2 (March 2009): 121–39.
7  Luna, "Elucidating the Concept of Vulnerability."
8  David R. Williams and Lisa A. Cooper, "COVID-19 and Health Equity—A New Kind of 'Herd Immunity,'" *JAMA: Journal of the American Medical Association* 323 (June 2020): 2478–80.
9  Renee Catacalos, "Black Residents Navigate an Unequal Food Landscape in Washington, D.C.," Review of *Black Food Geographies: Race, Self-Reliance, and Food Access in Washington, D.C.*, by Ashanté M. Reese, *Journal of Agriculture, Food Systems, and Community Development* 9 (spring 2020): 327–29.
10  United States Department of Agriculture, "Definitions of Food Security," September 9, 2020, https://www.ers.usda.gov/topics/food-nutrition-assistance/ food-security-in-the-us/definitions-of-food-security.aspx#ranges. (cited hereafter as USDA.)
11  During the COVID-19 pandemic, the Census Bureau has asked households about their ability to access food and feed their households during the preceding week.
12  USDA, "Key Statistics and Graphics of Food Security Status of U.S. Households in 2019," September 9, 2020, https://www.ers.usda.gov/topics/ food-nutrition-assistance/food-security-in-the-us/key-statistics-graphics. aspx#foodsecure.
13  Waxman and Gupta, "Food Insecurity Fell."
14  Kevin M. Fitzpatrick et al., "Assessing Food Insecurity among US Adults during the COVID-19 Pandemic," *Journal of Hunger and Environmental Nutrition* 16 (January 2021): 1–18; and Diane Schanzenbach and Abigail Pitts, "Estimates of Food Insecurity during the COVID-19 Crisis: Results from the COVID Impact Survey, *Week 2* (May 4–10, 2020)," Northwestern Institute for Policy Research, May 18, 2020, https://www.ipr.northwestern.edu/documents/ reports/food-insecurity-covid_week2_report-18-may-2020.pdf.
15  Waxman and Gupta, "Food Insecurity Fell."
16  Monica Hake et al., "The Impact of the Coronavirus on Child Food Insecurity," *Feeding America*, April 22, 2020, https://www.feedingamerica.org/sites/ default/files/2020-04/Brief_Impact%20of%20Covid%20on%20Child%20 Food%20Insecurity%204.22.20.pdf.
17  Hake et al., "Impact of the Coronavirus."

18　Hake et al., "Impact of the Coronavirus."

19　James P. Ziliak, "Food Hardship during the COVID-19 Pandemic and Great Recession," *Applied Economic Perspectives and Policy* 43 (March 2021): 132–52.

20　Anna M. Leddy et al., "A Conceptual Model for Understanding the Rapid COVID-19–Related Increase in Food Insecurity and Its Impact on Health and Healthcare," *American Journal of Clinical Nutrition* 112 (November 2020): 1162–69.

21　Leddy et al., "Conceptual Model."

22　"The History of Our Food System Is Rooted in Racism," *Freight Farms*, August 10, 2020, https://www.freightfarms.com/blog/history-food-system.

23　"Understand Food Insecurity," *Feeding America*, n.d., https://hungerand-health.feedingamerica.org/understand-food-insecurity/.

24　Leddy et al., "Conceptual Model."

25　Gregorio A. Millett et al., "Assessing Differential Impacts of COVID-19 on Black Communities," *Annals of Epidemiology* 47 (July 2020): 37–44.

26　Clyde W. Yancy, "COVID-19 and African Americans," *JAMA: Journal of the American Medical Association* 323 (May 19, 2020): 1891.

27　See United States Bureau of Labor Statistics, "Table A-2 Employment Status of the Civilian Population by Race, Sex, and Age," July 2, 2021, https://www.bls.gov/news.release/empsit.t02.htm; and Jhacova Williams, "Laid Off More, Hired Less: Black Workers in the COVID-19 Recession," *RAND Blog*, September 29, 2020, https://www.rand.org/blog/2020/09/laid-off-more-hired-less-black-workers-in-the-covid.html.

28　Ben Casselman, "The U.S. Added 1.4 Million Jobs in August as Unemployment Fell to 8.4 Percent," *New York Times*, September 4, 2020, https://www.nytimes.com/live/2020/09/04/business/stock-market-today-coronavirus/jobs-report-august-2020 United States Bureau of Labor Statistics, "The Employment Situation–April 2021," May 7, 2021, https://www.bls.gov/news.release/archives/empsit_05072021.pdf; United States Bureau of Labor Statistics, "The Employment Situation–February 2021," March 5, 2021, https://www.bls.gov/news.release/archives/empsit_03052021.pdf.

29　Lauren Bauer et al., "Who Are the Potentially Misclassified in the Employment Report?," *Brookings*, June 30, 2020, https://www.brookings.edu/blog/up-front/2020/06/30/who-are-the-potentially-misclassified-in-the-employment-report/; Steven Brown, "The COVID-19 Crisis Continues to Have Uneven Economic Impact by Race and Ethnicity," *Urban Institute*, July 1, 2020, https://www.urban.org/urban-wire/covid-19-crisis-continues-have-uneven-economic-impact-race-and-ethnicity.

30　United States Bureau of Labor Statistics, "The Employment Situation April 2021."

31　See Nicole Bateman and Martha Ross, "Why Has COVID-19 Been Especially Harmful for Working Women?," *Brookings*, October 2020, https://www.brookings.edu/essay/why-has-covid-19-been-especially-harmful-for-working-women/; Elise Gould and Valerie Wilson, "Black Workers Face Two of the Most Lethal Preexisting Conditions for Coronavirus—Racism and Economic Inequality" *Economic Policy Institute*, June 1, 2020, https://www.epi.org/publication/black-workers-covid/.

32　Feeding America, *Map the Meal Gap 2020* (Chicago: Feeding America, 2020).

33　"U.S. Home Ownership Rate in 2019, by Race," *Statista*, June 21, 2021, https://www.statista.com/statistics/639685/us-home-ownership-rate-by-race/.

34　Jung Hyun Choi, "Breaking Down the Black-White Homeownership Gap," *Urban Wire*, February 21, 2020, https://www.urban.org/urban-wire/breaking-down-black-white-homeownership-gap.

35  Sophia Weeden, "Black and Hispanic Renters Face Greatest Threat of Eviction in Pandemic," *Joint Center for Housing Studies of Harvard University*, January 11, 2021, https://www.jchs.harvard.edu/blog/black-and-hispanic-renters-face-greatest-threat-eviction-pandemic.
36  Weeden, "Black and Hispanic Renters."
37  Weeden, "Black and Hispanic Renters."
38  Adam Macinnis, "Baltimore Pastor Sees Long-Term Solution to Food Insecurity: Black Church Farms", *Christianity Today*, August 3, 2020, https://www.christianitytoday.com/news/2020/august/food-security-hunger-covid-protests-black-church-farm.html.
39  Amy Frykholm and Heber Brown III, "The Black Church Food Security Network Aims to Heal the Land and Heal the Soul," *Christian Century*, November 10, 2020, https://www.christiancentury.org/article/interview/black-church-food-security-network-aims-heal-land-and-heal-soul.
40  See C. Eric Lincoln and Lawrence H. Mamiya, *The Black Church in the African American Experience* (Durham, NC: Duke University Press, 1990); and Henry Louis Gates, Jr., *The Black Church: This Is Our Story, This Is Our Song* (New York, NY: Penguin Press, 2021).
41  Stephanie Boddie, "Creating an Oasis Food Ecosystem in a Post-'Faith-Based Initiative' Environment," in *Urban Ministry Reconsidered: Contexts and Approaches*, ed. R. Drew Smith, Stephanie Boddie, and Ronald E. Peters, 176–84 (Louisville, KY: Westminster John Knox Press, 2018).
42  Boddie, "Creating an Oasis."
43  Heber M. Brown III, "The Genesis of the Black Church Food Security Network," *Princeton Theological Seminary*, July 11, 2019, https://www.ptsem.edu/news/the-genesis-of-the-black-church-food-security-network.
44  Monica M. White, *Freedom Farmers: Agricultural Resistance and the Black Freedom Movement* (Chapel Hill, NC: University of North Carolina Press, 2018).
45  Brown, "Genesis of the Black Church Food Security Network."
46  Stephanie Clintonia Boddie and Lakia M. Scott, "Food Insecurity Is an Equity Issue," *Hunger News and Hope* 19 (fall 2019): 2–3.
47  *Negro Migration in 1916–17: Reports by R. H. Leavell, T. R. Snavely, T. J. Woofter, Jr., W. T. B. Williams and Francis D. Tyson* (Washington: Government Printing Office, 1919); Joe William Trotter, Jr., ed., *The Great Migration in Historical Perspective: New Dimensions of Race, Class, and Gender* (Bloomington: Indiana University Press, 1991); Isabel Wilkerson, *The Warmth of Other Suns: The Epic Story of America's Great Migration* (New York, NY: Vintage Books, 2010).
48  Brown, "Genesis of the Black Church Food Security Network."
49  "Food Waste in America in 2020: Statistics and Facts," *Nutrition Connect*, n.d., https://nutritionconnect.org/resource-center/food-waste-america-2020-statistics-and-facts.

# 7  Setswana Medicinal Practices and Tensions with Western Healthcare Perspectives

*Itumeleng Daniel Mothoagae*

## Introduction

This essay focuses on past encounters between the London Missionary Society (LMS) and the Batswana people who lived in the Northwestern part of South Africa as well as in Botswana.[1] The theo-politics and the geo-politics of space, health, religion, and knowledge characterized the LMS missionary enterprise in southern Africa. Missionaries, as a core part of their endeavors and vigor to convert the Batswana, introduced Western medication, tobacco, agricultural skills, and schools.[2] Those introductions functioned collectively as a discursive tool to affect cultural change, including conversion to Christianity.

As part of the theo-politics and geo-politics of knowledge, missionaries engaged in spatial contestation with local *dingakas*, or diviners-healers.[3] Through literary works, the missionaries constructed an intentionally obscure characterization of *dingakas* as well as traditional medicines. In this essay, I map the intersectionality of traditional herbal medicine, Western medicine, and the spatial contestations of black bodies. In particular, I contend the introduction of Western medicine among the Batswana needs to be located within the "colonial matrix of power," a concept based on Walter Mignolo's articulation of Anibal Quijano: "The 'colonial matrix of power' is the specification of what the term 'colonial world' means both in its logical structure and in its historical transformation."[4] Relative to Setswana, Western medicine as a technology of power continues to function as a form of gaze and dominance over the health system and is expressed in cultural practices, especially religion.

Long-standing debates among Batswana about the use of traditional herbs/plants such as *lengana* (Artemisia afra/African wormwood) and *ser-okolo* (wilder ginger/African ginger/*Siphonochilus aethiopicus*) for medicinal purposes is evident in health discourses that took place during the late nineteenth century. Such discourses found their way into newspapers such as *Mahoko a Becwana*, where the broader technology of the colonial matrix of power was expressed through the condemning of traditional herbs/plants, which Westerners deemed to be heathenism. In one letter published in

DOI: 10.4324/9781003214281-9

*Mahoko a Becwana*, Michael Tshabadira Moroka addressed the following remarks to a fellow Batswana:

> [Are] you saying that traditional medicine is sinful or heathenism? Or it is against the laws of God or of the Europeans? Or are you simply feeling pity for them? I am asking you. If you say it is sinful or perhaps heathenism, have you abandoned small medicinal treatments for children? ... For goodness sake! When you see that which is new, you want to imitate it and you forget your past... . I don't know, Batswana, what we are, because we are not doing the practices of either Tswana or European culture.[5]

Moroka's statement illustrated the extent to which the debate on the use of traditional medicine dominated the discourses of the time. Such discourses intensified during the COVID-19 pandemic. Furthermore, black bodies continue to be the subjects of colonial/Western/patriarchal/capitalist/Christian gazes, norms, and standards as parts of a continual negotiation of the extent to which African traditional herbs/plants can be utilized. The gaze is evident in the regulatory bodies that apply Western standards and norms in determining the efficacy of such medicinal herbs/plants. Doing so, I contend, negates indigenous knowledge systems.

Similar to human immunodeficiency virus and to acquired immunodeficiency syndrome, the COVID-19 pandemic and the use of antiretroviral drugs and vaccines in the context of South Africa have highlighted the depth of the tensions between Western and traditional African medicines and/or Western knowledge system and indigenous knowledge system. Such tensions illustrate how the matrix of power continues to exist within a structure Walter D. Mignolo terms "coloniality."[6]

## African Worldviews, Missionary Mindsets, and Contested Power Over Black Bodies

Efforts to convert indigenous people to Christianity was an act of disciplinary power that missionaries performed to advance colonialism and cultural revolution. Those affiliated with the LMS, through the colonial matrix of power, employed image ontology as a technology to erode the cultural tenets of the Batswana. Michel Foucault believed people did not exercise power via means of episodic or sovereign acts of domination or coercion.[7] Instead, power pervaded society and was in a constant flux of negotiation.[8] Foucault's analysis of power is useful in examining the alteration and erosion of cultural tenets, politics, indigenous knowledge, and health systems that missionaries sought to change through their constructions of the black body within the Western health system.

In the context of healthcare, performance of power functioned on the level of ontology and spirituality, rendering black bodies in need of salvation and also as objects of study. Therefore, Western Christian ideas of salvation and healthcare systems functioned collectively as a disciplinary power.[9] Achille Mbembe outlines effects of conversion: "the act of conversion is also involved in the destruction of worlds. To convert the other is to incite him or her to give up what she or he believed. [Conversion] distances the convert from family, relatives, language, customs, even from geographical environment and social contacts—that is, from various forms of inscription in a genealogy and an imaginary."[10] Converting to Christianity therefore implies a reconstructed way of being and also requires an embrace of canons and regimes of truth. Abandoning one's belief systems and taking on new ones leads to spiritual and epistemological dislocations.

Another dimension of missionary dislocation of African life was at the level of what Mbembe terms "image ontology," or perceptions and prejudices one has about another based on facial appearance, skin color, and related items.[11] Image ontology is central in the process of the construction of the black body and to prejudices necessitating the need to discredit and convert indigenous people to a different spiritual belief. It is through image ontology that political erasure and spiritual epistemicide become actualized.

Missionary image ontologies regarding Africans are evident within missionary literature. In an 1842 publication, LMS missionary Robert Moffat described African diviner-healers and Batswana cosmology as satanic. "In every heathen country," he wrote, "the missionary finds, to his sorrow, some predominating barriers to his usefulness, which require to be overcome before he can expect to reach the judgements of the populace. Sorcerers or rain-makers, for both offices are generally assumed by one individual, are the principal with whom he has to contend in the interior of Southern Africa. They are," Moffet continued, "our invertebrate enemies, and uniformly oppose the introduction of Christianity amongst their countrymen to the utmost of their power. [They] constitute the very pillars of Satan's Kingdom in all places where such impostors are found. By them is his throne supported and the people kept in bondage."[12]

Moffat's characterization of the diviner-healer and the rainmaker, or *dingaka tsa dinaka* and *moroka*, respectively, as a sorcerer and an agents of darkness highlights the colonial mindset and the discursive practices of Moffat's time. Discrediting *ngaka wa morokas* and labeling them as demons associated their traditional healing practices (e.g., using indigenous herbs for medicinal purposes) as evil. Claiming African healers were possessed by evil spirits was one of the mechanisms that missionaries used to facilitate the process of conversion. Western forms of medicines constituted part of the technologies the missionaries utilized as vehicles of cultural change and conversion to Western cultural practices.

## The Construction of the African Body
## within the Colonial Matrix of Power

The arrival of missionaries in South Africa during the nineteenth century was characterized by conversion of the indigenous people. Conversion was premised on the notion of image ontology and disciplinary power—what Michel Foucault termed biopower, a major source of societal discipline and conformism. He moved attention from supreme power to life-giving power that could be observed in the organizational systems and in communal services created in eighteenth-century Europe. Prisons, schools, as well as religious institutions and movements were foremost. Eventually, through systems of surveillance and assessment, missionaries no longer required violence to secure power.[13]

Following Foucault's argument, I argue the missionary movement bordered on sovereign power and disciplinary power. Sovereign power came in the performance of medicinal experimentation. Disciplinary power came in the form of the life-giving, or the improvement thereof, in health conditions of indigenous people.

During the 1880s, Humphreys Williams pointed to a social technology that missionaries performed. It utilized not only preaching but also Western medicine as a form of evangelizing: "It is surprising how soon an isolated case of sickness will become an epidemic, as soon as it has become known that the 'Moruti' [missionary, teacher] has dispensed medicine. At one place a man came to saying he was suffering from certain pains in the stomach. I treated him for indigestion. On the morrow I was amazed to find some dozen or more people coming to my wagon. They all wanted medicine, and strange to say, for the same complaint as that I had treated the previous day."[14] At the same time, indigenous people viewed the presence of missionaries and the use of medicines as beneficial to them, so the question I ask is: Who used whom?

Missionary clinics and hospitals performed power over traditional medicines and black bodies in ways Alexander Butchart outlined: "The theatre of healing had deployed the tactics of clinical medicine upon infirm African bodies as a vehicle of visibility to broadcast outwards and towards the watching the sovereign power of God and 'civilization'. Installation of the hospital reversed this relationship of visibility, and the dominant power vesting in the work of the medical missionary switched from that of conspicuous sovereign to silent surveyor of African suffering and superstitions that 'rudely and barbarously destroy the last remnants of decency and modesty.'"[15]

Butchart's nineteenth-century observation illustrated how Western medicines, in the context of South Africa, functioned as a theatre of healing. The notion of surveillance, a concept that Foucault applied later in his analysis of power, was key to Butchart's argument. For Foucault, one should not have viewed surveillance in isolation from power relations; instead, surveillance was interconnected with power relations, especially governmentality.

In other words, the technologies of power, and how people exerted it, demonstrated the complexity of how power could be used to produce subjectification.[16] Both the missionary theatre of healing and the geo-spatial location of hospitals functioned as what I term the *thingification* of black bodies aimed at the subjectification or production of docile individuals. One should view both technologies of power, as argued by Butchart, as complementary to one another, as the technologies functioned to make spectacles of black bodies.

A 1973 observation by P.J. Kloppers captured the intersection between colonial image ontology and the African body. He stated, "When I do a ward round at the White hospital and then walk over to the Bantu hospital, I truly have to change over in my way of thinking; I have to take one computer program out of my mind and substitute another marked 'Bantu' to work there."[17] Kloppers evidenced a deep-seated racial profiling based on image ontology, where the African body could not be equal to a European body.

Klopper's comment reflected a notion of epistemological superiority and a Western medical perception that dehumanized African bodies, treating them literally as lumps of flesh. There are consequences within such a view, namely, that an African body can be penetrated, dislodged, and disposed of. Furthermore, it points to the medical matter of perceiving and advancing the Western medical system based on the notion of guinea pigs. Western health systems not only reduced black bodies to objects of study but also colonized African medicinal herbs/plants, devalued the indigenous knowledge system, and universalized Western medicine.

## Colonial Missionary Healthcare Paradigms and Indigenous Healthcare Paradigms

Despite colonial machinations, indigenous Africans never abandoned their indigenous health systems. Rather, they performed a technology of resistance in their continual use of such systems. It is within this context, particularly in South Africa, that tensions focus between an emergent Western/missionary health systems and traditional health systems.

Indigenous African people continue to utilize their indigenous medicinal herbs/plants and consult with diviner-healers (*dingakas*) for diagnoses. Their approach to health problems always has been holistic. In addressing the question of recognition of diviner-healers, however, I must examine certain tendencies of the South African government. As Mosa Moshabela, Thembelihle Zuma, and Bernhard Gaede contend, the "current body of evidence demonstrates much progress in the way that traditional healing is perceived in South Africa, having shifted from a derogatory 'witchcraft paradigm' supported by the Witchcraft Suppression Act (3 of 1957), to a more tolerant, and in some instances reconciliatory, discourse of a 'healing paradigm' now protected under the Traditional Health Practitioners Act (22 of 2007)."[18]

The move by the South African government to recognize the role of diviners-healers no doubt was a move towards pluriversality, or pluralism. This movement toward seeing the world in a more pluralistic way challenges the norms of Western medicine. Pluralism is not without its own challenges, however, given that biomedical paradigms operate within the colonial matrix of power.

The COVID-19 pandemic has further opened up the question of epistemic privilege that continues to reside within the colonial missionary/Western health system. Furthermore, COVID has intensified the call for complete recognition of complementary medicines such as the indigenous herbs/plants. Sarah Wild points out disagreements over how traditional remedies should be analyzed. Scrutiny, she notes, remains tied to Western methodologies and protocols: "Scientists, public officials, and traditional healers all seem to agree that traditional medicines must be shown to be safe and effective. The sticking point is how this should happen. And despite a newfound willingness to engage with traditional medicines, Sahpra's evaluation unit will face practical difficulties in evaluating African traditional medicines—including the lack of written records."[19]

The clinical gaze of colonial missionary health systems operates through a Western lens of scientific knowledge, while traditional health systems of many African people employs an indigenous knowledge lens. The former exercises epistemic privilege, while the latter operates within a space Frantz Fanon referred to as the zone of nonbeing.[20] Contemporary South African debates persist about the value assigned to the two systems. Even how best to respond to COVID has been a bone of contention among Africans.

A decolonization of knowledge begins with a recognition by colonial missionary/Western health systems of indigenous knowledge systems as valuable and legitimate. That step will be required to move toward pluriversality of knowledge. The COVID pandemic has raised further awareness on the role of indigenous medicinal plants such as *lengana* (*Artemisia afra*/African wormwood) and *serokolo* (wilder ginger/African ginger/*Siphonochilus aethiopicus*) and the roles of such plants in treating illnesses such as asthma, hysteria, the common cold, and flu. Africans also have used *Serokolo* to treat malaria and painful menstruation.

Instead of giving due credit (including commercial benefits) to the indigenous African medical sector that generates medicinal plants and traditional usages, the colonial missionary health system continues to apply technologies of subversion while exploiting these medicinal plants for its own advancement. Nevertheless, I am confident that local communities in South Africa will continue to recognize and utilize indigenous knowledge related to traditional medicines. They will continue to use and administer medicinal plants for basic healthcare, with traditional medicinal approaches enduring as an integral part of their socio-cultural life. In this way, indigenes will continue to challenge and defy Western epistemic privilege and its associated clinical gaze.

## Notes

I dedicate this essay to my late son, Moagi Mothoagae (2016–2019).

1 Batswana refers to a tribe. Within the tribe, however, there are various clans with different dialects. Each dialect illustrates the richness and the diversity of the tribe and forms part of a language called Setswana. My essay locates itself within two clans of Batswana people, the Setlhaping and the Bakwena.

2 According to John Mackenzie, a minister and missionary, "the ceremony of 'boguera' was administered at Shoshong in April 1865. Each man mustered his retainers, and, surrounded by his own sons and near relatives, marched daily to the camp of the neophytes. Proud is the Bechuana father who is surrounded by several sons on these occasions." Mackenzie, *Ten Years North of the Orange River: A Story of Everyday Life and Work among the South African Tribes from 1859 to 1869* (Edinburgh: Edmonston and Douglas, 1871), 378. In a subsequent work, Mackenzie wrote: "There is an honour connected with this which no distinction of rank can supply. Sekhome's mortification was therefore very great when he found himself marching to the camp alone—with none of his five eldest sons accompanying him. They were all at school instead, and every Sunday they were in their places at church. They themselves resolved that they would not go through this heathen ceremony. Here began a period of trouble for our mission. Sekhome, in inviting missionaries to his town, had evidently not anticipated opposition of this kind. He had hoped to be able to regulate all matters connected with the Word of God . . . as he exercised control over everything else." Mackenzie, *Day-Dawn in Dark Places: A Story of Wanderings and Work in Bechwanaland* (New York, NY: Cassell and Company, 1884), 227.

3 In 1842, Robert Moffat had the following to say about the *dingaka*, whom Moffat characterized as labeled a "rain-maker [who possessed] an influence over the minds of the people superior even to that of their king, who is likewise compelled to yield to the dictates of this arch-official." Moffat, *Missionary Labours and Scenes*, 306.

4 Walter D. Mignolo, "Delinking: The Rhetoric of Modernity, the Logic of Coloniality and the Grammar of De-Coloniality," *Cultural Studies* 21 (March/ May 2007): 476.

5 *Words of Batswana: Letters to Mahoko A Becwana, 1883–1896*, P.T. Mgadla, and Stephen C. Volz, trans. and comps. (1918; repr., Van Riebeeck Society: Cape Town, 2006), 203.

6 Mignolo, "Delinking (the term *coloniality* appears in the subtitle).

7 See, for example, Michel Foucault, "The Eye of Power," in Foucault, *Power/ Knowledge: Selected Interviews and Other Writings, 1972–1977*, ed. Colin Gordon and Colin Gordon et al., trans. (New York, NY: Pantheon Books, 1980), 146–65.

8 See Michel Foucault, *Discipline and Punish: The Birth of the Prison*, ed. Alan Sheridan (1975, repr., New York: Vintage Books, 1995); Foucault, "Why Study Power? The Question of the Subject," *Beyond Structuralism and Hermeneutics*, Herbert L. Dreyfus and Rabinow, eds., 208–28 (Chicago: University of Chicago Press, 1982); and John Gaventa, *Power After Lukes: A Review of the Literature* (Brighton: Institute of Development Studies, 2003).

9 See, for example, Michel Foucault, *The Birth of the Clinic: An Archaeology of Medical Perception*, trans. A.M. Sheridan (1963; repr., New York, NY: Routledge, 2003).

10    Achille Mbembe, *On the Postcolony: Studies on the History of Society and Culture* (Berkeley, CA: University of California Press, 2001), 229.

11    Achille Mbembe, "The Dream of a World Free from the Burden of Race," *Workshop on Theory and Criticism*, June 29 to July 11, 2014, https://jwtc.org.za/volume_8/achille_mbembe_2.htm.

12    Moffat, *Missionary Labours and Scenes*, 305–6.

13    Foucault, *Discipline and Punish*; Michel Foucault, *The History of Sexuality*, trans. Robert Hurley (New York, NY: Pantheon Book, 1978).

14    Humphreys Williams, "First Experiences in the Kuruman District," *The Chronicle of the Church Missionary Society for the Year 1887* (London: Church Missionary Society, 1887), 115.

15    Alexander Butchart, *The Anatomy of Power: European Constructions of the African Body* (Pretoria: Unisa Press, 1998), 82–83.

16    Foucault, *Discipline and Punish*, Foucault, *History of Sexuality*; Michel Foucault, *The Order of Things: An Archaeology of the Human Sciences* (1966; repr., New York, NY: Routledge, 2002); Michel Foucault, "The Subject and Power," *Critical Inquiry* 8 (summer 1982): 787.

17    P. J. Kloppers. "The Aims of the Transkei and Ciskei Research Society," *South African Medical Journal* 47 (February 1973): 287.

18    Mosa Moshabela, Thembelihle Zuma, and Bernhard Gaede, "Bridging the Gap Between Biomedical and Traditional Health Practitioners in South Africa," *South African Health Review* (January 2016): 83.

19    Sarah Wild, "Bringing Traditional Healing under the Microscope in South Africa: Traditional and Mainstream Medicine Have Long Been at Adds. But Covid-19 May Be Driving a New, Evidence-Based Reckoning," *Undark*, December 30, 2020, https://undark.org/2020/12/30/covid-19-south-africa-traditional-medicine/.

20    Frantz Faon, *The Wretched of the Earth* (New York, NY: Grove, 1968).

# 8 Racism and Clinical Trials of COVID-19, Tetanus, and Malaria Vaccines in Kenya

*Elias O. Opongo*

## Introduction

The speed with which a number of medical scientists, pharmaceutical companies, and researchers moved to create and try possible COVID-19 vaccines raised ethical concerns about trial procedures and the viability of drugs administered. Vaccine developers, government officials, physicians, researchers, and other individuals targeted multiple African countries for trials, renewing the debate over the use of black bodies for medical experiments.

On April 1, 2020, French researchers Jean-Paul Mira and Camille Locht proposed Africa was an ideal place to test a possible COVID vaccine because the diverse health challenges of Africans made them extremely vulnerable to COVID.[1] Mira related the pandemic to certain acquired immunodeficiency syndrome (AIDS) "studies, where among prostitutes, we try things because we know that they are highly exposed and don't protect themselves."[2] Countless Africans and humanitarians people around the world reacted to his statement with immediate criticism and indignation. Several renowned Africans expressed their outrage publicly. "Africa," one person declared, "isn't a testing lab."[3]

Facing pressure from a France-based association called SOS Racisme, Mira apologized on April 3 for what he stated even though his employer alleged that people took the original remark out of context. In any event, Mira's April 1 comment reflected a long and horrific record of medical experimentation in Africa. Government officials collaborated with pharmaceutical companies based in Europe or in the United States to develop drugs for trials that physicians and other professional perform on the most vulnerable people in African society.

Oftentimes, medical professionals have conducted experiments in Africa under the guise of the greater good concept, meaning they wish to treat or to find cures for potentially fatal diseases such as tuberculosis, meningitis, malaria, human immunodeficiency virus (HIV), and AIDS to help the entire continent. Many experiments have raised moral and ethical concerns for decades. Matters related to informed consent has been a foremost concern, as some patients have been "forced" to participate in trials.[4] For example, in

DOI: 10.4324/9781003214281-10

a clinical trial conducted during the 1990s to test azidothymidine (a cancer drug developed in the 1960s but used ultimately to prevent a mother from transmitting HIV/AIDS to a child), more than 17,000 women in Zimbabwe underwent clinical experimentation without informed consent.[5] Likewise, those conducting the trials did not inform the women properly about all possible short- or long-term health effects; consequently, 1,000 babies contracted HIV/AIDS.[6]

In another 1990s instance, Pfizer pharmaceutical company conducted a clinical trial to test the effectiveness of trovafloxacin mesylate, an antibiotic known commonly as Trovan.[7] Often used to treat meningitis, among other conditions, Pfizer tested the drug on 200 children in Kano, Nigeria, as a possible preventative of HIV, but neither the Nigerian government nor the parents of the children gave informed consent.[8] Eleven children died, and others suffered blindness, deafness, or brain damage.[9] In 2009, Pfizer agreed out of court to pay $75 million to the Kano government to settle a lawsuit the government brought against the company.[10] Three years later, the government and several survivors of the trials filed an additional suit, whose subsequent verdict also favored the plaintiffs and caused Pfizer to shell out additional money.[11] In 2020, as the transnational company prepared to conduct trial vaccines during the COVID-19 pandemic, Kano residents were apprehensive because of the Trovan ordeal.[12]

Medical institutions and pharmaceutical companies such as Pfizer tend to target disadvantaged, marginalized, stigmatized, or otherwise vulnerable populations as trial subjects disproportionately to affluent populations. Prisoners, orphans, mentally ill, poor, or disabled people, as well as people of color are regular trial subjects.[13] Deeply rooted in slavery, racism, ethnic bias, and other immoral or unethical occurrences, the medical experiments about which I write in this essay have used black bodies as subjects routinely.[14] Such practices require ethical critique, and this essay does so by using global perspectives to examine racial/ethnic connotations of vaccine trials in Africa.

## Common Trends regarding Medical Experimentation on Black Bodies

Exploitative medical experimentation on black and other people of color has been a common practice for centuries in the US, Europe, the Caribbean, and elsewhere in the world. Two well-known examples will suffice. In Tuskegee, Alabama, the state public health agency launched a syphilis study in 1932 amid the Great Depression. The agency gave each participant an assurance of medical treatment but for forty years did not provide it.[15] Worse exploitation occurred in Germany during the late 1930s and the early 1940s. Leaders of the Nazi regime subjected undesirable women to population reduction practices ostensibly reserved for those who were sick.[16]

Africa has not been exempt from cruel practices. On many occasions, the US National Institutes of Health (NIH), the US Centers for Disease Control and Prevention, and the World Health Organization (WHO) have helped fund clinical trials. For instance, from 2018 to 2019 the NIH conducted trials in fourteen South African localities for an HIV/AIDS vaccine called HVTN 702, or Uhambo, involving 5,400 hundred HIV-negative people between ages eighteen and thirty-five. Participants believed they received vaccine protection from HIV. An analysis found 129 HIV infections among vaccinated people and 123 infections among people whom the NIH gave a placebo without their knowledge. Ultimately, NIH officials ended the trials, citing the ineffectiveness of the vaccine.[17]

Europeans conducting unsuccessful medical experiments in Africa is not a new occurrence. In a 2014 scholarly essay about European colonialism and biomedicine, Patrick Malloy examined how colonial authorities collected specimen samples from African subjects to research malaria to other plague-like diseases.[18] Collection was nonconsensual during that process to appropriate African blood to feed colonial medical research. In Tanganyika, on which Malloy concentrated in his essay, as well as in other colonized African localities, colonial officials forced indigenes to surrender tissue samples, literally portions of themselves, to researchers.[19]

The colonizers about which Malloy wrote were not alone. From the sixteenth through the nineteenth centuries, doctors affiliated with the international slave trade collected specimen sample for scientific research, taking advantage of the network of ships that transported human cargo from Africa to Europe, North America, and other continents. As Sam Kean noted in 2019, samples from humans, both alive and dead, were as prevalent as samples from plants and nonhuman animals.[20] Researchers removed polyps from the hands of enslaved people, extracted patches of dried skin, and took fetuses after miscarriages, among other black body parts.[21]

The problems I have addressed thus far result in part from some Westerners' belief that people in the Global South (Africa, Asia, Latin America, Oceania) are second-class residents of the international community.[22] That belief, I contend, has undergirded medical experimentations on the African continent for centuries, as Malloy demonstrated.[23] Accordingly, Western medical researchers and pharmaceutical company executives have used black bodies without proper consent or authorization. This "grim history," to quote Amanda Lichtenstein, has caused innumerable Africans of yore to have a deep mistrust of vaccinations, medical trials, and experiments.[24] Because such mistrust continues, it has grave implications for COVID-19 vaccine trials in Africa, particularly Kenya.

## Vaccine Trials in Kenya

A number of vaccine mishaps are prefaces to the COVID story. For example, in November 2014 the Kenya Council of Catholic Bishops opposed a vaccine campaign the World Health Organization was sponsoring and the Kenyan Ministry of Health was implementing to inoculate as many as 2.4 Kenyan women aged fourteen to forty-nine, or those in their childbearing years. The campaign began secretly in October 2013 and proceeded in phases. Council spokespersons said they submitted sample vials of the vaccine for independent testing, and at least 30 percent contained the human hormone chorionic gonadotropin, which was linked to anti-fertility vaccines.[25]

According to council, "when the ordinary tetanus vaccine is combined with b-HCG and given in five doses every six months, the women develop immunity for both tetanus and HCG, a hormone necessary for pregnancy. Subsequently, the body rejects any pregnancy, causing repeated miscarriages and eventually sterility."[26] Aware of those ideas in November 2014, the council and other Kenyan Catholics criticized the government for its lack of due diligence in ensuring that vaccines for a sizeable portion of the Kenyan female population was safe. "What is immoral and evil," one member of the Catholic Doctors Association of Kenya proclaimed, "is that the tetanus laced with HCG was given as a fertility regulating vaccine without disclosing its contraceptive effect to the girls and mothers."[27]

Meanwhile, numerous people worldwide became familiar a January 2014 report by the Wemos Foundation, a public organization headquartered in the Netherlands. The report indicated Kenya and other African countries had "unique" profiles that interested "many life science companies. Of all emerging locations or regions, Africa has arguably the least access to quality care, ensuring a steady stream of dedicated patients to fill trial enrolments."[28] By January 2020, the foundation predicted, markets in Kenya and its fellow continental localities could "represent a $45 billion opportunity for drug makers, spurred in part by robust economic growth and demographic changes."[29]

In April 2019, months before anyone could test the Wemos Foundation's prediction, the World Health Organization initiated malaria vaccine trials in Kenya, Ghana, and Malawi for children aged six months to two years.[30] The WHO carried out the trials using cluster-randomized studies with 720,000 children.[31] Bioethicists from across the globe criticized the trials because the WHO relied on the implied, as opposed to the formal consent, of parents.[32] In addition to the consent issue, the WHO presented the vaccine as part of a routine preventative scheme for children rather than as a vaccine trial program. As Lisa Winters wrote in February 2020, "The trial was set to follow in the footsteps of a Phase 3 test that involved giving multiple doses of the vaccine to close to 15,500 children between ages six weeks and 17 months over a five-year period. While malaria cases decreased by about one-third, there were some worrisome side effects. Children who received the vaccine were 10 times more likely to develop meningitis in cerebral malarial cases compared to those who didn't get the shots. Girls in the test cohort, overall, were twice as likely to die from any cause compared to girls in the control group."[33]

Kenyan counties involved in the 2019 malaria vaccine trials included Homa Bay, Kisumu, Migori, Siaya, Busia, Bungoma, Vihiga, and Kakamega.[34]

According to WHO Regional Director for Africa Matshidiso Moeti, the trials would provide "key information and data to inform a WHO policy on the broader use of the vaccine in sub-Saharan Africa. If introduced widely, the vaccine has the potential to save tens of thousands of lives."[35] Moeti, however, did not reveal possible side effects of the vaccine on the children, whom I contend the WHO used as guinea pigs despite representatives of the organization claiming otherwise. For instance, on the day the WHO launched its program in Homa Bay, a WHO representative to Kenya named Rudi Eggers said: "This is a day to celebrate as we begin to learn more about what this vaccine can do to change the trajectory of malaria though childhood vaccination."[36]

The positive presentation of the malaria vaccine by Eggers and the acknowledgement of using children find out more about potential effects of the vaccine demonstrated the WHO was involved full-fledged trial research and not simply a pilot. Therefore, the organization should have ensured that every administrator followed customary protection protocols, including warning participants and their parents about potential dangers of the vaccine. Part of those lapses rests with the Kenyan government, whose officials were known for being friendly to businesses. Furthermore, many officials were and remain ready for their country to become a worldwide leader in clinical research. Therefore, they have made tremendous efforts to fight infectious and tropical diseases, such as malaria, with the hope of generating a permanent cure. Pursuant to achieving that goal, the government established a full-fledged Kenya Medical Research Institute in 1989. Working in collaboration with other agencies, the institute has conducted a number of vaccine trials. Many target HIV/AIDS, which numerous foreign research organizations, universities, and charities in Kenya have sought to eradicate since the late 1970s.[37]

Foreigners continue to perform active roles in clinical studies and in other medical research activities in Kenya. Some, however, operate questionably because their activities (e.g., trials) do not meet proper disclosure criteria. As stated earlier in this essay, some trial administrators do not tell participants the truth about which vaccines they administer or provide information about side effects of the vaccines. Other administrators conduct trials without securing appropriate consent. Fortunately, the Kenyan government to date has done a relatively solid job managing the vaccination process for COVID-19.

In April 2020, national regulatory authorities and ethics committees from across Africa agreed to combine expertise "to expedite clinical trial review and approvals for new multinational preventive, diagnostic and therapeutic interventions to the COVID pandemic."[38] The African Vaccines Regulatory Forum, a continental technical committee of the African Medicines Regulatory Harmonization Initiative, consented to overseeing reviews. Kenya was a center of trial activity. Officials looked to the Pharmacies and Poisons Board as its national medicines regulatory authority in ensuring all clinical trials were sound both scientifically and ethically. Moreover, all administrators were to adhere to established protocols of the International Conference on Harmonization on Good Clinical Practice.[39]

With pharmaceutical companies working hard to develop effective COVID vaccines, Kenyan officials, working through the Ministry of Health, committed the country to providing the highest standard of health to all citizens. The officials also pledged to support and participate in several global clinical trials designed to treat COVID, such as allowing some citizens to undergo Remdesivir drug inoculations.[40] All the same, I believe firmly that the pandemic can be overcome only through multisectoral engagements that bring together myriad stakeholders (academicians, government officials, independent businesspeople, executives of multinational conglomerates) who are committed to following established international guidelines, and ethical considerations for conducting clinical trials.

The Kenyan government in April 2020 issued a report in which it acknowledged possible challenges to overseeing effectively COVID vaccine trials. An adequate number of staffers to supervise trials was one concern. Additionally, COVID protocols often require trial participants to isolate, "which introduces difficulties for Investigators to maintain their medical oversight. These challenges could have an impact on the conduct of trials, such as the completion of trial assessments, completion of trial follow-up visits and the provision of Investigational Medicinal Products."[41] While the government report provided standard procedures for vaccine trials, including participants' consent and freedom to continue or to withdraw from trials, the government only advised participants to pay attention to unexpected serious adverse reactions; the government did not reveal in advance some of the possible side effects of the vaccine.

### Race and Ethical Evaluations of Vaccine Trials

Medical experimentation on black bodies always has been a controversial issue to people worldwide, but the issue has become more controversial during the COVID pandemic. Questions persist about how pharmaceutical companies recruit their participants for vaccine trials. Because many companies have histories of targeting weak or otherwise vulnerable people, especially people of color, people are monitoring the acts of pharmaceutical companies very closely. In Africa, poverty and inadequate government protection for citizens against medical manipulation have made Africans easy targets for ambitious companies seeking subjects for clinical trials that serve as steps toward marketing their products primarily, if not solely, to generate revenue instead of helping people.

Despite guidelines from the Council for International Organizations of Medical Sciences and the from the World Medical Association, among other groups, intended to guarantee ethical standards for clinical trials, developing countries often lack structures and resources required to adhere to such guidelines.[42] Furthermore, some developing countries with established ethics panels (e.g., institutional review boards) experience technical challenges due to limited training about identifying ethically questionable practices. In relation to some African countries, regulatory authorities choose not to conduct thorough reviews to retain research funding. Consequently, high-risk trials take place.[43]

According to Wemos, "Few people would argue that medical research and the search for cures for debilitating and deadly diseases are not necessary or beneficial. And if taking part in a study enables poverty-stricken people to access much-needed treatment without any cost, some would describe the collaboration between participant and trial sponsor as 'win-win' situation."[44] All the same, the concealments of information characteristic of African participant recruitment raises serous moral and ethical concerns. Withholding critical information run counter to the premise of informed consent. According to a report by public health organization Wemos, comprehensive understanding of the consent procedure is undermined where the ability to analyze or to interpret the meaning of what is contained in a consent form is not present—and not simply because a participant lacks the capability to understand something but also because the agent conducting the trial is not transparent.[45]

## Conclusion

In medical research involving people capable of giving informed consent, each person must be adequately informed of the aims, methods, sources of funding, possible conflicts of interest, institutional affiliations of the researcher, the anticipated benefits, and potential risks of the study; any discomfort the study might entail; post-study provisions; and all other relevant aspects of the study.[46] Additionally, experts, including government agents, such develop professional, credible, and effective guidelines for clinical trial processes.[47] Such practices and procedures are proven ways to proceed.

In the case of black bodies on the African continent, the abovementioned schemes theoretically help rogue pharmaceutical companies with vested interests in making money from conducting unethical clinical trials. As the COVID-19 pandemic has shown, humanitarian people worldwide should recognize the indignities of such companies and take steps to reduce vile behaviors. I believe private and public medical facilities, government agencies, and civil society institutions, including faith-based institutions, should be at the forefront of preventing immoral and unethical abuses.

## Notes

1  Amanda Lichtenstein, "COVID-19 Revives Grim History of Medical Experimentation in Africa," *Global Voices*, https://globalvoices.org/2020/04/11/covid-19-revives-grim-history-of-medical-experimentation-in-africa/.

2  Lichtenstein, "COVID-19."
3  Lichtenstein, "COVID-19."
4  Lichtenstein, "COVID-19."
5  Lichtenstein, "COVID-19."
6  Lichtenstein, "COVID-19."
7  See "Lichtenstein, "COVID-19"; Patrick I. Okonta, "Ethics of Clinical Trials in Nigeria," *Nigerian Medical Journal* 55 (May–June 2014): 189; Jose Stephens, "Where Profits and Lives Hang in the Balance," *Washington Post*, December 17, 2000, https://www.washingtonpost.com/archive/politics/2000/12/17/where-profits-and-lives-hang-in-balance/90b0c003-99ed-4fed-bb22-4944c1a98443/; and Jacqui Wise, "Pfizer Accused of Testing New Drug without Ethical Approval," *British Medical Journal* 322 (January 27, 2001): 194.
8  See Lichtenstein, "COVID-19"; Peter Lurie and Sidney M. Wolfe, "Unethical Trials of Interventions to Reduce Perinatal Transmission of the Human Immunodeficiency Virus in Developing Countries," *New England Journal of Medicine* 337 (September 12, 1997): 853–56; and Wise, "Pfizer Accused of Testing New Drug."
9  Lichtenstein, "COVID-19."
10  See Okonta, "Ethics of Clinical Trials in Nigeria," 189; "Pfizer Lawsuit (Re Administration of Experimental Drug in Nigeria, Filed in Nigeria)," *Business and Human Rights Resource Centre*, May 30, 2007, https://www.business-human-rights.org/en/latest-news/pfizer-lawsuit-re-administration-of-experimental-drug-in-nigeria-filed-in-nigeria/; "Pfizer Settles Drug Testing Case with Nigerian State for $75 Million," *Business and Human Rights Resource Centre*, August 3, 2009, https://www.business-humanrights.org/en/latest-news/pfizer-settles-drug-testing-case-with-nigerian-state-for-75-million/; and Cassandra Willyard. "Pfizer Lawsuit Spotlights Ethics of Developing World Clinical Trials," *Nature Medicine* 13 (July 2007): 763.
11  Ibrahim Shuaibu, "Nigeria: The Day Pfizer's Trovan Victims Got Compensation," *AllAfrica*, November 26, 2014, https://allafrica.com/stories/201411261368.html.
12  See Ibrahim Garba and Danielle Paquette, "In this Nigerian City, Pfizer Fears Loom Over the Vaccine Rollout," *Washington Post*, March 20, 2021, https://www.washingtonpost.com/world/2021/03/20/nigeria-pfizer-kano-coronavirus-trovan/; Lichtenstein, "COVID-19"; and Wise, "Pfizer Accused of Testing New Drug."
13  Stephen Kenny, "How Black Slaves Were Routinely Sold as 'Specimens' to Ambitious White Doctors," *Conversation*, June 11, 2015, https://theconversation.com/how-black-slaves-were-routinely-sold-as-specimens-to-ambitious-white-doctors-43074.
14  Kenny, "Black Slaves."
15  See United States Centers for Disease Control and Prevention, "The Tuskegee Timeline," April 22, 2021, https://www.cdc.gov/tuskegee/timeline.htm; Joel D. Howell, "Trust and the Tuskegee Experiments," in *Clio in the Clinic: History in Medical Practice*, ed. Jacalyn Duffin, 213–25 (New York, NY: Oxford University Press, 2005); Kenny, "Black Slaves"; and Londa Schiebinger, *Secret Cures of Slaves: People, Plants, and Medicine in the Eighteenth-Century Atlantic World* (Stanford: Stanford University Press, 2017).
16  Henry P. David, Jochen Fleischhacker, and Charlotte Höhn, "Abortion and Eugenics in Nazi Germany," *Population and Development Review* 14 (March 1988): 81–112, esp. 89.

17 UNAIDS, "Press Statement: HVTN 702 Clinical Trial of an HIV Vaccine Stopped," February 4, 2020, https://www.unaids.org/en/resources/presscentre/pressreleaseandstatementarchive/2020/february/20200204_vaccine.

18 Patrick Malloy, "Research Material and Necromancy: Imagining the Political Economy of Biomedicine in Colonial Tanganyika," *International Journal of African Historical Studies* 47 (September 2014): 425–43.

19 Malloy, "Research Material and Necromancy."

20 Sam Kean, "Historians Expose Early Scientists' Debt to the Slave Trade," *Science*, April 4, 2019, https://www.sciencemag.org/news/2019/04/historians-expose-early-scientists-debt-slave-trade.

21 Kean, "Historians Expose Early Scientists' Debt."

22 Nour Dados and Raewyn Connell, "The Global South," *Contexts* 11 (winter 2012): 12–13.

23 Malloy, "Research Material and Necromancy."

24 Lichtenstein, "COVID-19."

25 World Health Organization, *Fertility Regulating Vaccines: Report of a Meeting between Women's Health Advocates and Scientists to Review the Current Status of the Development of Fertility Regulating Vaccines*, Geneva Switzerland, 17–18 August 1992 (Geneva: World Health Organization, 1993), 7, 12, 15–22, 24, 26–27, 30, 35, 40–42, 45, 49.

26 Fredrick Nzwili, "Kenya's Catholic Bishops: Tetanus Vaccine is Birth Control in Disguise," *Washington Post*, November 11, 2014, https://www.washingtonpost.com/national/religion/kenyas-catholic-bishops-tetanus-vaccine-is-birth-control-in-disguise/2014/11/11/3ece10ce-69ce-11e4-bafd-6598192a448d_story.html.

27 Nzwili, "Kenya's Catholic Bishops."

28 Wemos, *The Clinical Trials Industry: Realities, Risks and Challenges* (Amsterdam: Wemos, 2014), 17.

29 Wemos, *Clinical Trials Industry*, 18. Because of the COVID-19 pandemic, the African market—and hence potential for revenue growth—about which Wemos wrote in January 2014 has expanded further than Wemos predicted.

30 Shawna Williams, "Distribution of World's First Malaria Vaccine Begins," *Scientist*, April 23, 2019, https://www.the-scientist.com/news-opinion/distribution-of-worlds-first-malaria-vaccine-begins-65777.

31 Lisa Winter, "Bioethicists Criticize WHO's Malaria Vaccine Trial," *Scientist*, February 28, 2020, https://www.the-scientist.com/news-opinion/bioethicists-criticize-whos-malaria-vaccine-trial-67195.

32 Winter, "Bioethicists Criticize WHO's Malaria Vaccine Trial."

33 Winter, "Bioethicists Criticize WHO's Malaria Vaccine Trial."

34 World Health Organization Regional Office for Africa, "Malaria Vaccine Launched in Kenya: Kenya Joins Ghana and Malawi to Roll Out Landmark Vaccine in Pilot Introduction," September 13, 2019, https://www.afro.who.int/news/malaria-vaccine-launched-kenya-kenya-joins-ghana-and-malawi-roll-out-landmark-vaccine-pilot (hereafter cited as WHOROA).

35 WHOROA, "Malaria Vaccine Launched."

36 WHOROA, "Malaria Vaccine Launched."

37 See Wemos, *Clinical Trials Industry*, 19; and WHOROA, "Malaria Vaccine Launched."

38 WHOROA, "African Regulatory Agencies, Ethics Committees to Expedite COVID-19 Clinical Trial Reviews," April 20, 2020, https://www.afro.who.int/news/african-regulatory-agencies-ethics-committees-expedite-covid-19-clinical-trial-reviews.

39  WHOROA, "African Regulatory Agencies, Ethics Committees to Expedite COVID-19 Clinical Trial Reviews."
40  Aga Khan University Hospital, Nairobi, "AKUH Participates in Global Clinical Trial for Potential Treatment for COVID-19 Associated Pneumonia," July 21, 2020, https://hospitals.aku.edu/nairobi/AboutUs/News/Pages/Clinical-trial-for-COVID-19.aspx.
41  Ministry of Health Pharmacy and Poisons Board, *Guidance to Sponsors and Investigators for Conduct of Clinical Trials During the COVID-19 19 Pandemic in Kenya* (Nairobi: Ministry of Health, 2020), 9.
42  Willyard. "Pfizer Lawsuit."
43  Willyard, "Pfizer Lawsuit."
44  Wemos, *Clinical Trials Industry*, 21.
45  Wemos, *Clinical Trials Industry*, esp. 11, 14, 24, 32.
46  Wemos, *Clinical Trials Industry*.
47  Wemos, *Clinical Trials Industry*.

# Part II

# Ecclesial Responses to Black Health Vulnerabilities

# 9 The African Methodist Episcopal Church and Its Reckonings with Deadly Plagues, 1793–2020

*Dennis C. Dickerson*

## Introduction

The African Methodist Episcopal (AME) Church has reckoned with deadly plagues for centuries. From the bold public health intervention of denominational founder Richard Allen and fellow clergyman Absalom Jones during a 1793 yellow fever outbreak in Philadelphia, Pennsylvania, through a vigorous acquiescence to governmental guidance in 2020 and 2021 during the COVID-19 pandemic, the AME Church has validated a ready acceptance of the latest science in dealing with potentially fatal plagues. This essay discusses AME responses to large-scale public health emergencies from the denomination's creation during the late eighteenth century to its global maturity during the twenty-first century as the oldest African American denomination in the United States.

## African Methodist Episcopal Responses to Yellow Fever Outbreaks

Yellow fever periodically afflicted cities throughout the United States from the 1790s through the 1800s. Though scientists did not learn a specific mosquito species was the primary virus carrier until 1901, public health practitioners in earlier periods knew unsanitary settings somehow incubated the mysterious malady and spurred its spread. Quarantine, evacuation, and urgent disposal of corpses and contaminated items in the homes of ill people were common responses of those who tried to control the virus, which inflicted fever, jaundice, hemorrhaging, and damage to vital organs and usually resulted in the death of the afflicted.[1]

At the height of the 1793 yellow epidemic in Philadelphia between August and November, some 5,000 city residents succumbed to the virus. Allen and Jones answered a newspaper solicitation to aid white people who were sick on the mistaken white assumption that nonwhite people were immune to the virus.[2] Despite receiving tutorials in bleeding (a procedure embedded in ineffectual humoral theory) by white Philadelphian Benjamin Rush, a well-known physician, civil leader, and signer of the US Constitution, Allen

DOI: 10.4324/9781003214281-12

and Jones exhibited a practiced public health consciousness in providing services to dead and dying populations in the city. Similar to Rush and to many other informed individuals, Allen and Jones not only recognized the rapid transfer of dead bodies to coffins for burial was a pressing duty but also realized several "colored nurses" they hired were crucial to bringing relief to those suffering with serious illnesses.[3]

Allen and Jones chronicled their activities in *A Narrative of the Proceedings of Black People, during the Late Awful a Calamity in Philadelphia, in the Year 1793: And Refutation of Some Censures, Thrown Upon Them in Some Publications.*[4] Though some detractors questioned the financial integrity of Allen and Jones regarding expenses, the empirical project Allen and Jones managed showed their keen sensibility about public health practice and yielded vital information to objective professionals.[5] In each public health involvement, they compiled numerical evidence about mortality from yellow fever gleaned from their personal experiences treating hundreds of patients and burying dead victims. In so doing, Allen and Jones belied conventional white wisdom regarding nonwhite invincibility to the disease. When Allen contracted it in 1793, his experience proved black people were susceptible. He perhaps believed his recovery conferred on him some protection against the affliction, as did many other people, but his actual belief regarding the matter is unknown.[6]

Recurring outbreaks of yellow fever in the nineteenth-century US had a tremendous impact on the AME Church. Affecting the southern region of the country most heavily after 1822, the disease disrupted AME meetings and sickened members, some fatally.[7] The official denominational newspaper, the *Christian Recorder* (founded in 1848 as the *Christian Herald*), published testimonies about various spates of the epidemic and the etiology of the disease.[8] The *Recorder* also tracked health emergencies and provided accounts about clergy who eschewed escape from the epidemic to remain with their afflicted communities. The effects on travel by church leaders within a busy black ecclesia whose multiple meetings and interdenominational commitments required ministers to reckon with uncertainty.

In February 1878, the Rev. J.C. Waters, an AME leader in Jacksonville, Florida, reported suffering from a "severe attack of this dreaded malady," yellow fever.[9] Waters surmised it was the "most virulent and fatal fever of the bilious type that afflicts the human family."[10] He described how a yellowish color appeared on various parts of the body as well as how chills and pains accompanied the illness. He advised the best treatment lay with bed rest, hot tea, blankets, and castor oil. A small tube of mustard water for a patient's feet produced copious perspiration. The sweating helped until the fever broke, but survival was uncertain.[11] The fever was not contagious, Waters went on to state, but it was infectious, especially to "any locality highly charged with malarial poison."[12]

Waters's child and sister contracted yellow fever, but his wife's case was among the most severe in Jacksonville. Even so, he empathized with others in the city. A family residing near the parsonage of The Church he pastored experienced three deaths in a single week. "What I know" about the yellow fever, Waters concluded, was "learned in that school which I trust you will never have occasion to attend—the school of experience."[13] His associate, the Rev. William B. Johnson also had such experience: Johnson witnessed his wife die from the disease in 1876.[14]

As yellow fever spread throughout Jacksonville and other parts of the South in 1878, AME correspondents filled the *Christian Recorder* with careful chronicles of the epidemic's effects. In August, approximately six months after Waters reported on conditions in Jacksonville, a correspondent observed "the yellow fever is making desolate many a fireside at New Orleans," Louisiana.[15] The same correspondent commended the Rev. James H. Madison, pastor of the St. James Church, for staying with his congregants, affirming "a sense of duty will not allow him to leave."[16] During the next few months, the "fearful rider" (yellow fever) struck the Union Bethel Church of New Orleans as well.[17] In November, the Rev. Lazarus Gardner, a foremost leader in the southern region of the AME Church, said many individuals who attended Union Bethel fell victim to the disease and others were ill.[18]

The AME Church continued to wrestle with various impacts of yellow fever on clergymen, their families, and other congregants during the early 1880s. Floridian church leaders interrupted numerous denominational operations. For example, in late 1882 along the western coast of the state, especially around Pensacola, they ordered quarantines. As officials prepared for the annual state conference in Monticello, located about 144 miles west of Jacksonville, Pastor B.W. Roberts informed delegates he could not attend because the disease had "left destitution, poverty and death in its wake."[19] In Pensacola, meanwhile, 2,350 people were ill and 197 died.[20]

A resurgence of yellow fever in 1888 affected W.W. Sampson, a Jacksonville, Florida, pastor, founder of the East Florida Divinity High School, cofounder and onetime traveling agent of the Scientific, Normal and Divinity Institute (later Edward Waters College), and incorporator of Brown's Theological Institute.[21] In September, the *Christian Recorder* indicated Sampson's wife was "smitten by the scourge," though the newspaper did indicate whether she survived or perished.[22] The paper also noted the Rev. W.P. Ross "bravely declines coming North to escape the awful scourge."[23] Instead, he remained with "his people," including two congregants who contracted the disease.[24]

Bishop Henry M. Turner of Abbeville, South Carolina, provided additional news about yellow fever in 1888. While speaking at a meeting in Trenton, New Jersey, he discussed a prominent Florida pastor who contracted the disease. Turner and his fellow attendees sang a hymn and offered a prayer of recovery, but he said nothing further about the condition of the man for whom they sang and pray. The ultimate condition of Bishop Benjamin W. Arnett, a native of Brownsville, Pennsylvania, is certain. Elevated to the episcopacy at the 1888 AME general conference and assigned to both South Carolina and Florida, Arnett was "prevented by the yellow fever from entering his own field."[25] He thus joined Bishop Turner in his diocese. Arnett, the *Christian Recorder* announced, "has led in urging brethren to generosity in aiding the yellow fever sufferers."[26]

As Arnett assisted Turner in 1888, a prescient AME pastor in Jacksonville, Florida, named W.P. Ross discussed the racial dimensions of the yellow fever epidemic. Similar to Richard Allen in Philadelphia, Pennsylvania, a century earlier, Ross observed a massive evacuation of Jacksonville with "conveyances crowded with excited, anxious men and women leaving the city."[27] The exodus left numerous abandoned businesses and unemployed black citizens "now suffering for want of the necessaries of life," Ross professed.[28] Even though many black people did not contract the fever, its presence nonetheless spurred an "unvarnished falsehood" among white people regarding their black contemporaries "breaking open stores and robbing houses" to make ends meet or simply because they were thieves.[29] Ross demurred, "No such lawlessness among the colored people is going on at all. Jacksonville was never more orderly than now, and the colored people are doing just what they did in war times—looking after the white people's property."[30] Ross expected divine judgment to be visited on white people who peddled such libel, but he hoped they would come to accept the "grand Bible truth—God our Father and man our Brother" found in the AME motto and stop libeling black people.[31]

Several AME leaders in Jacksonville were less optimistic than Ross in 1882 about the various consequences of yellow fever. Three pastors left their posts on account of the epidemic. Regardless of possible health consequences, Ross and four other AME pastors remained in the city. "I can't run and leave my people," Ross declared.[32] "From morning until late at night," he pledged, "I am going [to] look ... after the poor and suffering."[33]

## Combatting Influenza

By the opening of World War I in 1914, sanitary campaigns to rid watery breeding environments for mosquito carriers and the development of a vaccine in 1901 had become effective methods to reduce the threat of yellow fever. However, a deadlier pandemic, influenza (often misnamed the Spanish flu), emerged by the close of war in 1918. Former epidemics paled in comparison to the fatal impact influenza, which undermined the human respiratory system. Transnational in its impact, the virus caused approximately 675,000 deaths in the US and more 50 million globally.[34]

Members of the AME Church, not like other denominationalists, realized the ubiquity of influenza in 1918. So pervasive was the scourge that the Pittsburgh Annual Conference branch of the Women's Parent Mite Missionary Society referred to it as a disease "that swept the universe and claimed so many of our loved ones."[35] Other members of the AME Church were similarly cognizant the pandemic was hard to escape and disruptive to both church and state. A committee report from the annual conference of the North Georgia AME Church recognized "the country is now being menaced by an epidemic known as Spanish influenza." The report showed the disease seemed omnipresent, ravaging people in army camps to those in urban areas and rural hamlets. The virulence of the disease, the report elaborated, created circumstances that were "sufficiently alarming to cause local boards of health in many places to close schools, churches, and other indoor public gathering places as a precautionary effort to prevent [the further] spread of the disease." The individuals who authored the report prayed local, state, and national initiatives "will soon overcome this deadly malady and restore the people of the country to their normal state of health and vigor."[36]

The perspectives above contrasted with the facile 1918 analysis of Joseph S. Flipper, a Georgian AME Church bishop who "urged the brethren to not be alarmed at the epidemic of Influenza, since epidemics" tended to follow wars—in this instance, World War I.[37] Speaking at the annual conference in southwestern Georgia, he reminded delegates that smallpox outbreaks occurred following the Civil War and the Spanish-American War. An occasional epidemic "is God's way," Flipper told delegates, "and we must have hearts filled with empathy for our brethren, and pray God to spare the lives of those who are stricken."[38]

Members of the temperance committee at the 1918 meeting of the Southwestern Georgia Conference of the AME Church were less casual than Bishop Flipper about the Spanish flu. They admonished their denominationalist peers to ignore those who peddled easy remedies to address the disease. Committee members also criticized some physicians for recommending whiskey "as the one and only cure for this dreaded disease."[39] Just as Richard Allen and Absalom Jones discredited the myth of black people contracting yellow fever, the temperance committee said credible evidence indicated "those who drank whiskey died in larger numbers than those who did not."[40]

The early twentieth-century toll of sickness and death from influenza, as in earlier epidemics of yellow fever, was palpable among AME congregants. C. Emery Allen, a presiding elder in Michigan, reported in 1919 about the terrible scourge (influenza) that was killing hundreds of thousands of people. Not only were most AME churches in the state closed anywhere from three to six weeks at a time, Allen recalled, but many ministers, their families, and other congregants were ill. Allen himself contracted the disease. For seven weeks, he had to quarantine inside his home. Once recovered, he contracted pneumonia. North of Michigan, in Ohio, concurrently, another presiding elder noted how influenza, one of the severest epidemics of viral disease in US history, was interrupting livelihoods and ending lives. He lamented, "Scores of the members of our churches fell victims of the terrible plague, the 'Flu,' and today they sleep in Jesus."[41]

Delegates to the Augusta, Georgia, annual conference, like their denominational contemporaries elsewhere in the country, were mindful that influenza was "almost universal in its operation" and that "thousands have fallen beneath its fatal stroke."[42] Nonetheless, the Georgians chafed under "one of the new and startling methods employed for its suppression."[43] They questioned local officials for closing churches while allowing fairs, railroads, shows, and stores to continue operating. As a result of The Church closings, the delegates asserted, "ministers were deprived of their means of living," creating "untold suffering [among those] most useful citizens," ministers.[44] According to one delegate, AME churchgoers feared "the exercise of this new and unheard of power of the civil authority over the churches ... will finally result in still greater encroachments."[45]

Public health officials in Pennsylvania were no less emphatic in the exercise of their authority against the pandemic than those in Georgia. William H.H. Butler, a presiding elder in the Pittsburgh Annual Conference, said influenza killed thousands of people, causing state health officials to deploy full authority in combatting the disease. The state health mandate, as Butler understood it, would "impose such drastic restrictions upon public assemblages as to make practically prohibitive every form of church enterprise or gathering."[46] Consequently, Butler presumed church state officials in Pennsylvania would cancel the statewide meeting scheduled for Washington in the southwestern region about thirty miles southwest of Pittsburgh. Church officials communicated the cancellation to Bishop Cornelius T. Shaffer, who thereupon postponed the meeting for two weeks or until government officials lifted public meeting restrictions.[47]

Bishop Shaffer understood better than most clergy the actions of state health officials. In 1888, during his pastorate at the Mother Bethel Church in Philadelphia, he earned a degree from a local institution called Jefferson Medical College. As a trained physician, he was equipped in 1918 to weigh both health and ecclesiastical dimensions of his episcopal responsibilities in the midst of the pandemic. Shaffer, his three presiding elders, and the host pastor in nearby Washington agreed to seek information about which conditions would allow the annual conference to meet. They learned that "it would be impossible to obtain assurance of the lifting of the ban against public gatherings for many weeks." They also learned "that not even the bishop, officers and members of the conference could be allowed for business purposes only with the public of the community excluded from our sessions, as the number would be too great."[48]

AME officials such as Butler and Shaffer told state health officials the pressing business of their ecclesiastical jurisdiction required they continue minimal functions in 1918. Among acts, the collecting and disbursing of denominational allocations, as well as the assigning of pastors to more than eighty congregations centered in Western Pennsylvania, necessitated they hold the annual conference. A statewide committee on which Butler sat promised to abridge the conference schedule and to scale-down attendance. Whereas previous meetings had numerous session and averaged hundreds of conferees, the 1918 conference if allowed would have few sessions, and no more than twenty conferees would conduct church business. After a continual effort by the committee, Butler eventually reported, his associates and he secured permission to host the meeting in an abbreviated manner. Butler, Shaffer, and other denominational leaders promised to conform strictly to official mandates, forego any publicity about the meeting, cooperate with other concerned citizens who wished to control the spread of disease.

On October 30, 1918, Shaffer stood behind a rostrum at the St. Paul's AME Church in Washington, Pennsylvania, and gaveled the Pittsburgh annual conference into a limited session. He reminded delegates that their two-day meeting was taking place in accordance with strict orders by members of local and state boards of health who wished to contain influenza. People from across the US provided updates elsewhere in the country. In the end, AME denominational leaders in Washington, Pittsburgh, and various other Pennsylvania cities and towns believed their decisions to host pared down emergency conferences was prudent. According to them, they witnessed visible signs of influenza abating.

When the 1919 session of the Pittsburgh annual conference convened, Presiding Elder Butler said government officials lifted their bans on public gatherings sooner than other denominational heads he thought. Conventioneers rejoiced because they soon would be able to resume their normal church and secular routines. That welcome news really moved another presiding elder. Because yellow fever was receding, he could hold district meetings for the first time since 1917. The two-year ordeal showed AME acquiescence to modern public health protocols, especially those that pertained to the suspension of public gatherings. While some chafed at what they perceived as heavy-handed state and local government mandates banning church meetings, others complied, albeit grudging in some cases.

### African Methodist Episcopal Ecclesial Structuring of Modern Healthcare Responses

Because of the appreciable numbers of physicians and other individuals with medical training as well as a generally high level of respect for science in many AME congregations, denominationalists participated in sundry health care and missional projects on both sides of the Atlantic Ocean. In 1893, a physician named Thomas C. Unthank founded Douglass Hospital in Kansas City, Kansas, and under his supervision it became a premier facility in the Midwest. Decades later in South Africa, Bishop Richard R. Wright Jr. established the Crogman Community Clinic.[49]

In a 1942 publication titled *A Century of Missions of the African Methodist Episcopal Church*, Secretary-Treasurer of the Missionary Department Llewellyn L. Berry suggested the denomination endow scholarships to train professionals in "first aid, healthful living, the importance of fresh air, personal hygiene, proper feeding and nutrition, prevention of contagion, the birth of healthy off-springs, reduction of infant and maternity deaths."[50]

Such training, Berry explained, would help "dispel superstition … and undertake the treatment and prevention of endemic diseases."[51]

In 1948, while serving as a delegate to the General Conference, Leonidas H. Berry, Berry's son and an internationally recognized gastroenterologist, sponsored "a bill to create a permanent connectional health commission [to serve as] a central clearing house to supervise and assist in the development of health education programs and activities in local churches."[52] During the 1956 General Conference, Berry proposed to transform the AME-supported Douglass Hospital into a denominational sanitarium and facility for chronically ill people. Berry was medical director until he retired during the 1976 General Conference where, amid a standing ovation, he established the health commission he proposed twenty-eight years earlier.[53] Decades later, from late 2019 and into early 2020, the commission would provide frontline care to individuals affected by the COVID-19 pandemic.

In February 2020, a month after the US Centers for Disease Control and Prevention publicized the first travel-related COVID case in the country,[54] the AME Church International Health Commission released a four-page bulletin titled *Church Preparation and Response to Potential Pandemics.*[55] The commission's medical director, Miriam J. Burnett, a pastor and physician who earned graduate degrees in public health and divinity as well as a medical degree, proclaimed: "As members of the AME Church, we must work together, follow basic infection and behavior modification to decrease the spread of illness and disease."[56] In framing the AME response to the disease, Burnett cited the guidance from the Center for Disease Control and Prevention and the World Health Organization.[57] That congregations adhere to sanitary practices like washing hands and avoiding handholding were key pieces of advice.[58] Burnett also quoted various scriptures from Leviticus that complement twenty-first century protocols on physical, or social, distancing: "On the seventh day the priest is to examine him, and if he sees that the sore is unchanged and has not spread in the skin, he is to keep him in isolation another seven days… . As long as he has the infection he remains unclean. He must live alone; he must live outside the camp."[59] Burnett likewise encouraged congregants to disseminate health information through health-related, popular, religious media.[60]

In March 2020, the month the World Health Organization declared COVID a pandemic, its spread compelled the AME Council of Bishops and the AME General Conference Commission to postpone the general conference scheduled for Orlando, Florida, to July 2021.[61] Harry L. Seawright, president of the Council of Bishops, noted: "Our utmost concern is for the safety and health of the AMEC family as we would potentially gather for our quadrennial meeting, as well as an overarching concern for public health around the globe, especially as it pertains to the novel coronavirus."[62] In the interim months, churchgoers utilized online media platforms to maintain worship and to simulate fellowship, and they instituted protocols for shifting back to in-person services when such services were safe.[63]

Jeffrey N. Leath, a second member of the Council of Bishops, reminded ministers and members of the adage regarding a difference between faith and foolishness. Leath, bishop of the thirteenth district, encouraged congregations to wait before resuming in-person worship because COVID affected black Americans at disproportionately high rates compared with white Americans. Those in his diocese had to obtain authorization from their episcopal leadership before they resumed traditional in-person worship services. Even then, Leath declared, worshippers had to wear masks, sanitize, and follow related safety protocols until further notice.[64]

## Conclusion

From 1793 to 2021, normative AME responses to epidemics and pandemics lay in following the latest recommendations in public health protocols and showing deference to scientific and medical knowledge, especially when communicated by trained professionals within the denomination. Whether it was the empirical observations of Absalom Jones and Richard Allen that drove their activities during the 1793 yellow fever epidemic or AME compliance with 2020 and 2021 guidelines from local, state, and federal government health agencies regarding COVID, denominationalists believed their dual pursuit of prayer and public health could help defeat the scourge of disease.

## Notes

1  See L.O. Howard, "Insects as Carriers and Spreaders of Disease," *Yearbook of United States Department of Agriculture, 1901* (Washington: Government Printing Office, 1902), 177–92, esp. 190–92; and K. David Patterson, "Yellow Fever Epidemics and Mortality in the United States, 1693–1905," *Social Science and Medicine* 34 (April 1992): 855–65.
2  Richard Allen, *The Life, Experience, and Gospel Labors of the Rt. Rev. Richard Allen …* (Philadelphia, PA: F. Ford and M. A. Riply, 1880), 33.
3  Allen, *Life, Experiences, and Gospel Labors*, 37.
4  A.J. and R.A., *A Narrative of the Proceedings of Black People, during the Late Awful a Calamity in Philadelphia, in the Year 1793: And Refutation of Some Censures, Thrown upon Them in Some Publications* (Philadelphia, PA: William W. Woodward, 1794) (hereafter cited as Jones and Allen, *Narrative*).
5  Dennis C. Dickerson, *The African Methodist Episcopal Church: A History* (New York, NY: Cambridge University Press, 2020), 54–55.
6  See Allen, *Life, Experience, and Gospel Labors*, 47, 59, 61; Dickerson, African Methodist Episcopal Church, 54–55; Jones and Allen, *Narrative*; and Richard S. Newman, *Freedom's Prophet: Bishop Richard Allen, the AME Church, and the Black Founding Fathers* (New York, NY: New York University Press, 2008), 85.
7  Patterson, "Yellow Fever Epidemics and Mortality," esp. 855, 857–58.
8  The *Christian Herald* became the *Christian Recorder* in 1852.
9  J. C. Waters, "Communications," *Christian Recorder*, February 8, 1878.
10  Waters, "Communications."
11  Waters, "Communications."
12  Waters, "Communications."

13  Waters, "Communications."
14  In 1878, the Rev. William B. Johnson was one of two AME members who brought felicitations to the general conference of the predominantly white Methodist Episcopal Church, South, held in Atlanta, Georgia. Johnson previously pastored a church in Savanah, approximately 250 miles southeast of Atlanta.
15  "The Yellow Fever at N.O." *Christian Recorder*, August 8, 1878.
16  Reverend J.H. Madison died from yellow fever in September 1878. See "Recent Deaths," *Boston Evening Transcript*, September 5, 1878; and Jeremiah R.V. Thomas, "The Last Hours of Rev. J.H. Madison," *Christian Recorder*, October 17, 1878.
17  L. Gardner, "Word from New Orleans," *Christian Recorder*, November 7, 1878.
18  Gardner, "Word."
19  Larry Eugene Rivers and Canter Brown, Jr., *Laborers in the Vineyard of the Lord: The Beginnings of the AME Church in Florida, 1865–1895* (Tallahassee, FL: University Press of Florida, 2001), 134.
20  Rivers and Brown, *Laborers in the Vineyard of the Lord*, 134.
21  "An Act to Incorporate Brown's Theological Institute," February 10, 1872, *Acts and Resolutions Adopted by the Legislature of Florida, at Its Fifth Session, Under the Constitution of A.D. 1868. Also the Laws Adopted at an Extraordinary Session of the Legislature, Beginning April 22, 1872* (Tallahassee, FL: Tallahassee Sentinel, 1872), 68–69; Gary Dorrien, *The New Abolition: W.E.B. Du Bois and the Black Social Gospel* (New Haven, CT: Yale University Press, 2015), 56; Robert L. Hall, "Tallahassee's Black Churches, 1865–1885," *Florida Historical Quarterly* 58 (October 1979): 189n23; Vann R. Newkirk," Edward Waters College," in *New Life for Historically Black Colleges and Universities: A 21st Century Perspective*, ed. Vann R. Newkirk, 26–33, esp. 27 (Jefferson, NC: McFarland and Company, 2012); Daniel A. Payne, *History of the African Methodist Episcopal Church*, ed. C.C. Smith (Nashville, TN: Publishing House of the A.M.E. Sunday-School Union, 1891), 448; Charles Spencer Smith, *A History of the African Methodist Episcopal Church ...* (1922; repr., New York, NY: Johnson Reprint Corporation, 1922), 359; Alexander W. Wayman, *Cyclopaedia of African Methodism* (Baltimore, MD: Methodist Episcopal Book Depository, 1882), 144.
22  "Personal," *Christian Recorder*, September 20, 1888. Reverend W.W. Sampson died from yellow fever September 30. "Only Six Fever Victims," *York (PA) Gazette*, October 1, 1888.
23  "Personal."
24  "Personal."
25  *Christian Recorder*, October 4, 1888.
26  *Christian Recorder*, October 4, 1888.
27  W. P. Ross, "Yellow Fever in Jacksonville, Fla.," *Christian Recorder*, September 20, 1888.
28  Ross, "Yellow Fever,"
29  Ross, "Yellow Fever."
30  Ross, "Yellow Fever."
31  Ross, "Yellow Fever."
32  Ross, "Yellow Fever."
33  Ross, "Yellow Fever."
34  Regarding the 1918 to 1920 death of influenza, see Carol R. Byerly, *Fever of War: The Influenza Epidemic in the U.S. during World War I* (New York, NY: New York University Press, 2005), 5, 99.

35 *Minutes of the 23rd Annual Convention (of the) Women's Mite Missionary Society*, Pittsburgh Conference Branch, African Methodist Episcopal Church, held in St. James AME Church, Pittsburgh, PA, July 10-13, 1919 (privately printed, n.d.), 13.

36 *Minutes of the North Georgia Annual Conference, African Methodist Episcopal Church*, held in Bethel AME Church, Dalton, GA, November 1918, n.d., 30.

37 *Proceedings of the Twenty-Second Annual Session of the Southwest Georgia Annual Conference of the African American Methodist Episcopal Church Held in Payne Chapel AME Church, Cuthbert, Ga., December 11 and 12, 1918* (Nashville, TN: AME Sunday School Union, 1919) (hereafter cited as 1918 *Southwest Georgia AME Proceedings*).

38 *Southwest Georgia AME Proceedings*.

39 *Southwest Georgia AME Proceedings*.

40 *Southwest Georgia AME Proceedings*.

41 *Minutes of the Thirty-Third Annual Conference of the Michigan Conference, Fifteenth District of the African Methodist Episcopal Church*, held in Bethel AME Church, Detroit, Michigan, September 1–15, 1919 (Nashville, AME Sunday School Union Press, 1920), 55; *Minutes of the Thirty-Eighth Annual Session of the North Ohio Conference of the African Methodist Episcopal Church*, held in Payne's Chapel AME Church, Hamilton, Ohio, October 8–12, 1919 (Philadelphia, AME Book Concern, n.d.), 63.

42 Fifth Annual Year Book of the August Georgia Annual Conference of the African Methodist Episcopal Church Held at St. James AME Church, Tennille, Ga., December 5–9, 1918 (Nashville, TN: AME Sunday School Union, 1919), 7 (hereafter cited as *1918 Georgia AME Annual Conference Year Book*).

43 *1918 Georgia AME Annual Conference Year Book*, 7.

44 *1918 Georgia AME Annual Conference Year Book*, 7.

45 *1918 Georgia AME Annual Conference Year Book*, 7.

46 *Journal of Proceedings of the Emergency Executive Committee of the Fifty-First Annual Session of the [Pittsburgh] Conference of the African Methodist Episcopal Church Held in St. Paul AME Church, Washington, Pa., Wed., Thurs., Oct. 30–31, 1918* (Philadelphia, PN: AME Book Concern, [1918]), 21 (hereafter cited as *1918 Emergency Executive Committee Meeting*).

47 See *1918 Emergency Executive Committee Meeting*, 21.

48 Richard R. Wright, Jr., *The Bishops of the African Methodist Episcopal Church*, Nashville: AME Sunday School Union, 1963, 301.

49 See "Crogman Community [Clinic]," in Richard R. Wright, Jr., comp., *The Encyclopædia of the African Methodist Episcopal Church: Containing Principally the Biographies of the Men and Women, Both Ministers and Laymen, Whose Labors during a Hundred and Sixty Years, Helped Make the AME Church What It Is ...*, 2nd ed. (Philadelphia, PN: Book Concern of the AME Church, 1947), 363; and *Vanessa Northington Gamble, Making a Place for Ourselves: The Black Hospital Movement, 1920–1945* (New York, NY: Oxford University Press, 1995), 9.

50 L. L. Berry, *A Century of Missions of the African Methodist Episcopal Church* (New York, NY: Gutenberg Printing Company, 1942), 235.

51 Berry, *Century of Missions*, 235.

52 *Official Minutes of the Thirty-Third Session of the General Conference of the African Methodist Episcopal Church Held at Kansas City, Kansas, May 1948*, comp., Russell S. Brown (Nashville, TN: AMA Sunday School Union, n.d.).

53 *The Combined Minutes of the Fortieth Session of the General Conference of the African Methodist Episcopal Church Held in Atlanta, Georgia, June 16–26, 1976* (Nashville, TN: AME Sunday School Union, n.d.), 421.

54  United States Centers for Disease Control and Prevention, "First Travel-Related Case of 2019 Novel Coronavirus Detected in United States," January 21, 2020, https://www.cdc.gov/media/releases/2020/p0121-novel-coronavirus-travel-case.html.

55  Miriam J. Burnett, *Church Preparation and Response to Potential Pandemics* (Nashville, TN: AME Church International Health Commission, 2020), 1.

56  Miriam J. Burnett, *Church Preparation and Response to Potential Pandemics* (Nashville: AME Church International Health Commission, 2020), 1.

57  Burnett, *Church Preparation and Response to Potential Pandemics*, 1–2, 4.

58  Burnett, *Church Preparation and Response to Potential Pandemics*, 1.

59  Burnett, *Church Preparation and Response to Potential Pandemics*, 1, quoting Lev 13:5, 13:46, New International Version.

60  Burnett, *Church Preparation and Response to Potential Pandemics*, 2–3.

61  "WHO Director-General's Opening Remarks at the Media Briefing on COVID-19," *World Health Organization*, March 11, 2020, https://www.who.int/director-general/speeches/detail/who-director-general-s-opening-remarks-at-the-media-briefing-on-covid-19—11-march-2020.

62  Harry L. Seawright, statement to the Connectional Church, March 31, 2020, https://www.ame-church.com/news/covid-19-resources/.

63  African Methodist Episcopal members began developing protocols for a return to traditional in-person worship services in May and June of 2020.

64  See, for example, Jeffrey N. Leath, "Immediate Action—Authorizing Motions," November 30, 2020, https://leath128.blog/.

# 10 Pandemics, the Rev. Francis J. Grimké, and Life Lessons

*Kathryn Freeman, Elise M. Edwards,*
*Bertis D. English, and Stephanie C. Boddie*

## Introduction

Ecclesiastes confirms, "There is nothing new under the sun."[1] During the COVID-19 pandemic, countless people have wondered how their lives will be when it ends. Some have been optimistic, but many others have been pessimistic or outright fearful. In this essay, we use the lifework of the Rev. Francis J. Grimké, an African American humanitarian who pastored the Fifteenth Presbyterian Church in Washington, DC, as a guide to navigate old and new trials during the pandemic as well as to propose future navigational tools. Grimké's clerical leadership and his sustained fight against racism and ethnic bias, among religious and secular endeavors, are instructive; however, advice he gave during a sermon on November 3, 1918, amid the influenza pandemic, is especially sage.[2]

## From Slavery to Freedom to Pastorate

Francis Grimké was born on November 4, 1850.[3] He was the second biological son of Henry Grimké, a former attorney and widower from an affluent planter family in Charleston, South Carolina, and Nancy Weston, an enslaved wet nurse of African and European ancestry Henry forced to be his common law wife.[4] Before Henry died from yellow fever complications on September 28, 1852, he provided for the manumitting of Francis and his older enslaved sibling, Archibald.[5] According to Henry's instructions, his eldest son, E. Montague, a free white man whom Henry parented with his first wife, should ensure "the virtual freedom" of half-brothers Archibald, Francis, and John, who entered the world after Henry passed on from it.[6]

E. Montague complied with Henry's wish for approximately eight years before yielding to the desire of his spouse, Julia Catherine (née Bridges), to have additional personal bondservants at her disposal.[7] E. Montague thereupon delivered Archibald, Francis, and John to her.[8] All three servants rebelled, with E. Montague eventually apprenticing Francis to a white man whose cruel treatment included starvation and whipping.[9] After state officials in South Carolina seceded from the Union and laid

DOI: 10.4324/9781003214281-13

the cornerstone of the Confederacy on December 20, 1860, Francis sought a respite from E. Montague and Catherine by becoming a valet to a Confederate military officer.[10]

Francis's wartime events are unclear, but he in 1887 recalled being a valet for about two years prior to self-emancipating and joining thousands of "freedom's soldiers" by fleeing to the Union lines.[11] In Charleston "one day, while we were stationed in Castle Pinckney," a fortification in the harbor, Francis recounted, "I was suddenly arrested just as I was about to step into the boat on my return to the fort, and thrown into jail, or what is known as the 'workhouse.'"[12] During his detainment, which lasted several months, he recollected further in 1887, "I became dangerously ill from exposure and bad treatment, and came very near losing my life. It was only by being finally removed to my mother's house, and by the most skillful treatment, that I recovered. I had thus fallen into the hands of this half-brother and guardian [E. Montague]; he, fearing that I would go away again, sold me, before I was well enough to go out, to [another Confederate] officer, and again I went back into the Army, where I remained until" war's official end in 1865.[13]

At the onset of postwar Reconstruction, a white female schoolteacher arranged for Francis and Archibald Grimké to go north to receive formal education. Their hosts treated them badly, though the two siblings did learn about shoemaking, among other trades. Once the teacher learned of such treatment, she coordinated their admittance to Lincoln University near Oxford, Pennsylvania, in 1866. Abolitionist Presbyterians founded the original academy as the Ashmun Institute in 1853, and state lawmakers granted a chartered in 1854.[14]

As Francis and Archibald matriculated through the university, whose designation changed from institute to university the same year they enrolled, aunts Angelina and Sarah Grimké, two well-known abolitionist members of the Religious Society of Friends, began providing financial support. Both Francis and Archibald appreciated the assistance, which paid immense dividends. Without having to worry about covering all monetary needs by themselves, they were able to concentrate more fully on their educational and spiritual development than many other students. Francis made excellent grades, as exemplified by Lincoln administrators naming him valedictorian of the 1870 graduating class, and his brother and roommate, Archibald, amassed a sterling record as well. After completing Lincoln the same year as Francis, Archibald went to Harvard Law School in Boston, Massachusetts, earning a degree in 1874.[15]

Not long after Archibald commenced his legal training, Francis made a foray into the study of law. Frances began at Lincoln in 1871 but paused his coursework the next year to serve as financial agent of the university. He reentered the law school in 1873 but moved to Washington, DC, to attend Howard Law School one year later. Francis stayed at Howard until 1875, a time during which he decided to answer one of the divine calls to ministry he had ignored since his time at Lincoln. He thus relocated to Princeton, New Jersey, and enrolled in the Theological Seminary of the Presbyterian Church in the United States of America, familiarly Princeton Theological Seminary, earning a doctor of divinity degree in 1878.[16]

With the coveted doctorate in hand, Francis Grimké returned to Washington, DC, to pastor the Fifteenth Street Presbyterian Church, one of the oldest and most notable prominently black churches in the capital city.[17] He underwent ordination and commenced his pastorate officially on July 7, 1878.[18] Former and current educational and priestly endeavors were gratifying, but Grimké became ecstatic when he married Salem Normal School in Massachusetts alumna Charlotte L. Forten on December 19, 1878.[19] She was a black author from a prosperous family in Philadelphia, Pennsylvania, whom one newspaper described as "about the only colored contributor to magazines in this country, ... having been time to time a paid writer on the *Atlantic Monthly* and *Scribner.*"[20] Their "wedding in colored high life" took place in Washington, and papers from across the country reported on the nuptials.[21]

Under Rev. and Mrs. Grimké's leadership, Fifteenth Street Presbyterian Church's membership comprised by many affluent African Americans grew from 150 to more than 500.[22] As historian Brenda Stevenson would write in 1988, Grimké distinguished himself as one of the most talented, "sensitive, morally upright, and fiercely dedicated" preachers in Washington.[23] He was one of only a few clergymen of African descent in the city to be both university educated and seminary trained; moreover, his training took place at one of the foremost seminaries in the world, Princeton Theological.[24] Described by the renowned African American civil rights activist, educator, journalist, mathematician, and sociologist Kelly Miller as a "man of God in an age of gold," Grimké eschewed the trappings of wealth and power to faithfully preach the gospel, honor his beloved wife, Charlotte, and condemn white supremacy in every facet of American life.[25]

Besides possessing the abovementioned characteristics and traits, Rev. Grimké was an "outspoken defender of the rights of the Negro," to quote his and Miller's associate, Carter G. Woodson, a Harvard-educated scholar, organizer, and businessman.[26] As a testament to Grimké being an ardent "race man," he joined the Niagara movement Carter's fellow Harvard graduate and intellectual equal, William E. B. Du Bois of Great Barrington, Massachusetts, launched in 1905 to demand full citizenship for African Americans.[27] In 1909 and 1910, as Du Bois helped establish and incorporate, respectively, the biethnic National Association for the Advancement of Colored People (NAACP), Grimké was a "warm supporter" of the NAACP.[28] Grimké's enthusiasm for the NAACP increased in future years; however, Charlotte, their biological and church families, and putting what he preached into practice were three of Francis's primary concerns.[29]

## War, Pandemic, and Bias

As Reverend Grimké pastored the Fifteenth Street Presbyterian Church in Washington, DC, during the early twentieth century, several personal, national, and global events impacted his and other African Americans' health and welfare. For example, on July 23, 1914, Grimké's brilliant and devoted wife of thirty-five years, Charlotte, died.[30] Days later, on July 28, as he celebrated his beloved "Lottie,"[31] who lived to be seventy-six but "who never grew old in spirit—she was always young, as young as the youngest"— World War I erupted in Europe.[32] After the US entered the war officially in 1917, more than 350,000 African Americans served in segregated combat and supplemental units before the 1918 ceasefire.[33] Grimké, however, refused to purchase so-called liberty bonds or encourage his congregants to do so because, "in this boasted land of the free, the very men who are calling for a loan to defend liberty are the oppressors, are the ones who are trampling upon the rights of ten millions of colored people."[34] Grimké repudiated President Woodrow Wilson, a stanch racist and "clog on the wheels of progress," for re-segregating the federal government.[35] Grimké also refused to support the Red Cross because its white leaders and ordinary volunteers routinely discriminated against nonwhite health care workers, including physicians and nurses.[36]

Reverend Grimké was passionate about equality, often lamenting the existence of separate white and nonwhite churches, and chiding churchgoers of all complexions who said or who did nothing to fight inequality.[37] He was particularly vociferous about white ecclesiastical leaders. "The men who have been most active in promoting Jim-crow car legislation, in bringing about all forms of discrimination, in holding the race up to contempt, in saying the bitterest things against it, have not all been outside of the church," he once groused, adding: "many of them have not only been in the church, but have held high places in it."[38] Grimké was a principled man, and the power of the gospel to transform individual lives and entire societies was one of his core tenets.[39]

The explicit reemergence of the Ku Klux Klan, which members nicknamed the "invisible empire," during World War I was another topic about which Grimké spoke often.[40] The Klan's official 1915 rebirth atop Stone Mountain in Georgia symbolized a blitzkrieg of "white terror" that propelled the first of three twentieth-century waves of an eventual torrential migration of African Americans from the South to the North and to other regions of the country.[41] Wave one formed in 1916, a year after the Klan's "impressive" reestablishment, as the *Atlanta Constitution* newspaper characterized the Stone Mountain event.[42] During the next several years, approximately 1.2 million black and biethnic southerners moved north.[43] Some sought refuge from the Klan and other violent white paramilitary organizations, while others wanted to avoid less lethal manifestations of Jim and Jane Crowism, such as poll taxes, literacy tests, and cognate requirements for voting.[44] Yet others longed for better educational or professional opportunities than they had in the South.[45]

The North was no utopia for the majority of African Americans. Summer 1919 was particularly difficult. That season, as plenipotentiaries from across the globe signed a treaty in Versailles, France, to formally end World War I,[46] bigoted white people in the US provoked at least twenty-five riots, killing more than 250 nonwhite people.[47] Unfortunately, white brutality was not the only peril. Among others, influenza—misnamed the Spanish flu and the three-day fever, among others—was paramount.[48] Influenza struck the US stealthily circa August 1918, first against military service persons and soon against civilians.[49] By the time the pandemic ceased in April 1920, anywhere from 50 to 100 million people were dead, and more than 675,000 died in the US.[50]

Local officials in Washington, DC, where the Rev. Francis Grimké lived and labored, broadcast the first influenza-associated death in the city on September 21, 1918. Without swift public health measures because many physicians, nurses, and others in healthcare were serving abroad in military capacities, the flu reached crisis stage within a month. By November, the month during which most wartime combat ceased and Grimké delivered the poignant sermon about which we write more below, thirty persons were dying each day in Washington. He and other survivors worried, as neither the etiology of influenza nor an effective treatment were known. With seemingly few practicable options available to him, Washington Health Officer William Fowler ordered the closing of the Fifteenth Street Presbyterian Church that Grimké pastored along with other worship houses, libraries, public schools, and theaters. In an effort to reduce crowd sizes downtown, Fowler placed businesses on alternating timetables. Next, his fellow public officials and he shut the doors of government buildings. Protective measures notwithstanding, people countrywide began to refer to Washington as a "harvest field" of influenza due to more than 33,000 infections and 3,000 deaths by 2020.[51]

Relatively few scholarly publications were interested in studies about ethnic disparities in the US during its 1918 to 1920 influenza epidemic, but some of the individuals whose research or writing did appear in print found that black Americans had fewer incidences of influenza than white Americans. Blacks, however, had more fatalities than whites. Contributing factors included blacks being more likely than whites to have substandard or overcrowded housing and limited sanitation. Moreover, because of massive socioeconomic inequality in the country, the typical black person was at a greater risk than a white person to have chronic respiratory disease, malnutrition, or inadequate health care.[52]

Ethnic tension spread across the US as fast as influenza during the near year and a half epidemic from 1918 to 2020, and neither Rev. Grimké nor his African American contemporaries in Washington, DC, were immune to either one of the two diseases. Many white people in the capital city and elsewhere in the country alleged that nonwhite people threatened their job security or, among other things, were influenza vectors who should live in segregated neighborhoods and seek treatment in segregated hospitals. In a seemingly perpetual irony, African American health professionals worked day and night to care for patients of every ancestry group despite official or unofficial color lines in many places throughout the US.[53]

While biased white people spewed vitriol from 1918 to 1920, Grimké injected love. In both religious and secular settings, he placed "relentless emphasis on the primacy of the preaching the gospel and of living the gospel in any effort to engage the world."[54] As scholars C. Eric Lincoln and Lawrence H. Mamiya would note in 1990, serving as cultural brokers or mediating institutions to help rural emigrants acclimate to urban environments were primary functions of many early 1900s congregations, and the Fifteenth Street Presbyterian Church that Grimké pastored was a center of such activities.[55]

Similar to other turbulent experiences in Grimké's life, he used the influenza epidemic to promote godliness. Among other acts, he encouraged biased white Americans, including "so-called professing Christians," to repent by not only acknowledging but also valuing the inherent dignity of nonwhite Americans dealing with influenza.[56] As during more pleasant times, Grimké assailed bigotry wherever and whenever he saw it from 1918 to 1920, often speaking about human and civil rights using religious overtones. Comparing the plight of black and biethnic Americans and Israelites, as discussed in the Old Testament, was a recurrent act.[57] For him, the gospel and discrimination could not coexist; wherever one was present, the other was absent.

Patience, positivity, and obeying reasonable public policies were three additional lessons Grimké taught during the influenza epidemic. Among other acts, he tried to remain upbeat as government restrictions on religious facilities and other places where churchgoers often gathered posed serious challenges for many people of faith. Grimké knew state-ordered closings would affect Fifteenth Street Presbyterian and the noble work its members performed, but he also knew legitimate concerns about health and safety underlay the decision to close Fifteenth Street and other worship houses, educational facilities, and public buildings in Washington, DC.[58]

### Reflections: Influenza and COVID-19

On Sunday, November 3, 1918, after weeks of government orders restricting public and private gatherings such as school sessions and religious events, Grimké was able to hold worship services at Fifteenth Street Presbyterian without violating any municipal prohibition. "Some Reflections, Growing Out of the Recent Epidemic of Influenza that Afflicted Our City" was the title of his sermon, and we believe its message is relevant during the COVID-19 pandemic.[59] He opened with 2 Samuel 24 in the Old Testament:

"So Jehovah sent a pestilence upon Israel from the morning even unto the time appointed; and there died the people from Dan even unto Beersheba seventy thousand men. And when the angel stretched forth his hand toward Jerusalem to destroy it, Jehovah repented him of the evil, and said to the angel that destroyed the people, It is enough; now stay they hand."[60]

Not long after in the sermon, Grimké asked: "What ought [the pandemic] to mean to us? Is it to come and go and we be no wiser, or better for it? Surely God had a purpose in it, and it is our duty to find out, as far as we may, what that purpose is, and try to profit by it."[61] Grimké provided his answer in the conclusion of the sermon. He enjoined Christians to be "more determined than ever to run with patience the race set before us.... Let us all draw near to God [and] be better Christians."[62] Such words resonate during the COVID pandemic, which claimed almost 600,000 human lives in the US from late 2019 to mid-2021.[63] For us that death toll, which is approximately 75,000 fewer than the influenza epidemic caused from late 1918 to early 1920,[64] is a reminder that life is too precious to allow the "twin crises" of disease and bigotry to provoke unnecessary chaos and death.[65]

## Conclusion

Grimké, in his November 1918 sermon, contended influenza "shattered the theory, so dear to the heart of the white man ... that a white skin entitles its possessor to better treatment than one who possesses a dark skin."[66] Any white person who believed that nonsense, Grimké continued, harbored a belief "that God utterly repudiates, as He has shown during this epidemic scourge; and [with whom] He will ... deal [at their times of] solemn account. The lesson taught is clear and distinct," Grimké continued; nevertheless, he wondered if those who carried the virus of white supremacy would "seek to mend [their] evil ways" and adhere to the "great law of Love."[67] Clarifying what he meant, Grimké said ethnic "prejudice, colorphobia, runs directly counter to" loving God and to loving thy neighbor.[68]

We believe a similar principle applies to COVID. Despite the high level of misery, the disease has generated since the World Health Organization announced the pandemic in March 2020, consequent hardship has given people around the globe an opportunity to become more understanding, wiser, and unified. Those who do so will help advance the color-neutral progress Grimké advocated in November 1918.[69]

## Notes

1 Eccl. 1:9, New International Version.
2 Francis J. Grimké, *Some Reflections, Growing Out of the Recent Epidemic of Influenza that Afflicted Our City: A Discourse Delivered in the Fifteenth Street Presbyterian Church, Washington, D.C., Sunday, November 3, 1918* (Washington, DC: Francis J. Grimké, 1918).

3  Francis Grimké stated November 4, 1850, was his date of birth in *The Works of Francis J. Grimké*, vol. 3, ed. Carter G. Woodson (Washington, DC: Associated Publishers, 1942) (94). Similar to countless other people of African descent born in the United States of America during the nineteenth century, especially before the Civil War, some resources suggest a different birthdate. See, as an example, Thabiti M. Anyabwile, *The Faithful Preacher: Recapturing the Vision of Three Pioneering African-American Pastors* (Wheaton, IL: Crossway, 2007), 113 (indicating Grimké entered the world on October 10, 1850).

4  Francis Grimké wrote often about his lineage.

5  Anyabwile, *The Faithful Preacher*, 113; Clifton E. Olmstead, "Francis James Grimké (1850–1937): Christian Moralist and Civil Rights," in *Sons of the Prophet: Leaders in Protestantism from Princeton Seminary*, ed. Hugh T. Kerr (1963; repr., Princeton, NJ: Princeton University Press, 2019), 161–75, esp. 165–66; Sean Michael Lucas, "Meet Francis Grimké (1850–1937), Faithful Minister of Grace," *Gospel Coalition*, September 11, 2018, https://www.the-gospelcoalition.org/article/francis-grimke/.

6  Anyabwile, *Faithful Preacher*, 113.

7  Anyabwile, *Faithful Preacher*, 113; Lucas, "Meet Francis Grimké."

8  Anyabwile, *Faithful Preacher*, 113; Lucas, "Meet Francis Grimké"; William J. Simmons, *Men of Mark: Eminent, Progressive, and Rising* (Cleveland, OH: G. M. Rewell and Company, 1887), 608.

9  Lucas, "Meet Francis Grimké."

10  *Declaration of the Immediate Cause Which Induce and Justify the Secession from the Federal Union; and the Ordinance of Secession* (Charleston, SC: Evans and Cogswell, 1860); Frances J. Grimké, *The Works of Francis J. Grimké*, vol. 1: *Addresses Mainly Personal and Racial*, ed. Carter G. Woodson (Washington, DC: Associated Publishers, 1942), viii; Simmons, *Men of Mark*, 608.

11  Ira Berlin, Joseph P. Reidy, and Leslie R. Rowland, eds., *Freedom's Soldiers: The Black Military Experience in the Civil War* (New York: Cambridge University Press, 1998). See also Grimké, *Works*, vol. 1, viii; Charlotte Forten Grimké, *The Journals of Charlotte Forten Grimké*, ed. Brenda Stevenson (New York, NY: Oxford University Press, 1988), 51; and Simmons, *Men of Mark*, 608.

12  Grimké, *Works*, 1: viii.

13  Grimké, *Works*, 1: viii.

14  "An Act to Incorporate the Ashmun Institute," April 29, 1854," in Langston Hughes Memorial Library Special Collections Department, Lincoln University in Lincoln University, Pennsylvania (hereafter cited as Lincoln University Special Collections); Anyabwile, *Faithful Preacher*, 114; "The Ashmun Institute," in Lincoln University Special Collections; William H. Ferris, *The African Abroad or His Evolution in Western Civilization: Tracing His Development Under the Caucasian Milieu* (New Haven, CT: Tuttle, Morehouse and Taylor, 1913), 2:888–97; Grimké, *Journals*, 51–52; Grimké, *Works*, vol. 1, *passim*; Simmons, *Men of Mark*, 609–10.

15  Anyabwile, *Faithful Preacher*, 114; "Commencements," *Boston Post*, June 25, 1874, 6; Ferris, *The African Abroad*, 2:888–97; "Kelly Miller Writes about Dr. Francis J. Grimke, Exemplar of the College Bred Negro," *New York Age*, October 30, 1937, 6 (referring to the Grimkés and other who finished Lincoln University in Pennsylvania in 1870 as "the first regular college class to be graduated from any Negro college or university in the US, or for that matter, in that world"); Simmons, *Men of Mark*, 609–10.

16  Grimké, *Works*, 1:x, viii–xi, 217; Simmons, *Men of Mark*, 609–10. Several contemporaneous newspapers suggested Francis Grimké completed Princeton Theological Seminary in 1877 rather than 1878. See, as an example, "Personal."

17 John F. Cook Sr. organized the *Fifteenth Street Presbyterian Church in Washington, DC, formally on November 21, 1841. Cook, a onetime African Methodist Episcopal denominationalist, and eighteen other persons made up First Street.* See, for example, John W. Cromwell, "First Negro Churches in the District of Columbia," *Journal of Negro History 7 (1922): 64–106,* esp. *69, 80–82.*

18 Grimké, *Works,* 1: xi–xii *(noting he was not at the helm of the Fifteenth Street Presbyterian Church in Washington, DC, from late* 1885 to late 1889; instead, he was the Laura Street Presbyterian Church in Jacksonville, Florida, to which Charlotte and he moved because of his health concerns); "Pastor Tomorrow: Rev. Dr. H.B. Taylor to be Associate at Fifteenth St. Presbyterian," (Washington, DC) *Evening Star,* June 20, 1925, 8 (announcing Rev. Grimké resigned recently; instead of accepting his resignation, parishioners elected to make him a salaried pastor for life, an office in which he served until dying on October 11, 1937).

19 Grimké, *Works,* 1:xxxiii, 51; "Personals," *Hartford (CT) Courant,* December 23, 1878, 2.

20 "Personal," *Lancaster (PA) Intelligencer,* December 23, 1878, 2.

21 "Current Matters," *New Orleans Daily Democrat,* December 23, 1878, 7 (one of several newspapers in which the quotation appeared).

22 Kerr, *Francis Grimké,* 165.

23 Grimké, *Journals,* 52.

24 Regarding historical literacies of African American clergymen, including those who entered the ministry after Francis Grimké, see C. Eric Lincoln and Lawrence H. Mamiya, *The Black Church in the African American Experience* (Durham, NC: Duke University Press, 1990), esp. 1.

25 Kelly Miller, "Man of God in an Age of Gold," June 6, 1925, in box 16, folder 4, subseries 2.1: Writing by Miller, Kelly Miller Family Papers, 1890–1989, Stuart A. Rose Manuscript, Archives, and Rare Books Library, Emory University, Atlanta, Georgia. See also Frances J. Grimké, *The Works of Francis J. Grimké,* vol. 4: *Letters,* ed. Carter G. Woodson (Washington, DC: Associated Publishers, 1942), 405; and C.G. Woodson, "Kelly Miller," *Journal of Negro History* 25 (January 1940): 137–38.

26 Carter G. Woodson, *Negro Orators and Their Orations* (Washington, DC: Associated Publishers, 1925), 690n2.

27 Craig R. Prentiss, *Staging Faith: Religion and African American Theater from the Harlem Renaissance to World War II* (New York, NY: New York University Press, 2014), 113.

28 Grimké, *Works,* 1: xviii.

29 Grimké, *Works,* 1: xviii, 19n1, 518–19, 618–27.

30 Francis Grimké, in the third volume of his *Works,* indicated Charlotte Grimké died on July 23, 1914 (5, 34, 50, 80, 93, 100, 107, 114, 126, 220, 267, 330, 543); however, Brenda Stevenson suggested July 22 in both the chronology for and introduction to Grimké, *Journals,* xl, 55, citing "Dr. Grimké's Obituary, July 23, 1914," in Francis Grimké Papers, Moorland-Spingarn Research Center, Howard University. See also "Death of Mrs. F.K. Grimke" and "Died," (Washington, DC) *Evening Star,* July 24, 1914, 7, 10.

31 Francis Grimké often referred to his wife, Charlotte, as "Lottie."

32 Francis Grimké, as quoted by Brenda Stevenson in the introduction to Grimké, *Journals,* 1–56 (quotation on 55).

33 Emmett J. Scott, *Scott's Official History of the American Negro in The World War* (Chicago, IL: Homewood Press, 1919), 9 (indicating more than 4,00,000 African Americans fought in the war).

34 Grimké, *Works,* 3:72.

35   Grimké, *Works*, 3:65 (quotation), 118, 138–39, 294.
36   Grimké, *Works*, 3:25–26.
37   Anyabwile, *Faithful Preacher*, 119.
38   Grimké, "Christianity and Race Prejudice," 18.
39   Anyabwile, *Faithful Preacher*, 119.
40   "Klan Is Reestablished with Impressiveness," *Atlanta Constitution*, November 28, 1915, 2.
41   Allen W. Trelease, *White Terror: The Ku Klux Conspiracy and Southern Reconstruction* (1971; repr., Baton Rouge: Louisiana State University Press, 1995).
42   "Klan Is Reestablished with Impressiveness."
43   Jacqueline Jones, *Labor of Love, Labor of Sorrow: Black Women, Work, and the Family from Slavery to Present*, rev. ed. (New York, NY: Basic Books, 2010), 132; Stewart E. Tolnay, Robert M. Adelman, and Kyle D. Crowder, "Race, Regional Origin, and Residence in Northern Cities at the Beginning of the Great Migration," *American Sociological Review* 67 (June 2002): 456–75; Isabel Wilkerson, *The Warmth of Other Suns: The Epic Story of America's Great Migration* (New York, NY: Vintage Books, 2011).
44   Lincoln and Mamiya, *Black Church*, 118; Wilkerson, *Warmth of Other Suns*.
45   Jim Crow is familiar nomenclature. For a representative qualification regarding Jane Crow, or gender- and sex-based discrimination, see Pauli Murray, *Song in a Weary Throat: Memoir of an American Pilgrimage* (1987; repr., New York, NY: Liveright, 2018), 315–16, 472, 474–75, 507.
46   *The Treaty of Peace Between the Allied and Associated Powers and Germany, the Protocol Annexed Thereto, the Agreement Respecting the Military Occupation of the Territories of the Rhine, and the Treaty between France and Great Britain Respecting Assistance to France in the Event of Unprovoked Aggression by Germany. Signed at Versailles, June 28th, 1919* (London: His Majesty's Stationery Office, 1919).
47   DeNeen L. Brown, "Remembering 'Red Summer,' When White Mobs Massacred Blacks from Tulsa to D.C.," *National Geographic*, June 19, 2020, https://www.nationalgeographic.com/history/article/remembering-red-summer-white-mobs-massacred-blacks-tulsa-dc; Allan H. Spear, *Black Chicago: The Making of a Negro Ghetto, 1890–1920* (Chicago: University of Chicago Press, 1967); United States National Archives and Records Administration, "Racial Violence and the Red Summer," June 28, 2021, https://www.archives.gov/research/african-americans/wwi/red-summer, (hereafter cited as NARA).
48   Countless post–World War I sources employed inaccurate terminology such as Spanish flu and three-day fever. See, as examples, "To Fight the Spanish Flu," (Anadarko, OK) *American Democrat*, October 10, 1918, 1; and "Influenza; What It Is and What to Do When It Comes—Rupert Blue," *Decatur (IL) Herald*, October 6, 1918, 15.
49   Carol R. Byerly, *Fever of War: The Influenza Epidemic in the U.S. during World War I* (New York: New York University Press, 2005); NARA, "The Deadly Virus: The Influenza Epidemic of 1918," n.d., https://www.archives.gov/exhibits/influenza-epidemic/.
50   Influenza killed approximately one fifth of the world population and a fourth the US population. See Byerly, *Fever of War*, 5, 99; Alfred W. Crosby, *America's Forgotten Pandemic: The Influenza of 1918*, 2nd ed. (New York, NY: Cambridge University Press, 2003); Lakshmi Krishnan, S. Michelle Ogunwole, and Lisa A. Cooper, "Historical Insights on Coronavirus Disease 2019 (COVID-19), the 1918 Influenza Pandemic, and Racial Disparities: Illuminating a Path Forward," *Annals of Internal Medicine* 173 (June 5, 2020): 474–81; and Soraya Nadia McDonald, "In 1918 and 2020, Race Colors America's Response to Epidemics:

A Look at How Jim Crow Affected the Treatment of African Americans Fighting the Spanish Flu," *Undefeated*, April 1, 2020, https://theundefeated.com/features/in-1918-and-2020-race-colors-americas-response-to-epidemics/.

51 Krishnan, Ogunwole, and Cooper, "Historical Insights," 39. See also Sarah Alverson, "Washington D.C. and the Influenza Outbreak of 1918," *Health Emergency and Disaster Nursing* 7 (February 13, 2020): 39–41; CDC, "1918 Pandemic (H1N1 Virus)," March 20, 2019, https://www.cdc.gov/pandemic-resources/1918-pandemic-h1n1.html; "Death Here from Spanish Influenza," (Washington, DC) *Evening Star*, September 21, 1918, 2; Grimké, *Works*, 3:70; "Influenza Claims Victim in Capital," *Washington Times*, September 21, 1918, 1; "Makes Appeal to D.C. Doctors," *Washington Herald*, September 21, 1918, 9.

52 Vanessa Northington Gamble, "'There Wasn't a Lot of Comforts in Those Days:' African Americans, Public Health, and the 1918 Influenza Epidemic," *Public Health Reports* 125, supplement 3 (April 2010): 114–22 (placing the quotation mark outside the colon); Krishnan, Ogunwole, and Cooper, "Historical Insights"; Helene Økland and Svenn-Erik Mamelund, "Race and 1918 Influenza Pandemic in the United States: A Review of the Literature," *International Journal of Environmental Research and Public Health* 16 (July 2019): 1–18, https://doi.org/10.3390/ijerph16142487.

53 Carol Anderson, *White Rage: The Unspoken Truth of Our Racial Divide* (New York: Bloomsbury, 2017), 55–58; Krishnan, Ogunwole, and Cooper, "Historical Insights"; McDonald, "Race Colors America's Response"; John P. Turner, "Epidemic Influenza and the Negro Physician," *Journal of the National Medical Association* 10, no. 4 (1918): 184.

54 Anyabwile, *Faithful Preacher*, 120.

55 Lincoln and Mamiya, *Black Church,* 121.

56 Francis J. Grimké, "Christianity and Race Prejudice," pt. 2, June 5, 1910, in *Christianity and Race Prejudice: Two Discourses Delivered in the Fifteenth Street Presbyterian Church, Washington, D.C[.,] May 29th and 5th* (Washington, DC: W. E. Cobb, 1910), 18.

57 Exodus, 1–20, NIV; Grimké, *Works*, 1:82, 236, 347–63.

58 See, among other sources, Grimké, *Reflections*, 3; Grimké, *Works*, 3:70; and "Official Notices," (Washington, DC) *Evening Star*, October 5, 1918, 10.

59 Grimké, *Reflections*.

60 Grimké, *Reflections*, 3 (quoting 2 Samuels, 15–16, from an unidentified version of the Judeo-Christian Bible).

61 Grimké, *Reflections*, 3.

62 Grimké, *Reflections*, 12.

63 United States Centers for Disease Control and Prevention, "Daily Updates to Totals by Week and State: Provisional Death Counts for Coronavirus Disease 2019 (COVID-19)," July 13, 2021, https://www.cdc.gov/nchs/nvss/vsrr/COVID19/index.htm. (hereafter cited as CDC).

64 CDC, "1918 Pandemic (H1N1 Virus)."

65 Michael D. Barber, "The Twin Crises of Covid-19 and Racism: Pragmatic Mastery, Theory, Religion, and Ethics," *Open Theology* 7 (January 2021): 69–82.

66 Grimké, *Reflections*, 6.

67 Grimké, *Reflections*, 7–8.

68 Grimké, *Reflections*, 8.

69 "WHO Director-General's Opening Remarks at the Media Briefing on COVID-19," *World Health Organization*, March 11, 2020, https://www.who.int/director-general/speeches/detail/who-director-general-s-opening-remarks-at-the-media-briefing-on-covid-19. March 11, 2020.

# 11 Collins Chapel Hospital and the Christian Methodist Episcopal Church Responses to Healthcare Disparities in Memphis, Tennessee

*Raymond Sommerville and George W. Coleman Jr.*

## Introduction

Nestled inconspicuously in the thriving medical district of Memphis, Tennessee, is a two-building complex called the Collins Chapel Connectional Hospital (CCCH). Though located in the shadows of larger healthcare providers such as the St. Jude Children's Research Hospital, Le Bonheur Children's Hospital, and Regional One Health, the original CCCH building—a two-story house-turned-medical facility known as the Collins Chapel Old Folks' Home and Hospital (CCOFHH)—predates the larger providers and continues to stand as a landmark institution in Memphis. A team of black doctors trained at the Meharry Medical Department of Central Tennessee College in Nashville, approximately 210 miles northeast of Memphis, founded the CCOFHH in 1905. The doctors operated a surgical center, maternity ward, and outreach ministry under the auspices of the Collins Chapel Colored Methodist Episcopal (CME) Church, the oldest African American congregation in Memphis.[1]

As Memphis' first medical facility for black patients the CCOFHH provided needed healthcare services when the city's white hospitals refused services because of skin color. Through deadly epidemics and glaring health disparities affecting black communities in the Mississippi Delta, the CCOFHH responded with a faith-based holism representative of pioneering white Briton John Wesley's founding mission for Methodism. This essay recovers his holistic approach to healthcare in the eighteenth-century Atlantic and then shows how Methodists in North America adopted the approach. The essay gives special attention to the masses of formerly enslaved people who organized the CME Church in 1870 and how the CCCH continues to embody Wesley's holistic mission.

### The Wesleyan Holistic Vision and Mission

Innumerable people have celebrated Wesley for being an energetic evangelist, innovative organizer, practical theologian, and antislavery proponent. He and his younger brother, Charles Wesley, started Methodism as a "holy club" for liked-minded students at Christ Church, Oxford University, in

DOI: 10.4324/9781003214281-14

Britain.[2] The Wesleys led their fellow students in devotional practices of prayer, scriptural meditation, and fasting, as well as in acts of mercy, to include ministering to the sick, the incarcerated, and the poor.[3] The Wesleys expanded their mission from the university to the streets, intending "to spread scriptural holiness over the land."[4] Pursuant to realizing that grand vision, John sailed to the British colony of Georgia in 1735 as a missionary to Native Americans and to British settlers. He, however, aborted the endeavor within a year. That setback led to a decades-long spiritual and emotional crisis for him, but through the mediation of Charles and a group of Moravians in London, John underwent a reconversion experience in 1784 that resulted in a second wave of missional activity and personal growth.[5]

Holistic healthcare was an essential component of John Wesley's mission, even while in crisis. During the late 1730s he renewed his emphasis on regular visitation of the sick by lay leaders, including some preachers, whom he referred to as assistants. Wesley instructed them see every person within their district thrice per week.[6] Then, beginning with the publication of *A Collection of Receits [Receipts] for the Use of the Poor* in 1745, Wesley produced a steady stream of medical resources that offered advice on medications, treatments, and other services.[7] *Primitive Physic*, a volume on healing, was the most popular resource.[8] Published originally in 1747, it underwent twenty-one editions by his death in 1791.[9] In the preface, he encouraged readers to take responsibility for others as well as for themselves.[10]

A third way Wesley expanded his holistic care of the sick was by opening two free public clinics, one at his headquarters in London and the other in Bristol. Combined with a dispensary, those faith-based facilities provided medical care to urban poor who did not have access to the private, and often expensive, services that privileged citizens enjoyed.[11] In retrospect, Wesley's clinics were models for numerous future healthcare and healthcare training institutions, including historically black facilities such as the CCOFHH in Memphis and the Meharry Medical Department (formerly the Meharry Medical Department of Central Tennessee College) in Nashville.[12]

Named after an Egyptian metropolis, Memphis is a Mississippi River hub connecting Tennessee, Arkansas, Mississippi, and Missouri. Similar to the ancient African site, black people were central to Memphis, also known as the Bluff City, from its 1819 founding.[13] Cotton grown primarily by enslaved men, women, and children made the Tennessee locality (Memphis) a major commercial hub and transportation center through which millions of unfree people moved before traders, owners, and other free people relocated them to other places in the South. After the Civil War began officially in 1861, Tennessee seceded from the Union, and Memphis became a Confederate stronghold. Matters changed a year later, however, when Union forces seized Memphis, established a supply base and hospital, and occupied the city for the duration of the war.[14] Although jubilant when emancipated in 1865, thousands of black people in Memphis bore in their bodies

the somatic-psychological trauma of more than two centuries of enslavement since English colonists settled at Jamestown, Virginia, in 1607.[15]

## Collins Chapel Connectional Hospital as
## Case Study of Wesley's Vision

During the 1870s, just as CME Church leaders asserted their independence
by creating the first autonomous black denomination founded in the former
Confederacy, a yellow fever epidemic struck the Memphis area.[16] Carried by
individuals traveling on waterways, the epidemic peaked in 1878. Various
sources reported 17,600 cases and 5,150 fatalities during that year.[17] Many
affluent white citizens fled in panic, relocating to "healthier sites" and leaving black and poorer white citizens to fend for themselves.[18] Throughout the
"long, deep draught of sickness and of death," as the *Daily Memphis Avalanche*
described the epidemic, the Collins Chapel CME Church allied with other
congregations and medical organizations to provide relief.[19] Regrettably, the
Collins church family was unable to save one of its most beloved members:
Pastor J.H. Ridley, a leading education advocate as well as a minister, succumbed to the fever in 1879.[20] He "died with this harness on, while carrying
out the duties of his sacred office," the *Avalanche* memorialized.[21]

Fortunately for many other black Memphians during the yellow fever epidemic of 1878 to 1879, one of the best health services training facilities for
their ethnic group, the Meharry Medical Department of Central Tennessee
College, was located in Nashville. The Northern-based Methodist Episcopal
Church established Meharry in 1876, three years before the epidemic took
the life of Ridley. Hundreds of students matriculated through the medical department during the next several decades, and their formal learning
helped prepare them to assist thousands of people, including Ridley before
he passed away. By 1906, according to historian David McBride, 733 doctors, 85 pharmacists, 74 dentists, and 15 nurses had finished Meharry, one
of the finest institutions of its type in the country.[22]

At least two of the 907 Meharry graduates whom McBride references,
Mattie Howard Coleman and Charles Henry Phillips, were affiliated with
the CME Church. In fact, they belonged to the first generation of college-
educated individuals to emerge as leaders of the denomination. Coleman,
one of the earliest black female licensed physicians in the US, also was a religious organizer and a suffragette. In 1918, she cofounded and was inaugural
president of the CME Church Women's Missionary Council. Simultaneously,
Coleman advocated for women to vote. In 1925, as she extended her council
presidency (which did not end until 1939), fellow Meharry graduate Phillips
served as a CME bishop. The same year, 1925, the CME Church published
the third edition of his definitive *History of the Colored Methodist Episcopal
Church in America*.[23]

As Phillips's *History* circulated throughout the US during the latter half
of the 1920s, the CCOFHH continued to be a primary medical services

provider for African Americans in Memphis, Tennessee. In 1928, as the already economically receding South plummeted further toward abyss, a gradual process in the region that commenced several years before the stock market crash in 1929 signaled the traditional beginning of the Great Depression, churchgoers raised $30,000 to refurbish equipment and to build an annex at the CCOFHH. W.S. Martin, a Meharry alumnus and licensed physician, CME Church stalwart, and baseball executive, cofounded the CCOFHH and served as its chief officer. His brother and fellow funds raiser, J.C. Martin, a CME bishop with a doctorate of divinity, was pastor of Collins Chapel from 1901 to 1905.[24]

The money the Martin brothers and their associates collected in 1928 enabled them to offer sixty beds at the CCOFHH (the original number of beds in 1905 was fewer than twenty). The expanded accommodations were needed. African Americans comprised about 28 percent of the local population, a number that would swell to approximately 40 percent by 1940; but, as the National Association for the Advancement for Colored People would complain in 1952, African Americans had few healthcare facilities to treat their ailments. Furthermore, not one facility was public before 1956 even though African American tax dollars generated much revenue for the Bluff City.[25]

In 1954, as Memphis officials worked to finalize plans for the construction of a publicly operated nonwhite medical facility, which they ultimately named the E.H. Crump Memorial Hospital after longtime mayor Edward Hull (Boss) Jr., who passed away in 1954,[26] leaders of the Collins Chapel CME Church authorized the Old Folks' Home and Hospital to be rebuilt, relocated, and placed completely under the auspices of their newly styled denomination, the Christian Methodist Episcopal Church.[27] As the Jackson, Tennessee, *Sun* newspaper explained, numerous ministers and laypeople in the CME Church believed the term *colored* in the denominational name "is segregative and discriminative and causes some embarrassment on the West and East Coasts as well as in the north where the church is fast expanding."[28] In many regions, to include the South, numerous African American institutional leaders were thinking about similar name changes, and their desire to act on their thoughts sped when the US Supreme Court handed down its first of two *Brown* decisions in 1954 abolishing ethnically/racially segregated public educational facilities.[29]

In 1955 the Ford Foundation, a philanthropic organization headquartered in New York City, New York, made a half billion dollars available to colleges, universities, and medical facilities across the US.[30] As part of that initiative, the foundation offered grants totaling $958,000 to seventeen hospitals in eastern Tennessee.[31] The CCCH (formerly the CCOFHH) requested and received $25,700.[32] The CME Church and other supportive institutions, together with individual citizens, exceeded that amount in coming years. Nevertheless, the presence of the Crump Memorial Hospital and other larger facilities brought about the demise of the CCCH as the main healthcare provider for African Americans.

As a small faith-based server, the CCCH struggled to maintain its operational capacity once larger health management organizations and integrated healthcare systems emerged during the final quarter of the twentieth century. Owing to those occurrences, the CCCH faced dormancy when crack cocaine, human immunodeficiency virus (HIV), acquired immunodeficiency syndrome (AIDS), and other major crises arose in the 1980s. For decades, as the CCCH essentially deteriorated from lack of use, certain leaders of the CME Church wondered how to use the space without adequate denominational funds to sustain operations. As it turned out, the same COVID-19 pandemic that caused millions of deaths worldwide enable the CCCH to experience a rebirth.

## CME Church Responses to the COVID-19 Pandemic: Memphis Examples

Not unlike countless religious families across the globe, the CME Church's 800,000 members in the US, the Caribbean, and Africa were ill-prepared for the devastating impact of COVID-19 when the World Health Organization released a statement in January 2020 regarding Chinese officials having made a "preliminary determination of a novel (or new) coronavirus."[33] The subsequent pandemic caused CME Church leaders to close sanctuaries, cancel meetings, and revamp care plans for grieving or anxious congregants.[34] The precautions were sensible. Within a single month, from March to April 2020, government officials in the US attributed 56,246 deaths to COVID.[35] African Americans were especially vulnerable to COVID because of persistent racial/ethnic disparities in preventative healthcare, infection risks owing to employment types (e.g., domestic services), access to testing, and adequate insurance. In response to those and to other problems whose severity COVID increased, the CME Church pursued three overlapping approaches to dealing with the pandemic: pastoral-missional, ecumenical-collaborative, advocacy-action.[36]

Once state and municipal governments began encouraging and then ordering religious officials to shut church doors, CME Church officials scrambled to find alternative ways for parishioners to gather collectively. Lawrence L. Reddick III, senior bishop of the CME Church, and the College of Bishops, the executive branch of the denomination government, utilized online technologies to provide pastoral encouragement and counsel. Reddick and his fellow bishops also organized a series of training webinars to assist congregations in launching online worship services, teaching sessions, and church meetings. In addition to those bishops, Carmichael Crutchfield, a minister and academician in Memphis, Tennessee, connectional leader for Christian education, developed a weekly online Sunday morning seminary lesson, a seasonal vacation bible school, and a Zoom graduation service for students in the class of 2020.[37]

Even though many denominationalists navigated cyberspace terrain for the first time during the winter to spring in 2020, some realized within a short period that technology could expand their vision of church and help them reach new constituencies. For example, Twana A. Harris, senior pastor of the Carter Metropolitan CME Church in Detroit, Michigan, began livestreaming Sunday services so clergy and laity from other churches and denominations could participate.[38] Such decisions were more prudent than certain suggestions US President Donald J. Trump Sr. made during the spring months. In May, while giving a press briefing on COVID-19 in the US, he spoke prematurely about the need to lift local and statewide stay at home orders for religious organizations.[39] Deeming churches, mosques, synagogues, and other houses of worship as providers of "essential services,"[40] Trump said those places should reopen immediately despite the COVID death toll in the country nearing 100,000, roughly 40,000 above a prediction he made in April.[41] While the toll decreased in May,[42] the CME Church remained steadfast in its support for an April statement the Conference of National Black Churches and various civil rights leaders issued encouraging people to stay at home: "We regard this pandemic as grave threat to the health and life of our people, and as a threat to the integrity and vitality of the communities we are privileged to serve."[43]

The CME Church in Memphis, Tennessee, employed the Wesleyan concept of holistic health to serve local communities, especially vulnerable members, as COVID-19 swept across the Bluff City. Municipal officials reported 1,918 confirmed cases and thirty deaths in April alone.[44] Extending decades of godly service, parishioners at the Collins Chapel CME Church worked with those officials as well as with county and federal employees, local nonprofits, various businesspeople, and numerous other benefactors to design one of the most novel service projects in Memphis. Aware of persistent racial/ethnic and financial disparities in the city, Collins Chapel and Room In The Inn Homeless Ministry entered into a contractual agreement to construct a twenty-one-bed recuperative care center and "safe haven" for individuals who did not have permanent housing after they received treatment at a medical facility.[45]

Henry Williamson Sr., resident bishop at the CME Church's international headquarters in Memphis and chair of the CCCH Committee, was at the forefront of the effort to build the post-discharge recovery space. Under his leadership, patrons raised $5 in 2020 and 2021 to restore and outfit the historic facility. He and others involved in the fundraising campaign engaged in multilevel conversations about the possibility of the CCCH resuming its place as a vital partner in the healthcare community of Memphis. Speaking in 2021 about the fourteen rooms the CCCH had especially for multiple family members, the Rev. Lisa Anderson, executive director of the Room In The Inn, said the time people spent at CCCH would be a period of "stability where families can have breathing space to take advantage of the support as they move from homelessness to housing."[46]

## Conclusion

The development of the CCCH from an old folks' home and hospital in 1905 to a recuperative care center in 2021 is a fine representation of the Colored (later Christian) Methodist Episcopal Church as a living embodiment of Wesleyan and black Christian visions for holistic and just healthcare. As the CME Church continues to unify with global communities to deal effectively with the COVID-19 pandemic, the denomination should be equally as vigilante about developing strategies to grapple with continual dilemmas in healthcare in local places such as Memphis, Tennessee. The reported words of the Rev. Martin Luther King Jr., who took his last breath while lying in a Bluff City hospital bed in 1968, still resound: "Of all the forms of inequality, injustice in health is the most shocking and inhuman."[47]

## Notes

1 Several late 1870s resources employed the term *college* when referring to the Meharry Medical Department. Students attended classes in buildings of the Central Tennessee College, but Meharry was not a college per se. About those matters and others referenced in the main text, see *Acts of the State of Tennessee Passed by the Fifty-Fifth General Assembly 1907* (Nashville, TN: McQuiddy Printing Company, 1907), 2261 (identifying December 6, 1906, as the date of state incorporation for the Collins Chapel Old Folks' Home and Hospital); G.P. Hamilton, *The Bright Side of Memphis ...* (Memphis: G. P. Hamilton, 1908), 21, 210; Othal H. Lakey, *The History of the CME Church*, rev. ed. (Memphis TN: CME Publishing House, 1996), 375, 402; "Meharry Medical College," (Nashville, TN) *Daily American*, May 15, 1879, 4; *Memphis' African-American Historical Landmark Is Undergoing a Complete Renovation* (Memphis, TN: First Episcopal District, n.d.); Charles Victor Roman, *Meharry Medical College: A History* (Nashville, TN: Sunday School Publishing Board of the National Baptist Convention, 1934), esp. 29, 216; and Raymond R. Sommerville, Jr., *An Ex-Colored Church: Social Activism in the CME Church, 1870–1970* (Macon, GA: Mercer University Press, 2004), 95.

2 Jeffrey W. Barbeau, *The Spirit of Methodism: From the Wesleys to a Global Communion* (Downers Grove, IL: InterVarsity Press, 2019), 7, 26.

3 Barbeau, *Spirit of Methodism*, 3–36.

4 *John and Charles Wesley: Selected Prayers, Hymns, Journal Notes, Sermons, Letters and Treatises*, ed. Frank Whaling (Mahwah, NJ: Paulist Press, 1981), 34.

5 Barbeau, *Spirit of Methodism*, esp. 36–38, 60–65.

6 See James G. Donat and Randy L. Maddox, "Introduction to John Wesley's Practice and Publications Offering Medical and Health Advice," in John Wesley, *The Works of John Wesley*, vol. 32: *Medical and Health Writings*, James G. Donat and Randy L. Maddox, eds., 10–26 (Nashville, TN: Abingdon Press, 2018).

7 John Wesley, *A Collection of Receits for the Poor* (Newcastle upon Tyne: John Gooding, 1745).

8 John Wesley, *Primitive Physic* (London: James Nichols, 1747).

9 Publishers released multiple posthumous editions of *Primitive Physic*.

10 Wesley, *Primitive Physic*, iv–x.

11 Donat and Maddox, "Introduction."

12 According to Charles Roman, the Meharry Medical Department of Central Tennessee College became the Meharry College of Walden University in 1900, and Tennessee state lawmakers granted a new charter for an autonomous Meharry Medical College in 1915. Roman, *Meharry Medical College*, 29.

13 See Elizabeth Gritter, "To Regain the Lost Rights of a Growing Race': Black Political Mobilization, 1865–1916," chap. 1 in *River of Hope: Black Politics and the Memphis Freedom Movement, 1865–1954* (Lexington, KY: University Press of Kentucky, 2014), 13–50; Steven V. Ash, *A Massacre in Memphis: The Race Riot that Shook the Nation One Year after the Civil War* (New York, NY: Hill and Wang, 2013); G. Wayne Dowdy, *A Brief History of Memphis* (Charleston, SC: History Press, 2011). According to Memphis lore, the multiple bluffs along the Mississippi River adjacent to the city accounts for the nickname Bluff City. Phillip Jackson "Here Is Why Memphis is Called the Bluff City," *Memphis Commercial Appeal*, September 23, 2019, https://www.commercialappeal.com/story/news/2019/09/23/why-memphis-called-bluff-city-law-premiere/2425269001/.

14 See, for example, Thomas L Connelly, *Civil War Tennessee: Battles and Leaders* (1979; repr., Knoxville, TN: University of Tennessee Press, 2004).

15 Physicians and historians W. Michael Byrd and Linda A. Clayton have documented the health matters relating to Black people in the present-day US from the Middle Passage to emancipation, describing the conglomeration of healthcare problems attributed to enslavement as a "slave healthcare deficit." Byrd and Clayton, *An American Health Dilemma: A Medical History of African Americans and the Problem of Race*, vol. 1: *Beginnings to 1900* (New York, NY: Routledge, 2000), 184 (the first of many times Byrd and Clayton reference the slave health deficit). During the Middle Passage, Byrd and Clayton note, horrible sanitation and poor nutrition on slave ships led to outbreaks of diseases such as dysentery, malaria, smallpox, measles, and yellow fever in addition to wounds and to deaths from accidents, fights, and floggings (194–97). Bad conditions continued after the Thirteenth Amendment to the US Constitution abolished legal racial/ethnic slavery, Byrd and Clayton recount (347–416).

16 Sommerville, *Ex-Colored Church*, 1.

17 Gerald M. Capers Jr., "Yellow Fever in Memphis in the 1870's," *Mississippi Valley Historical Review* 24 (March 1938): 484, 486, 496.

18 Capers, "Yellow Fever in Memphis," 497.

19 "To the Dregs," *Daily Memphis Avalanche*, August 30, 1878, 1.

20 Multiple sources indicate the Rev. J.H. Ridley sat on an 1882 committee whose members designed a plan to raise funds to establish Lane College in Jackson, Tennessee. Ridley, J.K. Daniels, the Rev. C.H. Lee, Sandy Rivers, and Berry Smith made up the committee, but they formed it in 1878 at the behest of Daniels, a onetime pastor of the Collins Chapel in Memphis. Not much money was in the coffer when Ridley passed away in 1879; nonetheless, the CMEC expended $240 in 1879 to purchase the four acres of land in Jackson where the denomination placed the eventual college, which opened in 1882 as a high school. See, among other accurate sources, "Died at His Post: The Late Rev. J. H. Ridley," *Daily Memphis Avalanche*, August 12, 1879, 1; Hamilton, *Bright Side of Memphis*, 285; "History of Lane College," in *Afro American-Encyclopedia: Or, the Thoughts, Doings, and Saying of the Race* ... , comp. James T. Haley (Nashville, TN: Haley and Florida, 1895), 328–32; and "Memorial Services," *Daily Memphis Avalanche*, December 16, 1879, 4 (announcing CMEC bishop Isaac Lane [namesake of the future college] would direct the December 2, 1879, memorial service of Ridley).

21  "Died at His Post."
22  David McBride, *Caring for Equality: A History of African American Health and Healthcare* (Lanham, MD: Rowman and Littlefield, 2018), 29.
23  C.H. Phillips, *The History of the Colored Methodist Episcopal Church in America: Comprising Its Organization, Subsequent Development and Present Status*, book 1, 3rd ed. (Jackson, TN: Publishing House C.M.E. Church, 1925); Phillips, *History of the Colored Methodist Episcopal Church in America: Comprising Its Organization, Subsequent Development and Present Status*, book 2, 1st ed. (Jackson, TN: Publishing House C.M.E. Church, 1925). See also Ellen Carol DuBois, *Suffrage: Women's Long Battle for the Vote* (New York: Simon and Schuster, 2020), 270; and Lakey, *History of the CME Church*, 326–32, 401, 403, 531.
24  The Collins Chapel Old Folks' Home and Hospital served as a training center for African American nurses by September 1913. During that month the Nashville, Tennessee, *Globe* newspaper featured an image of the facility, declaring: "Its location overlooks the city from a striking eminence, and every convenience is at hand. [Moreover, the] hospital is equipped with every latest appliance invented to serve surgical skill." "Collins Chapel Home and Hospital," *Nashville (TN) Globe*, September 19, 1913, 7. For other matters discussed in the main text, see Letoshia Foster, "Beyond What We Know: Health and Disease among Blacks, with an Emphasis on Women in Memphis, from Slavery to Early Twentieth Century," PhD diss., University of Memphis, 2020,18, 214, 235, 272–76, 278, 281, 286, 289–90; Hamilton, *Bright Side of Memphis*, 248–51; Rebecca Harrison, Aurelia Harden, and Vera Clark, *The Making of a Church: A Historical Landmark* (Memphis, TN: [n.p.], 1993), 2, 13–14; Neil Lanctot, *Negro League Baseball: The Rise and Ruin of a Black Institution* (Philadelphia, PN: University of Pennsylvania Press, 2004), 124–25; Gloria Brown Melton, "Blacks in Memphis, Tennessee, 1920–1955: A Historical Study," PhD diss., Washington State University, 1982, 272–77.
25  G. P. Hamilton, *Beacon Lights of the Race* (Memphis, TN: E.H. Clarke and Brother, 1911), 337–41. See Campbell Gibson and Kay Jung, "Tennessee—Race and Hispanic Origin for Selected Large Cities and Other Places: Earliest Census to 1990" (table 43), in "Historical Census Statistics on Population Totals by Race, 1790 to 1990, and by Hispanic Origin, 1970 to 1990, for Large Cities and Other Urban Places in the United States" (working paper no. 76, US Census Bureau, Washington, DC, February 2005), n.p.; Laurie B. Green, *Battling the Plantation Mentality: Memphis and the Black Freedom Struggle* (Chapel Hill, NC: University of North Carolina Press, 2007), 189–90; Gritter, *River of Hope*, 190; and United States Department of Commerce Bureau of the Census, *Sixteenth Census of the United States: 1940—Population*, vol. 1: *Number of Inhabitants* (Washington: Government Printing Office, 1942), 32, 36, 59, 63, 1013–14, 1022, 1024–28.
26  On the development of Crump Memorial Hospital, which received scant attention from Memphis newspapers when the facility opened in 1956, see Gritter, *River of Hope*, 190; and Melton, "Blacks in Memphis," 308–12.
27  See Lakey, *History of the CME Church*, 375, 402; *Memphis' African-American Historical Landmark Is Undergoing a Complete Renovation*; and Sommerville, *Ex-Colored Church*; 95;
28  U. Z. McKinnon, "CME General Conference to Study Funds, Publishing House Removal from Jackson," *Jackson (TN) Sun*, May 2, 1954, 2 (in section 2 of the paper).
29  Oliver Brown, et al. v. Board of Education of Topeka, et al., 347 U.S. 483 (1954).
30  Geoffrey Gould, "Half Billion Total Given to Nation's Schools, Hospitals," *Knoxville (TN) Journal*, December 13, 1955, 1, 6.
31  "ET Hospitals Eligible for Nearly $1 Million," *Knoxville (TN) Journal*, December 13, 1955, 1, 6.

32  "ET Hospitals Eligible for Nearly $1 Million," 6; *The Ford Foundation Annual Report 1956* (New York: Ford Foundation, 1956), 187; "State Institutions Listed for Foundation's Awards," *Nashville Tennessean*, December 13, 1955, 2.

33  World Health Organization, "WHO Statement Regarding Cluster of Pneumonia Cases in Wuhan, China," January 9, 2020, https://www.who.int/china/news/detail/09-01-2020-who-statement-regarding-cluster-of-pneumonia-cases-in-wuhan-china.

34  "Statement by the Conference of National Black Churches and Civil Rights Leaders Encourage Communities to Stay at Home," *Christian Methodist Episcopal Church*, April 25, 2020, https://thecmechurch.org/2020/04/statement-by-conference-of-national-black-churches-civil-rights-leaders-encourage-communities-to-stay-at-home/ (hereafter cited as "Stay at Home Statement").

35  "Excess Deaths from COVID-19 and Other Causes, March–April 2020," *JAMA: Journal of the American Medical Association* 324 (August 4, 2020): 510.

36  "Stay at Home Statement."

37  "Rev. Dr. Carmichael Crutchfield," *Memphis Theological Seminary*, n.d., https://memphisseminary.edu/dr-carmichael-d-crutchfield/.

38  The Carter Metropolitan CME Church commenced the livestreams in spring 2020.

39  "White House Briefing," May 22, 2020, *C-Span*, https://www.c-span.org/video/?472429-1/president-trump-calls-reopening-houses-worship.

40  "White House Briefing."

41  "President Trump with Coronavirus Task Force Briefing," *C-Span*, April 19, 2020, https://www.c-span.org/video/?471340-1/president-trump-coronavirus-task-force-briefing; "White House Briefing."

42  Daniel M. Weinberger et al., "Estimation of Excess Deaths Associated with the COVID-19 Pandemic in the United States, March to May 2020," *JAMA: Journal of the American Medical Association* 180 (October 2020): 1340–42.

43  "Stay at Home Statement."

44  "COVID-19 Update from Mayor Strickland (5-12)," *City of Memphis*, May 12, 2020, https://covid19.memphistn.gov/covid-19-update-from-mayor-strickland-5-12/.

45  Kirstin Garriss, "Historic Collins Chapel Reopens as Safe Haven for Homeless after Renovations," *Fox13Memphis.com*, April 19, 2021, https://www.fox13memphis.com/news/local/historic-collins-chapel-reopens-safe-haven-homeless-after-renovations/PWJOFQSIJVDTRJIIRPDVL4S2LY/. See also Max Garland, "Former Memphis Hospital Building to Provide Recovery Space for People without Homes," *Commercial Appeal*, November 24, 2020, https://www.commercialappeal.com/story/news/2020/11/24/memphis-hospital-recovery-space-homeless-people-room-in-the-inn-collins-chapel/6393628002/.

46  Garriss, "Historic Collins Chapel Reopens." See also Christian Methodist Episcopal Church, "Historical African American Collins Chapel Connectional Hospital Reopens to Serve the Homeless," April 19, 2021, https://thecmechurch.org/2021/04/collins-chapel-reopens-to-serve-homeless/; and *Memphis' African-American Historical Landmark is Undergoing a Complete Renovation*.

47  Associated Press, "King Says AMA Discriminates," *Ironwood (MI) Daly Globe*, March 26, 1966, 2 (one of several newspapers that reported about the speech, which the Rev. Martin Luther King Jr. made during the second national convention of the Medical Committee for Human Rights in Chicago, Illinois, on March 25). A number of contemporary sources, including David M. Craig, contain a slightly different version of the King statement: "Of all forms of inequality, injustice in health care is the most shocking and inhumane." Craig, *Health Care as Social Good: Religious Values and American Democracy* (Washington, DC: Georgetown University Press, 2014), 59.

# 12 Black United Methodist Church Responses to COVID-19

*Cynthia M. Moore-Koikoi*

## Introduction

The novel coronavirus, or COVID-19, has brought to mainstream American consciousness some understanding of a metaphor that constitutes a lived experience among countless black people in the United States: when the country gets a cold, its black population gets pneumonia. Black Americans have experienced a disproportionate number of deaths, hospitalizations, and economic repercussions owing to COVID. Pew Research Center states: "When it comes to public health, black Americans appear to account for a larger share of COVID-19 hospitalizations nationally than their share of the population."[1] According to July 2021 data from the Centers for Disease Control and Prevention, as of June, black Americans were being hospitalized at 2.9 times the rate of non-Hispanic white people and were dying at two times the rate.[2] In many cases, the ability to pay for adequate healthcare is a significant factor in whether one lives or dies. A Pew Research Center report from earlier that year indicated 34 percent of adult black Americans had finances in good or in excellent shape compared with 53 percent of all adults.[3]

As devastatingly unique as COVID-19 has been, it simply is the latest countrywide crisis to impact black Americans differentially. Earlier recent crises include human immunodeficiency viruses, acquired immunodeficiency syndrome, housing devastations, and the economic recession of December 2007 to June 2009. Historically, black members and organizations of the United Methodist Church (UMC) and its predecessor denominations have tried to ameliorate differential impacts by working independently or by partnering with various community and governmental organizations to provide educational, healthcare, and related social services.

A primary reason black segments of the UMC traditionally have tried to calm societal unrest, including racial injustice, is because helping their fellow humans is in the proverbial deoxyribonucleic acid (DNA) of Methodism. Although black Methodist churches struggled initially to meet long-standing community needs that COVID-19 exacerbated, I submit the "social holiness" gene of black United Methodists is dominant; therefore,

DOI: 10.4324/9781003214281-15

their strength, resiliency, creativity, and flexibility will empower them to help mitigate the impact of racially differential elements of COVID.[4]

## Historical Crisis Mitigation by Black Methodists

During the nineteenth century, white siblings and Methodist cofounders Charles and John Wesley asserted that solitary religion was not found in the gospels. They wrote, "The Gospel of Christ knows no Religion but Social; no Holiness, but Social Holiness. Faith working by Love, is the Length, and Breadth, and Depth, and Height of Christian Perfection."[5] According to contemporary United Methodist theology, it is essential for disciples of Jesus the Christ to care for the physical needs of all creations.[6] This act, I contend, is social holiness.

The fact that Methodist preachers established organizations such as Goodwill Industries International and the Salvation Army is evidence of the social holiness DNA that has compelled Methodists to mediate the impact of myriad crises. Concordantly, numerous black Methodists have taken ownership for addressing the unique needs of black communities whose members seek to fight social and economic injustice. The novel coronavirus is a recent example of crisis; however, black Methodists such as Richard Allen and Absalom Jones of Philadelphia, Pennsylvania, experienced crises during the late eighteenth century and into the early nineteenth century. Before Allen and Jones separated from the Methodist Episcopal Church (a predecessor denomination of the UMC) because of the racism they experienced in the Methodist Episcopal Church, they worked as lay preachers within The Church structure to establish the Free African Society (FAS) in 1787. According to the Rev. Julius E. Del Pino, the society was "the first attempt to coordinate human and political efforts for improving living conditions for blacks" in the present-day US.[7]

The FAS work Allen and Jones performed caught the attention of their fellow Philadelphian, Benjamin Rush, a prominent white physician who signed the American Declaration of Independence in 1776. When yellow fever swept Philadelphia in 1793, Rush called on Allen and Jones to help. Even though many citizens viewed Rush as racially enlightened or progressive, he still fell prey to the sin of *othering* people of color. Rush believed erroneously that people of African descent were different constitutionally than persons of European descent and thereby were immune to yellow fever. Consequently, he asked Allen and Jones to use the networks they established through the FAS to organize black Philadelphians to care for sick white Philadelphians. Rush thought black people could secure white allies by providing such aid. In turn, whites would help blacks fight for freedom and justice.[8]

Allen and Jones contended it was their "duty to do all the good that we could to our suffering fellow mortals."[9] They also considered engaging with the white community in ways that drew attention to black suffering a step toward ending racism. Hence, Allen and Jones helped black Philadelphians become nurses, pastoral caregivers, gravediggers, and other essential workers.[10] Such endeavors equate to contemporary efforts by various good-hearted black and brown people during the COVID-19 pandemic who have provided essential services to all ethnic groups.

In an unfortunate prelude to the present, black Philadelphians who toiled hard to save the lives of their contemporaries in 1793 faced backlash from certain white people. Among other things, whites accused them of "causing needless death and even stealing from patients."[11] Fake news about FAS workers became so prevalent that Allen and Jones wrote *A Narrative of the Proceedings of the Black People, During the Late Awful Calamity in Philadelphia, in the Year 1793: And Refutation of Some Censures, Thrown Upon Them in Some Publications* to correct the record.[12] Allen and Jones gave a detailed accounting of the funds that relatives of survivors gave for burial costs. "It is rather to be admired," Allen and Jones declared, "that so few instances of pilfering and robbery happened, considering the great opportunities there were for such things: we do not know of more than five black people, suspected of anything clandestine, out of a great number employed."[13]

The abovementioned experiences of Allen and Jones are microcosmic. Generations of future black Methodists have attempted to mitigate the impact of various crises only to have white people of all denominations question their intensions and motives. But, because the desire to bring about social holiness is inherent to many black Methodists, unwarranted backlashes have not deterred them. Consider, for example, post-Civil War members of the Sharp Street Memorial UMC in Baltimore, Maryland. From 1867 to 1872, during the Reconstruction period, The Church housed the Centenary Biblical Institute (later Morgan State University) to educate African Americans. Of similar note, decades later Methodist activist and educator Mary McLeod Bethune of Mayesville, South Carolina withstood attacks on her womanhood as well as her ethnicity and religiosity when she in 1904 founded the Daytona Literary and Industrial Training School for Negro Girls (which ultimately became Bethune-Cookman University) in Daytona Beach, Florida. In 1911 or 1912, after a student became sick and white employees of a local hospital turned her away, Bethune raised enough money to open an infirmary for the black community.[14]

The environments in which the abovementioned Methodists lived were tumultuous. The present COVID-19 environment is tumultuous as well. The pandemic has curtailed many black Methodist churches' traditional sources of empowerment by, among other acts, interrupting networking made possible through physical fellowship. Local and state stay-at-home orders have prevented churches from collecting tithes, offerings, and other monetary gifts during in-person worship services. Nevertheless, black Methodists have made great efforts to respond to challenges presented by COVID.

## Dialectical Model of COVID-19 Response

In a 1990 book titled *The Black Church in the African American Experience*, acclaimed scholars C. Eric Lincoln and Lawrence H. Mamiya helped popularize a dialectical model of the Black Church.[15] Although black congregations in predominantly white denominations were not central to the analysis, the Lincoln and Mamiya dialectical model continues to provide insight regarding why black United Methodists are meeting various needs of the black community during the coronavirus pandemic. Lincoln and Mamiya proposed several dialectical polarities of Black Church responses to struggle and change ranging along continuums of priestly to prophetic; other worldly to this worldly; particularism to universalism; privatistic to communal; bureaucratic to charismatic; and accommodationist to resistant. Lincoln and Mamiya explained, "The complexities of black churches as social institutions require a more dynamic and interactional theoretical perspective because they have played more complex roles and assumed more comprehensive burdens in their communities than is true of most white and ethnic churches."[16]

Many elements of the polarities about which Lincoln and Mamiya wrote remain in black UMCs and help explain how some churches have overcome COVID-19-related limitations to meet black community needs. For example, many black denominationalists have had to move between resistance and accommodation to survive in the UMC, which is predominately white. For example, as the COVID pandemic swept across the country, many white church leaders under my episcopal supervision had protracted conversations about resisting government restrictions concerning the size of social gatherings. In contrast, many Black Church leaders conversed briefly about restrictions and proceeded to create ways to accommodate the government. Their fast decisions allowed them to minister without breaking the law.

In addition to the acts above, some Black Church leaders employed the prophetic function of calling out the racial injustice of the pandemic when state governors, local health departments, or UMC bishops limited the priestly functions of in-person worship, fellowship, and Bible study during the COVID pandemic. In Dallas, Texas, a set of leading black United Methodists emphasized the deathly effects of COVID, especially on African Americans, but also worked collaboratively with city heads, the media, and other citizens to launch #WENEED2SURVIVE.[17] Organizers focused on distinctive vulnerabilities within communities of color, including the differential impact of the virus on the underinsured and those with preexisting conditions, and the roles that churches played in disseminating information in black communities. The campaign, begun in March 2020, was an important joint venture intended to reduce the differential impact of COVID in a city where black people comprised 23.6 percent of population but 35 percent of reported COVID cases as of March.[18]

Black United Methodists in Memphis, Tennessee, were as active as those in Dallas as COVID expanded across the South and the US in early 2020.

In May black denominational leaders in Memphis sponsored a videoconference titled "Ask the Docs: Preemptive Planning for Public Worship" designed to help pastors and laypeople plan for their returns to public worship.[19] Addressing a conference theme, health disparities, Methodist University Hospital Chief Medical Officer Robin J. Womeodu highlighted disproportionate rates of diabetes, hypertension, and end stage renal disease among Africans Americans.[20] Each one of the disorders, she emphasized, is an underlying condition that complicates COVID symptoms.[21] Womeodu and other presenters encouraged viewers, especially church leaders, to consider such risk factors when making decisions about in-person worship.

## Conclusion

Black UMCs have identified and, moreover, addressed the intersectionality of social, political, educational, and cultural impacts of COVID. In addition to the activities I discuss above, the UMC's Discipleship Ministries unit collaborated with a second unit, called Strengthening the Black Church for the Twenty-First Century, to organize a virtual summit in April 2020 for denominational leaders to provide information about COVID. Among other subjects, the summit addressed pandemic challenges, racial disparities, criminal justice issues, prison ministries, and reentry organizations.[22]

Black members of the UMC have helped make the denomination's response to COVID nimbler than it otherwise would have been. Leaders of the Multi-Ethnic Center for Ministry of the Northeastern Jurisdiction of the UMC dispensed with much of the usual bureaucracy involved in grant making within the larger denominational system and sent unsolicited funds to annual conferences. The leader also encouraged other members to donate funds to black and to brown churches whose financial conditions the pandemic affected adversely. Many other black United Methodists acted on social holiness convictions and formulated strategic responses to COVID. I and other black UMC members will do well to use the pandemic as an evolutionary inflection point to mark a change in how we use our particular giftedness to harness the resources of the broader denomination to address urgent needs within the black community during this season of crisis.

## Notes

1  Mark Hugo Lopez, Lee Rainie, and Abby Budiman, "Financial and Health Impacts of COVID-19 Vary Widely by Race and Ethnicity," *Pew Research Center*, May 5, 2020, https://www.pewresearch.org/fact-tank/2020/05/05/financial-and-health-impacts-of-covid-19-vary-widely-by-race-and-ethnicity//
2  Centers for Disease Control and Prevention, "Risk for COVID-19 Infection, Hospitalization, and Death by Race/Ethnicity," July 16, 2021, https://www.cdc.gov/coronavirus/2019-ncov/covid-data/investigations-discovery/hospitalization-death-by-race-ethnicity.html.

3 Khadijah Edwards and Mark Hugo Lopez "Black Americans Say Coronavirus has Hit Hard Financially, but Impact Varies by Education Level, Age," *Pew Research Center*, May 12, 2021, https://www.pewresearch.org/fact-tank/2021/05/12/black-americans-say-coronavirus-has-hit-hard-financially-but-impact-varies-by-education-level-age/.

4 United Methodist Communications, "United Methodist Beliefs: Social Holiness," September 7, 2017, https://www.umc.org/en/content/united-methodist-beliefs-social-holiness.

5 John Wesley and Charles Wesley, *Hymns and Sacred Poems*, 5th ed. (London: John and Charles Wesley, 1756), v.

6 "United Methodist Beliefs: Social Holiness."

7 Julius E. Del Pino, "Blacks in the United Methodist Church from Its Beginnings to 1968," *Methodist History* 19 (October 1980): 5.

8 Anna Louise Bates, "'Give Glory to God before He Cause Darkness': Methodists and Yellow Fever in Philadelphia, 1793–1798," *Methodist History* 58 (April 2020): 133–51.

9 A. Jones and R. Allen., *A Narrative of the Proceedings of the Black People, During the Late Awful Calamity in Philadelphia, in the Year 1793: And Refutation of Some Censures, Thrown Upon Them in Some Publications* (Philadelphia, PN: William W. Woodward, 1794), 3 (hereafter cited as Jones and Allen, *Narrative*).

10 Jones and Allen, *Narrative*.

11 Heather Hahn "Methodists Led Response in Earlier Epidemic," *United Methodist News*, May 12, 2020, https://www.umnews.org/en/news/methodists-led-response-in-earlier-epidemic.

12 Jones and Allen, *Narrative*.

13 Jones and Allen, *Narrative*, 14.

14 Audrey Thomas McCluskey and Elaine M. Smith, eds., *Mary McLeod Bethune: Building a Better World—Essays and Selected Documents* (Bloomington: Indiana University Press, 1999), 289n2 (recounting that some resources suggest that Mary McLeod Bethune established an infirmary in 1911); "A Normal School's Notable Progress," *Pittsburgh (PA) Courier*, July 26, 1912, 1.

15 C. Eric Lincoln and Lawrence H. Mamiya, *The Black Church in the African American Experience* (Durham: Duke University Press, 1990).

16 Lincoln and Mamiya, *Black Church*, 18.

17 A public announcement about #WENEED2SURVIVE dated March 27, 2020, is located at https://www.umcjustice.org/documents/141.

18 Jennifer Prohov and Tashara Parker, "Black COVID-19 Patients in Dallas County, Nationwide are Hospitalized at Higher Rates, Data Shows," *WFAA–TV*, April 9, 2020, https://www.wfaa.com/article/news/health/coronavirus/black-covid-19-patients-dallas-county-nationwide-higher-rates-hospitalized/287-8eacaf04-e7dd-48d5-a204-f053215b3098; United States Census Bureau, "Quick Facts: Dallas County, Texas," n.d., https://www.census.gov/quickfacts/dallascountytexas.

19 Memphis Conference Black Methodists for Church Renewal, "Ask the Docs: Preemptive Planning for Public Worship," *Vimeo*, May 19, 2020, https://vimeo.com/420431114.

20 Memphis Conference Black Methodists for Church Renewal, "Ask the Docs."

21 Memphis Conference Black Methodists for Church Renewal, "Ask the Docs:

22 United Methodist Church Discipline Ministries, "COVID-19 and the Black Church Online Summit," April 16, 2020, https://www.umcdiscipleship.org/articles/covid-19-and-the-black-church-online-summit.

# 13 The Redeemed Christian Church of God's Responses to Contemporary Health Urgencies in Nigeria

*Babatunde Adedibu and Adeleke Awojobi Olujobi*

## Introduction

Sub-Saharan Africa has witnessed significant changes in its religious space since the 1970s, particularly in Nigeria. There has been a rising tide of religious fanaticism and terrorism as well as an expansion of the vital role that religion performs as a succor and a social resource among adherents. The growing importance of neo-Pentecostal churches in addressing socioeconomic and health inadequacies has contributed to a characterization of those churches as progressive social forces "inspired by the Holy Spirit and the life of Jesus, [seeking] to address holistically the spiritual, physical, and social needs of people in their community."[1] Such beliefs reposition the churches as "development actors across borders."[2]

## Redeemed Christian Church of God Responses to Health Challenges

This essay focuses on the Redeemed Christian Church of God (RCCG), one of several Nigerian Pentecostal denominations that has achieved influence through a transnational network of churches during the previous five decades. Scholars have written extensively about the history,[3] missiology,[4] developmental strategies,[5] Weberian economic dynamics,[6] innovations, and creative leaders of the RCCG.[7] Its founder and general overseer, the Rev. Josiah Olufemi Akindayomi, established the wholly indigenous denomination in Lagos, the capital of Nigeria, in 1952. The RCCG had thirty-nine branches in southwestern Nigeria when Akindayomi died on November 30, 1979. The next general overseer, the Rev. Enoch A. Adeboye, began his tenure on January 20, 1980. He was thirty-nine. Under his leadership, the RCCG has expanded from a national church to a transnational church, with networks in 197 countries and territories worldwide.[8]

The RCCG began responding to diverse health challenges in its early years of operation, mostly through acts of kindness by members toward one another but without "centrally organised interventions from the church to its immediate environment," as The Church was very poor at the time.[9] By the

DOI: 10.4324/9781003214281-16

early 1990s, however, the ineffectiveness of the 1980s Structural Adjustment Program along with Nigeria's dwindling economy led churches and other faith-based organizations to commence broad-based socioeconomic palliatives to their communities.[10] Such acts era birthed holistic theology within RCCG, as the denomination began to "respond not only to the spiritual needs of people but also their physical and material needs ... through the demonstration of love which positively impacts communities and individuals."[11] Eight areas are paramount for the denomination: social, healthcare, education, media, business/economy, arts/culture/entertainment, government/politics, and sports.[12]

In relation to health, a central topic of this essay, the interventionist approach of the RCCG is redefining the role of faith-based organizations in Nigerians. In 2010, for example, the RCCG established the Healing Stripes Hospital in the Apapa region of Lagos. Organizers created specialist clinics for nephrology, cardiology, obstetrics and gynecology, pediatrics, urology, general surgery, diagnostic services, as well as for dental and eye care. From 2010 until 2021, the hospital attended to at least 13,400 patients, serving almost 5,500 without charge via a church welfare program. The hospital also provided free cancer screenings and a broad range of therapies to more than 17,500 patients and carried out approximately thirty free dialysis procedures per day.[13]

Via initiatives such as the Healing Stripes Hospital, the RCCG has harnessed and maximized the professional competencies of its members in the medical sector to ameliorate challenges in primary and secondary healthcare delivery in Nigeria. Drawing on social capital and material resources, to include a large number of medically skilled professionals and volunteers, the RCCG has been changing the face of healthcare delivery in the country. The RCCG response to human immunodeficiency virus (HIV) and to acquired immunodeficiency syndrome (AIDS) is especially noteworthy.

## HIV/AIDS

Seventy-seven million people have been infected with the HIV since 1981. Many developed AIDS, resulting in more than 35 million deaths. As of 2020, there were 37.7 million people living with HIV, and 1.5 million infections were new.[14] During the same year, about 680,000 people died from illnesses associated with AIDS.[15]

The devastation that HIV/AIDS has wrought is pronounced in Africa, due largely to poor health infrastructures, poor research facilities, and general leadership ineptitudes. In Nigeria, the RCCG and other faith-based organizations have stepped into the gap, utilizing various interventionist approaches to help treat and, moreover, to help prevent HIV/AIDS.[16] Mandating RCCG members who are engaged to be married receive HIV/AIDS tests before the solemnizing of their nuptials is one effort. The RCCG also sponsors the Redeemers *Aids* Initiative for People and Community (formerly the Redeemed Aids Programme Action Committee), which since 1997 has included "education, production of behavioural communication resources on HIV/AIDS, advocacy of moral restraint, creating and offering assistance to members of the church and the larger communities."[17] In addition to HIV/AIDS specifically, the initiative has programs devoted to tuberculosis prevention for general and at-risk population, especially orphans and vulnerable children, as well as for reproductive health and family planning, among other items. Responsiveness to such health-related phenomena has positioned the RCCG well to help Nigerian communities deal with COVID-19.

## The COVID-19 Pandemic

On December 12, 2019, the municipal health commission of Wuhan, Hubei Province, China, announced that twenty-seven persons had viral pneumonia and that seven were critically ill.[18] Unbeknownst to anyone at the time, they suffered from a novel coronavirus. On February 11, 2021, the International Committee on Taxonomy of Viruses named their condition severe acute respiratory syndrome coronavirus 2, or SARS-CoV-2 for short.[19] Exactly one month later, on March 11, the World Health Organization declared COVID a pandemic.[20]

An Italian businessman flying from Milan, Italy, to Lagos, Nigeria, on February 24, 2020, became the first known case of COVID in sub-Saharan Africa.[21] Aware of the growing COVID-related death toll in China and the Global North, as well as elsewhere in the world, the Nigerian federal government essentially placed the country on a two-week lockdown, beginning March 30.[22] Inadequate healthcare facilities and systematic poverty in Nigeria, together with outward economic migration of Nigerian medical personnel, heightened potential effects of the pandemic in the most populous country in Africa, Nigeria, which had approximately 206,140,000 people in 2020.[23]

Religion is a factor in how many Nigerians view COVID. As per a 2004 poll the research company Independent Communications and Marketing conducted for the British Broadcasting Company, more than nine out of ten Nigerians indicated they believed in God, prayed frequently, and were willing to die for their religious convictions.[24] Based on that research, which the company also conducted in nine other countries, pollsters suggested Nigeria was the most religious country in the world.[25] But Nigerian Pentecostal leaders have had diverse reactions to COVID. Conspiracy theories are commonplace. Claims of divine judgment on the West, as evidenced by high COVID-related death tolls in that hemisphere, is a frequent occurrence. Yet other leaders have proposed that God will protect believers from COVID. In a videotaped speech delivered in March 2020, RCCG General

Overseer Enoch Adeboye stated: "I want to assure you that there's no virus that is going to come near you at all because it is written that they that dwell in the secret place of the Most High shall abide under the shadow of the Almighty."[26]

Adeboye did not speak for the RCCG as a whole, which in some respects has differed from many Nigerian Pentecostal groups in relation to COVID. Among other things, the RCCG has chosen to focus on practical responses to the pandemic, such as donations of healthcare resources, including 8,000 units of hand sanitizer, 8,000 surgical facemasks, and 200,000 gloves to Mainland Hospital in Lagos.[27] In April, not long after Adeboye made the statement quoted above, he donated twenty million naira (about $51,546 in US currency) to Osun State and provided two ventilators to Ogun State.[28]

The responses of the RCCG and, ultimately, its general overseer, Adeboye, drew on an explanatory and a predictive model of health behavioral change to which the Nigerian federal government subscribed in an effort to limit the effects of COVID. The RCCG provided public health information through its media outlets (e.g., Dove Television, Live Way Radio) while emphasizing in sermons and prayers various psychological aspects of health behavioral change. Adeboye, someone whom many Nigerians respect highly, utilized his sermons to stress the urgent need for social distancing and for personal hygiene as essential expressions of health behavioral change. That message aligned with public health protocols of the federal government to minimize the spread of COVID. Adeboye and other RCCG leaders also have striven to make people aware of mental, emotional, and related tolls of COVID.[29]

On December 31, 2020, as the RCCG worked to reduce the effects of COVID, the World Health Organization approved Comirnaty COVID-19 mRNA vaccine for emergency use.[30] Approval made "the Pfizer/BioNTech vaccine the first to receive emergency validation from WHO" and, I contended, ushered in a new era of hope for humanity.[31] Nigerian healthcare providers administered the first such vaccination in Nigeria on March 15, 2021.[32] Physician Yunusa Thairu, a medical consultant associated with the United Nations Nigeria Isolation Center at Durumi in Abuja and with the University of Abuja Teaching Hospital in Gwagwalada, was one of the first persons inoculated.[33] As with other counties, the Nigerian government authorized healthcare providers to administer vaccines in phases, with Thairu and more than 1 million other health and allied workers participating in phase one.[34]

A conversation Thairu had with his mother was a representation of the concern a sizeable portion of the Nigerian population had about inoculation. "She got super worried and gave me a call," Thairu recollected in March 2020.[35] "I had to drive down to go see and assure her that I am fine, [that] there is nothing wrong with taking the vaccine. Upon seeing how healthy I was, she agreed to take the vaccine when it is available."[36]

Fears about the unknown and conspiracy theories drove hesitance or apathy about COVID-19 vaccination. Nevertheless, the Nigerian federal government pus measures in place to educate and to sensitize citizens about the safety and the efficaciousness of vaccines. The RCCG, however, did not take a public stance on vaccines. Even so, given the commitment of the RCCG to health-related matters since its founding, members likely will welcome vaccines, especially if the public health department of the denomination openly embraces vaccinations.

## Conclusion

The COVID pandemic will have a long-lasting effect on the entire world but especially in Nigeria. Beyond the general health of the citizenry, the comparatively weak economy of the country doubtless will become worse still. In April 2020 the International Monetary Fund (IMF) noted the pandemic was "having a severe impact on economic activity. As a result of the pandemic, the global economy is projected to contract sharply by 3 percent in 2020, much more than during the 2008–09 financial crisis."[37] When the IMF made the projection, the toll the pandemic was having on poor and other vulnerable segments of Nigerian society was several times worse than those who occupied higher rungs.[38]

In April 2021, the IMF offered an improved outlook, projecting the global economy to grow at 6 percent for the rest of the year and moderating to about 4 percent in 2022.[39] Nevertheless, "great lockdown," as the IMF termed the downturn in worldwide economic activity that COVID caused or worsened from December 2019 to the April 2021 projection,[40] produced "divergent recoveries."[41] In Nigeria, there is much potential for a widening opportunity gap for public healthcare. Many wealthy Nigerians will continue to have access to reliable private services, and most poorer Nigerians will have less reliable services. Therefore, the need for the RCCG and other denominations to help meet the healthcare needs of Nigerians will remain essential for the foreseeable future.

## Notes

1  Donald E. Miller and Tetsunao Yamamori, *Global Pentecostalism: A New face of Christian Social Engagement* (Berkeley, CA: University of California Press, 2007), 2.
2  Babatunde Adedibu, "The Changing Faces of African Independent Churches as Development Actors across Borders," *HTS Teologiese Studies/Theological Studies* 74 (January 2018), https://doi.org/10.4102/hts.v74i1.4740; Adedibu, "Pentecostal Approaches to Transformation and Development: The Case of the Redeemed Christian Church of God, Nigeria," in Philipp Öhlmann, Wilhelm Gräb, Marie-Luise Frost, eds., *African Initiated Christianity and the Decolonisation of Development: Sustainable Development in Pentecostal and Independent Churches* (New York, NY: Rutledge, 2020), 136–50; Dena Freeman, ed., *Pentecostalism and Development: Churches, NGOs and Social Change in Africa* (New York, NY: Palgrave Macmillan, 2012).

3 Babatunde Adedibu, "Missional History and the Growth of the Redeemed Christian Church of God in the United Kingdom (1988–2015)," *Journal of European Pentecostal Theological Association* 36 (April 2016): 80–93; Asonzeh F.K. Ukah, *A New Paradigm of Pentecostal Power: A Study of the Redeemed Christian Church of God in Nigeria* (Trenton, NJ: Africa World Press, 2008); Ukah, "Reverse Mission or Asylum Christianity? A Nigerian Church in Europe," in Toyin Falola and Augustine Agwuele, eds., *Africans and the Politics of Popular Culture*, 104–32 (Rochester, NY: Rochester University Press, 2009).

4 Adedibu, "Missional History."

5 Richard Burgess, "African Pentecostal Spirituality and Civic Engagement: The Case of the Redeemed Christian Church of God in Britain," *Journal of Beliefs and Values* 30 (December 2009): 255–73.

6 Asonzeh Ukah, "Transformations of Contemporary Nigerian Pentecostalism," in Lionel Obadia and Donald C. Wood, eds., *The Economics of Religion: Anthropological Approaches*, 197–216 (Bingley, UK: Emerald, 2011).

7 Babatunde Adedibu, "Sacralisation of the Social Space: A Study of the Trans-Border Expansion of the Redemption Camp of the Redeemed Christian Church of God," *HTS Teologiese Studies/Theological Studies* 75 (April 2019), https://doi.org/10.4102/hts.v75i2.5428.

8 Johnson Odesola, interview by authors, May 15, 2020.

9 Olufunke Adeboye, "'A Starving Man Cannot Shout Halleluyah': African Pentecostal Churches and the Challenges of Promoting Sustainable Development," chap. 7 in Öhlmann, Gräb, and Frost, 115–35 (quotation on 124), *African Initiated Christianity and the Decolonization of Development.*

10 The Structural Adjustment Program consists of a series of loans the International Monetary Fund and the Work Bank provides to countries to better economic conditions. The Nigerian program commenced in 1986. The government "reformed its foreign exchange system, trade policies, and business and agricultural regulations. These changes brought economic incentives more into line with the country's underlying comparative advantage. Under the new policies, gross domestic product broke a six-year pattern of decline to grow by 5 percent a year throughout the six-year 1986–92 period." World Bank Western Africa Department Country Operations Division, "Foreword," *Nigeria Structural Adjustment Program: Policies, Implementation, and Impact* ([N.P.]: World Bank, 1994), ii.

11 Adeboye, "Starving Man," 125.

12 Adeboye, "Starving Man," 127.

13 See Adeboye, "Starving Man," 129; and the homepage of Healing Stripes Hospital, https://www.healingstripeshospital.com/.

14 UNAIDS, "Global HIV and AIDS Statistics—Fact Sheet," http://www.unaids.org/en/resources/fact-sheet.

15 UNAIDS, "Global HIV and AIDS Statistics."

16 See, for example, Daniel Akhazemea and Babatunde Adedibu, "The Redeemed Christian Church of God, A Missionary Global Player: What Is Her Message Regarding Human Development?," in *Encounter Beyond Routine: Cultural Roots, Cultural Transition, Understanding of Faith and Cooperation in Development*, 53–64 (Hamburg: Evangelisches Missionswerk in Deutschland, 2011).

17 Adedibu, "Pentecostal Approaches to Transformation and Development," 146.

18 Zhangkai J. Cheng and Jing Shan, "2019 Novel Coronavirus: Where We Are and What We Know," *PubMed.gov*, February 18, 2020, https://dx.doi.org/10.1007%2Fs15010-020-01401-y.

19 World Health Organization, "Naming the Coronavirus Disease (COVID-19) and the Virus that Causes It," n.d., https://www.who.int/emergencies/diseases/novel-coronavirus-2019/technical-guidance/naming-the-coronavirus-disease-(covid-2019)-and-the-virus-that-causes-it.

20 "WHO Director-General's Opening Remarks at the Media Briefing on COVID-19," *World Health Organization*, March 11, 2020, https://www.who.int/director-general/speeches/detail/who-director-general-s-opening-remarks-at-the-media-briefing-on-covid-19—11-march-2020.

21 Alexis Akwagyiram and Camillus Eboh, "Italian with Coronavirus was not Isolated for Almost 48 Hours," *Reuters*, February 27, 2020.

22 Olarewaju Kola, "COVID-19: Nigeria Announced Lockdown of Major Cities," March 29, 2020, https://www.aa.com.tr/en/africa/covid-19-nigeria-announces-lockdown-of-major-cities/1784358 (noting the lockdown applied specifically to major cities and to Ogun State).

23 "Population of Nigeria (2020 and Historical)," *Worldometer*, n.d., https://www.worldometers.info/world-population/nigeria-population/#:~:text=Nigeria%202020%20population%20is%20estimated,of%20the%20total%20world%20population.

24 "Nigeria Leads in Religious Belief," *BBC News*, February 26, 2004, http://news.bbc.co.uk/2/hi/programmes/wtwtgod/3490490.stm#:~:text=BBC%20NEWS%20%7C%20Programmes%20%7C%20wtwtgod%20%7C%20Nigeria%20leads%20in%20religious%20belief&text=A%20survey%20of%20people's%20religious,The%20World%20Thinks%20Of%20God.

25 "Nigeria Leads in Religious Belief."

26 Stephen Kenechukwu, "Adeboye: Coronavirus Won't Come Near You if You Serve God," March 18, 2020, *Cable*, https://lifestyle.thecable.ng/adeboye-coronavirus-wont-come-near-you-if-you-serve-god/. For a scholarly exploration of various critiques of Adeboye and other leading Nigerian Pentecostal leaders, see Asonzeh Ukah, "Prosperity, Prophecy and the COVI9-Pandemic," *Pneuma* 42 (2020): 430–59.

27 Mary Nnah, 'Nigeria: COVID-19—Adeboye Donates Medical Supplies to Lagos," April 9, 2020, *AllAfrica*, https://allafrica.com/stories/202004090381.html.

28 "Donated Equipment by RCCG, a Boost to Our Effort, *News Flagship*, April 7, 2020, https://newsflagship.com/donated-equipment-by-rccg-a-boost-to-our-efforts-ogsg/.

29 Regarding the federal government and the model behavioral change to which it subscribed vis-à-vis COVID-19, see Christopher J. Carpenter, "A Meta-Analysis of the Effectiveness of Health Belief Model Variables in Predicting Behavior," *Health Communication*. 25 (2010): 661–69; David Taylor et al., *A Review of the Use of the Health Belief Model (HBM), the Theory of Reasoned Action (TRA), the Theory of Planned Behaviour (TPB), and the Trans-Theoretical Model (TTM) to Study and Predict Health Related Behaviour Change* (London: National Institute for Health and Clinical Excellence, 2006), 1–215; and Robert Joseph Taylor and Linda M. Chatters, "Church Members as a Source of Informal Social Support," *Review of Religious Research* 30 (December 1998): 193–203.

30 "WHO Issues Its First Emergency Use Validation for a COVID-19 Vaccine and Emphasizes Need for Equitable Global Access," *World Health Organization*, December 31, 2020, https://www.who.int/news/item/31-12-2020-who-issues-its-first-emergency-use-validation-for-a-covid-19-vaccine-and-emphasizes-need-for-equitable-global-access.

31 "WHO Issues Its First Emergency Use Validation for a COVID-19."

32 World Health Organization Regional Office for Africa, "Nigerian Health Workers Take Country's First COVID-19 Vaccine," March 19, 2021, https://www.afro.who.int/news/nigerian-health-workers-take-countrys-first-covid-19-vaccine (hereafter cited as WHOROA).

33 WHOROA, "Nigerian Health Workers Take Country's First COVID-19 Vaccine."
34 WHOROA, "Nigerian Health Workers Take Country's First COVID-19 Vaccine."
35 WHOROA, "Nigerian Health Workers Take Country's First COVID-19 Vaccine."
36 WHOROA, "Nigerian Health Workers Take Country's First COVID-19 Vaccine."
37 International Monetary Fund, *World Economic Outlook: The Great Lockdown* (Washington, DC: International Monetary Fund, 2020), xiv (hereafter cited as IMF, *Great Lockdown*).
38 *Davide Furceri, Prakash Loungani, and Jonathan D. Ostry*, "How Pandemics Leave the Poor Even Farther Behind," *Gifted Analysts*, May 12, 2020, https:// giftedanalysts.com/how-pandemics-leave-the-poor-even-farther-behind/.
39 IMF, *World Economic Outlook: Managing Divergent Recoveries* (Washington, DC: International Monetary Fund, 2021), xvi (hereafter cited as IMF, *Managing Divergent Recoveries*).
40 IMF, *Great Lockdown*.
41 IMF, *Managing Divergent Recoveries*.

# 14 The Church of God in Christ, COVID-19, and Black Pentecostal Constructive Engagement

*David D. Daniels III*

## Introduction

A black Pentecostal engagement of COVID-19, health science, and race points to a rapport between religious and secular actors who offer valuable perspectives and resources to pivotal conversations about society. This essay uses the episcopal statements by Church of God in Christ (COGIC) Presiding Bishop Charles E. Blake Sr. to demonstrate the aforementioned rapport. Blake advanced public health by promoting scientifically informed and medically sound measures consistent with COGIC theology and scriptural interpretation. He also established a COVID taskforce of scientists, physicians, clergy, and attorneys who communicated ways to help inform the public about vaccines and other ways to curb the pandemic.

Intercessory praying, adhering to guidelines developed by the Centers for Disease Control and Prevention, familiarly the CDC, and developing partnerships between COGIC congregations and various entities responsible for COVID testing and vaccination distribution are three core elements of the engagement I reference above. Unlike competing perspectives that oppose science (e.g., vaccinations) or uncritically adopt government recommendations, COGIC engagement is grounded in science and acts on government recommendations only after critical investigation.

## The COGIC: Origin and Theological Perspective on Medical Science

Charles Harrison Mason of Shelby County, Tennessee, and Charles Price Jones of Floyd County, Georgia, founded the COGIC in 1897. When differences about Pentecostal teachings caused Mason and Jones to part ways in 1907, Mason acquired legal rights to the denominational name and its charter. He thereupon established the COGIC headquarters in Memphis, Tennessee, the county seat of Shelby. Early on, the sizeable number of physicians and related professionals in the denomination helped create a space to pursue constructive dialogues between faith and science.[1]

DOI: 10.4324/9781003214281-17

To this date, the COGIC acknowledges drugs and related medicines as parts of God's plan of healing. While some Pentecostal traditions reject such items on theological grounds, juxtaposing faith with belief and medicine with doubt, and limiting healing to divine agency, the COGIC understands the roles of both divine and human agencies in healing. The official denominational manual, published in 1973, states: "We believe that Christ, through his redemptive power, has enabled us and called us to help relieve human suffering created by sin, and we are to use whatever available resources in the restoration of man to physical, mental and spiritual health."[2] The manual furthermore encourages one to be dedicated to "principles and practices in wholesome living, as a sound mind must reside in a sound body."[3] While the manual recommends prayer as a spiritual treatment for illness, the manual also encourages medical treatment. Insofar as one can use prescription pharmaceuticals "under medical supervision for one's health and well-being," the COGIC supports members who wish to receive COVID-19 vaccinations.[4]

From March to December 2020, COGIC Presiding Bishop Charles Blake Sr. composed and posted online statements to the denomination. In the first statement, dated March 11, he informed members that, after considerable prayer and consultation with trusted medical professionals, the COGIC was issuing a formal response to questions about the COVID pandemic. Among other acts, the COGIC would continue encourage its members to pray and to follow CDC guidelines. He included a link to the CDC website so members could access guideline changes and other information about the pandemic. Blake saw a need for a joint effort between the 10,000-plus congregations that made up the international COGIC and the CDC to help reduce exposure risks but also acknowledged risky decisions that could hasten transmission.[5]

Blake's March 11, 2020, statement makes clear he respected reliable scientific advice regarding the COVID pandemic, but he was careful not to underplay the role if prayer. He asked those in the COGIC to "continue to pray for the speedy recoveries of all who have been affected by COVID-19. Please also pray for the many health care workers who faithfully serve in numerous patient care settings as essential personnel, for our Church, the nation and the entire world [as the] Church of God in Christ trusts in the miraculous healing and protective power of the Lord Jesus Christ. As He alone is our Keeper," Blake emphasized, "we will continue to wholly put our trust and faith in Him."[6]

Blake disseminated his second episcopal statement regarding COVID on March 18, 2020, inquiring, "What are the saints to do?"[7] He answered: "First, needless to say, we are living in perilous times, but certainly not without a divine remedy to survive, overcome and to emerge safely and victoriously. In fact, the same way God exercised His power to save Israel from every disease which struck the land of Egypt, even so did our Lord and Savior Jesus Christ demonstrate Himself to be the Son of God in accomplishing the healing of every widespread outbreak and pandemic affecting the regions wherever He traveled."[8] For those reasons, Blake continued, "it is my desire to share some practical guidelines for elevating our awareness while fully engaging our faith."[9] Among other acts, denominationalists should remain informed, prepared, and empowered by adhering to CDC recommendations, ignoring misinformation or disinformation, and avoiding risky behavior. "During this crisis," he proclaimed, "our faith in God is most responsibly exercised in trusting those voices whose entire lives and professions have been dedicated to the awesome task of ensuring our public health.... Strategic planning is the key to warfare. Therefore, to win, you must remain connected to good counsel."[10]

Blake, in his third episcopal statement, which he posted to the internet on March 25, 2020, issued a call for all COGIC members worldwide to observe midnight, Thursday, March 26, through 4 p.m. Friday, March 27, as a time of fasting and intercession. "We will intercede on behalf of all nations and people for Heaven's help in mitigating this dreaded disease— and for healing the bodies, minds and spirits of a fallen and fearful humanity," Blake announced, expounding: "Ultimately, we trust in the great physician, Jesus Christ."[11]

That state, national, and international servant-leaders would make wise decisions about COVID-19 was Blake's hope. He thus prayed for people of every in profession from government to teaching. Many such people comprised the "compassionate vanguard of those in harm's way."[12] People working in "the mission-critical manufacturing supply chain" also belonged to that vanguard, as did grocery, pharmaceutical, hospital, nursing home, and countless other workers.[13] With infection and death rates increasing, Blake asked God to provide divine comfort to anyone with COVID or with some other medical condition.

Blake issued yet another episcopal statement on April 23, 2020. In the statement, he made clear the COGIC did not condone any act or action that defied the collective wisdom of local, state, of federal government officials, including scientific experts. The leadership of the COGIC, Blake clarified, on multiple occasions had communicated directly with pastors and other church leaders encouraging them to abide by the stay-at-home orders and other guidelines of such officials. The COGIC, Blake communicated further, remained committed "to prioritizing the welfare of people over the economy" as certain private and public citizens debated whether to prioritize profit margins or human beings.[14]

The May 1, 2020, online episcopal statement of Blake included statements from physicians who belonged to the COGIC and dealt in part with the "premature" reopening of churches.[15] Until there was tangible evidence that the curve of ailments and deaths legitimately attributable to COVID-19 had flattened, neither Blake nor the physicians supported reopening sanctuaries and advised other denominationalists to be careful about gathering in person.[16]

On May 22, 2020, US President Donald J. Trump encouraged local and state officials to lift bans on in-worship at churches, mosques, and synagogues because such places provided "essential services."[17] The next day, Blake, the COGIC General Board, and the scholars, scientists, physicians, clergy, and attorneys who comprised a recently established denominational COVID advisory committee issued a joint episcopal statement.[18] It urged pastors to heed the recommendations of the CDC and the National Institute of Allergy and Infectious Diseases to refrain from opening churches, congregating in buildings, or performing similarly risky acts.[19] The statement also urged pastors to establish reopening safety protocols before church doors reopened.[20]

## COGIC Ecclesial Assessments and Approaches to Healthcare Infrastructure

The COGIC official manual supports the acts that Blake, the general board, and the advisory committee encouraged about the constructive engagement of religion and science to facilitate good healthcare. According to the manual, relieving human suffering is a church calling the redemptive power of God enables. Because sin produces suffering and redemption frees one from sin, one should utilize every godly resource to acquire or to retain good mental, physical, and spiritual health. In a December 29, 2020, joint statement from Blake and advisory committee co-chairs Elton Amos and Terence Rhone, a doctor of medicine and a doctor of osteopathic medicine, respectively, Blake acknowledged the unprecedented speed of the development and the approval of COVID vaccines caused some people to be uneasy about being inoculated.[21] He, however, expressed confidence in the abilities of Amos and Rhone to advise the COGIC in safe, scientifically reliable, and godly led manners.[22]

Amos and Rhone, in their portion of the joint statement, declared that inoculation was the only proven medical option to prevent COVID from being a deadly condition to the majority of the world population. They then refuted a myth about the COVID vaccine containing a live virus; therefore, contrary to what some individuals alleged, the vaccine could infect anyone with COVID. A vaccinated person, Amos and Rhone went on the report, had a 95-percent chance of eradicating COVID before feeling ill. Moreover, that person would helped the global population reach the 70 to 80 percent of vaccination that many scientists, physicians, and other informed people believed needed to be reached before herd immunity was possible. In short, Amos and Rhone concluded, the benefits of being vaccinated outweighed the risks of not being vaccinated.[23]

The constructive engagement of the health science by COGIC found expression in different congregations across the US in addition to the statements from Blake, the board, and the advisory committee. Congregations partnered with county health departments, hospital systems, and pharmacies to distribute COVID vaccines in underserved communities. In the Crenshaw neighborhood of Los Angeles, California, where Blake pastored

West Angeles Cathedral, The Church and the county public health department joined forced to ensure local residents had access to vaccinations. In Arkansas City, Kansas, St. James Church joined with Graves Drug, a regional pharmacy, to provide similar access, as did Nehemiah Church in Durham, North Carolina.[24]

The COGIC collaborated with other denominations in its effort to vaccinate people. In Durham, for example, Presbyterians, Catholics, and Baptists assisted. Of the approximately 150 vaccine recipients, 60 percent were black, 40 percent were Latino, and most were at least sixty-five years old.[25] Such coordinated efforts helped address the racial/ethnic disparities related to COVID healthcare about which doctors Elton Amos and Terence Rhone of the advisory committee wrote in May 2020.[26] Experts, Amos and Rhone affirmed, knew healthcare disparities results nonwhite people dying than white people: "The U.S. government's history of experimentation, disparate health care services, and willful blindness to the social determinants of health that contribute to people of color's health status" likely caused the COVID pandemic to affect African Americans, Latino Americans, and Native Americans the worst.[27]

In supporting the establishment of health clinics in communities that medical establishments customarily underserved, the COGIC illustrated the significance of combining faith and science to meet societal challenges—in this instance, COVID. The New St. Paul COGIC in Detroit, Michigan, and the Glad Tidings International COGIC in Haywood, California, are two of several churches whose congregants sponsored clinics in North America. throughout the Global South (Africa, Asia, Latin America, Oceania).[28] In Nairobi, Kenya, a clinic on the campus of Cornerstone Faith Assembly, began providing water and other health services to the community during the early spring months of 2020. According to Bishop Francis Kamau, pastor of Cornerstone and prelate of the jurisdiction, the effort was vital, as the community had limited resources.[29]

The Cornerstone Faith Assembly expanded its COVID outreach program during the late the spring and summer months of 2020. From May to July, the congregation held online worship and education services from Tuesdays to Fridays. Commencing at noon and broadcast in English, Kikamba, Kikuyu, Kijaluo, and Swahili, among other languages to reach a broad audience, the services devoted ten minutes to COVID health protocols from the Kenyan Ministry of Health. In addition to Kamau, who led the sessions, nurses and other healthcare professionals made presentations. As regards the jurisdiction for which Kamau served as prelate, his colleagues and he secured temperature guns for fifty congregations to use when they resumed gathering in person.[30]

## Conclusion

Concerted efforts of the COGIC in addressing COVID have helped contain the spread of the pandemic, thereby decreasing morbidity and mortality, among other hardships. As a twelve-member consortium in Australia known as Church Agencies Network Disaster Operations, or Can Do, proclaimed in April 2020, the faith motivations and worldviews of international denominations can facilitate constructive behaviors that in turn help reduce the effects of COVID.[31] Can Do also urged people to avoid mistakes of former pandemics, such as the Ebola crises of 2014 to 2015 and 2018, when government officials and other decision makers did not engage with local faith actors in timely manners.[32] Instead of acting separately, Can Do advised secular and religious communities to work together, designing relevant health messaging, providing needed medical services, and performing similar roles to halt the COVID pandemic.[33]

The COGIC has undertaken the work about which Can Do wrote in 2020. The COGIC, moreover, has done so by promoting scientifically informed and medically sound measures consistent with denominational theology and scriptural interpretation. In leading by example, the COGIC has been not only transformational religiously but also civically. Denominational leaders have created or followed best practices to help prevent COVID transmission by defusing fear and mistrust associated with vaccinations. In so doing, the leaders have engendered hope and fostered trust, constructively engaged science and promoted public health, and served as a global intermediary between local, state, and federal officials and their constituents. Such acts and actions illustrate the vital roles that church communities can perform in educating people locating reliable information and services to ensure sound minds and bodies pursuant to living wholesome lives.[34]

While the COGIC considers prayer the first treatment for illness and hence living wholesomely, the denomination encourages medical treatment when necessary to help one have a sound mind and body. Certified professionals aid in the latter process by assisting with counseling ministries and by referring congregants to other qualified healthcare providers. Those acts are consistent with the denominational commitment to "the equal access of all [humankind] to the goods and service of this earth," a notion that conceptually includes such access to health care services for people regardless of religion, race/ethnicity, income, or some other factor.[35]

By being located in communities that medical establishments and other healthcare institutions often have underserved, COGIC congregations have been valuable liaisons between governments and populaces during the COVID pandemic. Denominationalists not only worship proximately to people whom COVID has affected, both directly and indirectly, but the same denominationalists frequently live in the communities where they worship. In other words, because the COGIC is embedded in those places, its members are familiar with local customs and therefore are positioned well to build and, of equal significance, to maintain strong relationships rooted in respect and trust, as Church Agencies Network Disaster Operations advised in April 2020.[36]

Conferring credibility to legitimate public health initiatives is another piece of sage advice from Can Do the COGIC has heeded during COVID.

By allowing churches and other denomination-related facilities to serve as COVID testing and vaccination sites, the COGIC has been a central component of a healing infrastructure that connects prayer and medicine. Such acts demonstrate that Bishop Charles Edward Blake Sr. and the COGIC has offered a model of a Pentecostal engagement of science, public health, and faith that is theologically based, medically informed, scientifically sound, and vitally important to humanity.[37]

## Notes

Much of this essay appears as David D. Daniels III, "COVID-19, Science, and Race: A Black Pentecostal Engagement," *Spiritus* 6 (spring 2021): 141–55.

1  Calvin White Jr., "In the Beginning, There Stood Two: Arkansas Roots of the Black Holiness Movement," *Arkansas Historical Quarterly* 68 (spring 2009): 1–22; White, *The Rise of Respectability: Race, Religion, and the Church of God in Christ* (Fayetteville, AR: University of Arkansas Press, 2012).

2  *Church of God in Christ Official Manual* (1973; repr., Memphis, TN: Church of God in Christ Publishing House, 1991), 121.

3  *Church of God in Christ Official Manual*, 126.

4  *Church of God in Christ Official Manual*, 124.

5  Charles E. Blake Sr. March 11, 2020, open letter to members of the Church in God in Christ, https://www.cogic.org/covid19/files/2020/03/Bishop-Blake-letter-Covid-19-2.pdf (hereafter cited as Blake March 11, 2020, Open Letter).

6  Blake March 11, 2020, Open Letter.

7  "Presiding Bishop's Update on COVID-19," March 18, 2020, https://www.cogic.org/covid19/presiding-bishops-covid-19-update-3-18-20/ (hereafter cited as Blake March 18, 2020, Update).

8  Blake March 18, 2020, Update.

9  Blake March 18, 2020, Update.

10  Blake March 18, 2020, Update.

11  "Presiding Bishop's Update on COVID-19," March 28, 2021, https://www.cogic.org/covid19/presiding-bishops-covid-19-update-3-25-20/ (hereafter cited as Blake March 28, 2020, Update).

12  Blake March 28, 2020, Update.

13  Blake March 28, 2020, Update.

14  "Presiding Bishop's Update on COVID-19," April 23, 2020, https://www.cogic.org/covid19/presiding-bishops-covid-19-update-4-23-20/.

15  "COGIC Doctors Contribute Response to COVID-19," 1 May 2020, https://www.cogic.org/wp-content/uploads/2020/05/COGIC-COVID-FINAL-2.pdf.

16  "COGIC Doctors Contribute Response."

17  "White House Briefing," May 22, 2020, *C-Span*, https://www.c-span.org/video/?472429-1/president-trump-calls-reopening-houses-worship.

18  "Statement from Presiding Bishop, General Board and COVID-19 Advisory Committee," May 23, 2020, https://www.cogic.org/covid19/files/2020/05/COVID-Blake-9.pdf.

19  "Statement from Presiding Bishop, General Board and COVID-19 Advisory Committee."

20  "Statement from Presiding Bishop, General Board and COVID-19 Advisory Committee."

21  "Presiding Bishop Blake and Expert COGIC [Doctors'] Statement on COVID Vaccine," December 29, 2020, https://www.cogic.org/wp-content/uploads/2020/12/COVID-Newsletter-Dec-2020-2.pdf.

22 "Presiding Bishop Blake and Expert COGIC [Doctors'] Statement."

23 "Presiding Bishop Blake and Expert COGIC [Doctors'] Statement.

24 Herbert Davis, interview by David D. Daniels III, February 13 and April 24, 2021 (hereafter cited as Davis Interview with appropriate date); C. Edward Watson, interview by David D. Daniels III, February 17 and April 24, 2021.

25 Davis Interview, February 13, 2021.

26 "COGIC Doctors Contribute Response."

27 "COGIC Doctors Contribute Response."

28 Nour Dados and Raewyn Connell, "The Global South," *Contexts* 11 (winter 2012): 12–13.

29 Davis Interview, February 13, 2021.

30 Francis Kamau, interview by David D. Daniels III, April 24, 2021.

31 "Church Agencies and Faith-Based Organisations in COVID-19 Humanitarian Response," *Can Do* (April 2020), https://www.icvanetwork.org/system/files/versions/200401%20Role%20of%20Churches%20and%20FBOs%20in%20COVID%20response_FINAL%5B2%5D.pdf.

32 "Church Agencies and Faith-Based Organisations."

33 "Church Agencies and Faith-Based Organisations."

34 See "Church Agencies and Faith-Based Organisations"; and *Church of God in Christ Official Manual*, 126.

35 *Church of God in Christ Official Manual*, 126.

36 "Church Agencies and Faith-Based Organisations."

37 "Church Agencies and Faith-Based Organizations.

# 15 Richard Allen, Black Aid Workers, and Civil Rights Lessons of the First Great Epidemic in the United States

*Richard Newman*

## Introduction

In the fall of 1793, the famed black preacher Richard Allen confronted a scene of disease and devastation that remains striking more than two centuries later. Allen's adopted hometown of Philadelphia, Pennsylvania, was the infant nation's largest city as well as the home of the federal government. At the time, Philadelphia was under siege by a deadly epidemic, yellow fever. After first appearing in the summer, the disease spread across the city with horrible efficiency. By winter, when the disease abated, approximately 4,000 people, roughly 10 percent of the population, had perished. Though COVID-19, the novel coronavirus the United States began to experience during the winter of 2019–2020 is bad, I cannot fathom the misery Allen witnessed.[1]

Allen's struggle to confront a secondary disaster—the social contagion of racism and discrimination—is nearly as striking as his fight against yellow fever. Though he and black aid workers volunteered to help save the infected city and did heroic nursing and medical work when others fled, Allen and his black peers faced terrible backlash once the tragedy ended. Far from a story about the citizenry banding together to overcome a deadly situation, Philadelphia's yellow fever experience serves as a cautionary tale about the way natural disasters, including disease outbreaks, expose deep racial divides in American culture. Not unlike future catastrophes (such as the 1918 influenza pandemic countrywide, the 1927 flood in Mississippi, or Hurricane Katrina's devastation of Louisiana in 2005), Philadelphia's yellow fever epidemic of 1793 uncovered racial fault lines that had their own fatal consequences.

## Hope in a Time of Dread: Disease, Disaster, and Racial Reckoning in 1790s Philadelphia

A great irony of Allen's aid work in Philadelphia during the 1793 yellow fever epidemic is that, initially, he was filled with high hopes. The rising black minister wanted to strike a powerful blow for racial equality in the new nation's capital city, and he believed the disease offered a means to achieve

DOI: 10.4324/9781003214281-18

that goal. Though Pennsylvania lawmakers passed a gradual emancipation law in 1780, putting slavery on the road to extinction in the Quaker State, many white people were unsure about black freedom. Allen saw African Americans as civic equals and cocreators of a new democratic ethos steeped in interracial cooperation. The 1793 outbreak gave him a chance to illustrate African Americans' civic mindedness by forming a brigade of black aid workers who would rush to the ailing city's defense. Working with white leaders such as physician Benjamin Rush and Mayor Matthew Clarkson, Allen and a fellow black clergyman, Absalom Jones, led a host of African Americans into Philadelphia streets and homes. Together, they battled the nation's first major disease disaster since the struggle for independence from Great Britain ended officially in 1783. With the federal government meeting in Philadelphia between 1790 and 1800, Allen also knew black aid workers would have a powerful audience of governing officials watching them. With that fact in mind, he anticipated black aid work facilitating a national civil rights struggle that would flow outward from Philadelphia.

To be successful, Allen and other African Americans knew they had to overcome eighteenth-century forms of social, or physical, distancing. Unlike COVID-19, a stealthy pandemic, yellow fever marked victims in a highly visible way. Afflicted patients often had yellowish eyes and skin, which indicated the onset of jaundice (a liver condition that colored the body). Early national Philadelphians shunned anyone who looked symptomatic. After the first wave of yellow fever cases arose toward the end of August 1793, many Philadelphians went steps farther, literally, than social distancing; they distanced physically by fleeing the city altogether. With money and the means to travel, wealthier Philadelphians led the way out of town. By late fall, perhaps half the population was gone. In the hollowed out city, sickness dominated the streets and people's attentions. Some governing and health officials wondered if the city would recover. Others worried that death and dislocation had undercut the country's purported moral sense—that is, the idea that democratic citizens would help each other create a better society through mutual cooperation and civic-minded benevolence. The yellow fever epidemic blasted apart that notion.

Allen's black brigade bravely stepped into Philadelphia's crumbling world. Risking their lives to help hundreds of sick and dying citizens, they sought not only to aid people medically but also to fill a civic void. In volunteering to aid the city, Allen and his fellow black Philadelphians shattered racial taboos. For example, they entered white homes not as indentured servants or enslaved workers but as free medical aids and caretakers. Allen learned how to bleed people from Benjamin Rush, who sought to purge the contagion and to balance precious bodily fluids. Grateful white Philadelphians ravaged by disease did not scream when they saw Allen, Absalom Jones, and other black health care professionals unpack their blades; instead, they saluted them for responding to the crisis. For Allen, this appreciation indicated some white people could overcome racial prejudice.

More than two centuries later, from late 2019 and into early 2020, COVID-19 created a similar sense of interracial possibility. Black and brown aid workers who risked their lives to respond to the pandemic believed their efforts would create a racial reckoning about health disparities in the United States. Experience, however, would undercut such hopes, as was the case with Allen in the 1793. Similar to many aid workers today, he was fired up by a fierce sense that yellow fever would cause people to change the racial status quo. Black aid work and civil rights activism would go hand in hand. Or so Allen hoped.

### Reckoning with Racial Illness in the Nation's Capital City

I doubt Allen imagined a racial reckoning might result from a major disaster before the yellow fever epidemic. A rising black preacher who purchased himself from bondage, Allen experienced another form of social distancing at St. George's Methodist Church where white leaders placed black congregants in segregated areas. Though Allen helped build St. George's base of black parishioners and the church's financial coffers, white Methodists treated African Americans as second-class members. In response to such abuse, Allen and his great friend, Absalom Jones, staged the nation's first documented sit-in by marching out of St. George's in 1787. As Allen put it triumphantly, neither he nor his black associates ever returned to segregated pews.[2]

After the St. George's sit-in and walkout, Allen began building his own house of worship, Mother Bethel African Methodist Episcopal (AME) Church. Christened during the summer of 1794, Mother Bethel became a longtime home of black autonomy, black educational and protest initiatives, and Black Power. After he and other leaders formed the AME denomination in 1816, Allen's church expanded nationally and became famous for fostering freedom struggles everywhere. Not only would the AME Church nurture Jarena Lee, *Télémaque* (Denmark Vesey), Morris Brown, and other black freedom fighters of the nineteenth century, but the denomination also would spawn a host of prominent civil rights leaders, including A. Philip Randolph and Rosa M. Parks, of the twentieth century. In South Africa, meanwhile, numerous anti-apartheid activists in South Africa were members of the AME Church. Their efforts were microcosms of the denominational commitment to human equality.

Allen had no way of knowing the future impact of the AME Church, but throughout his life he believed he was building a denomination dedicated to freedom and justice—an icon of racial healing. Hoping to enlist the support of white Philadelphians, from abolitionists to politicians to religious leaders, he made sure the AME Church served as a bridge of understanding between black and white Philadelphians. A visionary religious leader, Allen thought the denomination would model the brand of loving Christianity, emancipatory politics, and egalitarianism that came to define the doctrine of social holiness. Allen also believed black people would model interracial citizenship for doubting white people. His aid work during the 1793 yellow fever crisis flowed from those twin ideals.[3]

Ironically, yellow fellow almost derailed Mother Bethel when Allen contracted the dreaded disease in the fall of 1793. He spent time recovering inside Bush Hill, a makeshift hospital on the outskirts of Philadelphia. What would have become of the AME Church—which had yet to be consecrated formally—if Allen died? Thankfully, Allen survived his bout with the yellow fever. Once the epidemic abated, Allen presumed white people would treat black people equally because they had risked their lives to save the infected city and hence proved their civic worth.

The future Allen anticipated never materialized. While Mayor Matthew Clarkson and other white reformers hailed Allen and black aid workers in 1793, many other white citizens pictured African Americans as unruly residents who exploited the yellow fever epidemic for personal gain. The famous white printer Mathew Carey, who left the infected city, circulated some of those stories in his best-selling history of the yellow fever, *A Short Account of the Malignant Fever … in Philadelphia*, printed before the fever disappeared fully. Based on a mix of research, gossip, and interviews he conducted, Carey depicted a city gripped not only by disease but also by fear. While he saluted Allen's aid work, Carey castigated the broader African American population as disruptive and somewhat sinister during the epidemic. Referring to the "plundering" of private homes, Carey pictured African Americans as villains instead of heroes.[4]

Carey's villainizing black aid workers contributed to the secondary disaster Allen confronted in 1793. But cultural historians also have underscored the social meaning of secondary disasters: racial backlashes, acts of religious intolerance, and political retributions that flow from the original calamity.[5] By falsely accusing African Americans of nefarious behavior, Carey injected racism into the public sphere, contributing to a secondary disaster of racial animus against black aid workers. For Carey and others, black people remained a problematic and unruly element whose base character the yellow fever epidemic revealed.

Outraged, Absalom Jones and Richard Allen wrote their own history of the tragedy, *A Narrative of the Proceedings of the Black People, During the Late Awful Calamity in Philadelphia, in the Year 1793* (1794). The first copyrighted written work by black authors in the United States, *Narrative* surveyed African American aid work during the epidemic while also pointing to deeper racial disparities in health, politics, education, and social life. Jones and Allen noted African Americans risked their lives to aid white people whom yellow fever devastated. Furthermore, black people died in roughly the same proportion as white people, though few in the Philadelphia leadership class seemed to notice or to care about that fact. Of equal importance to historical memory, *Narrative* helped usher in a modern understanding of civil rights. In a section focusing specifically on slavery and racial injustice,

Jones and Allen defined black equality as a civic birthright and not as a gift from white lawmakers. Jones and Allen spent the rest of their lives fighting for that brand of freedom, justice, and equality.[6]

Jones and Allen's yellow fever story remain instructive in the twenty-first century. Among other lessons, their story shows that disease often transcends the medical realm, inspiring important social and cultural discussions about discrimination, medical policy, and other iniquities. Jones and Allen wanted their fellow American citizens to approach racial injustice as seriously as they did yellow fever. That reckoning is similar to recent calls to examine the disparate impact of COVID-19 on people of color, who face major disparities in the American healthcare system. Additionally, Jones and Allen's focus on black economic sacrifice during the yellow fever epidemic encourages contemporary Americans to think about the need for more equitable wages for low-income workers on the frontlines of the COVID pandemic. Likewise, the aid work of Jones, Allen, and other African Americans during the yellow fever epidemic demonstrates the chaos of disaster elides the daily sacrifices that marginalized people make to keep society going. Now, as during the 1790s, American citizens should not forget marginalized people's heroic efforts on the frontlines of tragedy.

As regard Allen's individual activism, his protest against racial injustice continues to inspire. He not only attempted to reform society but also create a brand of racial healing that would transcend the yellow fever saga. Indeed, from 1793 onward, he sought to mobilize Americans against all forms of racism, from the South's characteristic black enslavement to the North's black employment discrimination. Viewing racism as a virulent pathogen that attacked communities of color, he constantly challenged Americans to overcome it, to heal themselves from a diseased way of thinking. Allen continued to make similar pleas even while approaching death in 1831. Days before his demise, he instructed his son to reprint the yellow fever *Narrative* in his forthcoming autobiography. By republishing his and Absalom Jones' searing condemnation of racism in Philadelphia, the nation's founding city, Allen sought to inspire a new generation of civil rights activists during the antebellum era.[7] Sadly, it is all too easy to imagine that if Allen were alive today, he would feel a terrible sense of déjà vu in the racial iniquities the COVID pandemic has highlighted. Then, I suspect, he would get to work mobilizing anew against the disease of racism still vibrantly alive in the twenty-first century.

## Notes

1  Richard S. Newman, *Freedom's Prophet: Bishop Richard Allen, the AME Church and the Black Founding Fathers* (New York, NY: New York University Press, 2008), esp. 27–52, 78–127. Unless I note otherwise, my book is the source of information for this essay. Regarding Allen's adopting Philadelphia, Pennsylvania, as his hometown, I address the matter in chapter one, "For Zion's Sake … I Will Not Rest" (27–52). Allen himself once wrote: "I was

born in the year of our Lord 1769, on February 14th, a slave to Benjamin Chew, of Philadelphia. My mother and father and four children of us were sold into Delaware state, near Dover; and I was a child and lived with him until I was upwards of twenty years of age." Allen, *The Life, Experience, and Gospel Labors of the Rt. Rev. Richard Allen* ... (Philadelphia, PN: Martin and Boden, 1833), 5.

2 One the revolutionary character of the 1787 church sit-in Richard Allen and Absalom Jones led, see *Freedom's Prophet*, 63–66.

3 Regarding the African Methodist Episcopal Church and social holiness, see especially Dennis C. Dickerson, *The African Methodist Episcopal Church: A History* (New York, NY: Cambridge University Press, 2020), 23.

4 Mathew Carey, *A Short Account of the Malignant Fever, Lately Prevalent in Philadelphia; With a Statement of the Proceedings that Took Place on the Subject in Different Parts of the United States* (Philadelphia, PN, Mathew Carey, 1793), 77.

5 On the cultural meaning of natural disasters, see especially Ted Steinberg, *Acts of God: The Unnatural History of Natural Disasters in America* (New York, NY: Oxford University Press, 2006).

6 A. J. and R. A., *A Narrative of the Proceedings of the Black People, During the Late Awful Calamity in Philadelphia, in the Year 1793: And Refutation of Some Censures, Thrown Upon Them in Some Publications* (Philadelphia, PN: William W. Woodward, 1794) (hereafter cited as Jones and Allen, *Narrative*). Allen authored "To Those Who Keep Slaves, and Approve the Practice," an antislavery missive appended to the main pamphlet, *Narrative*.

7 For a reprint of the yellow fever pamphlet, see Allen, *Life, Experience, and Gospel Labors*.

# 16 Caribbean Churches, Capacities, and Responses to the COVID-19 Pandemic

*Ronald A. Nathan*

## Introduction

The Caribbean stretches from the Florida Keys in the North to the mainland territories of Venezuela, Guyana, Belize, and Suriname in the South. The Caribbean's history of colonialism and imperialism includes the decimation of the first peoples of the region, the transatlantic slave trade, and East Indian indentureship. Those cataclysmic inheritances provide the framework for Caribbean's contemporary demographics, which reflect the region's ethnic, cultural, linguistic, religious, social, and political diversity. For example, the Caribbean political landscape is comprised of liberal democracies, authoritarian states, overseas territories, associated and dependent states of France, Netherlands, the United Kingdom, and the United States. Ninety percent of the almost 44 million people who populated the Caribbean islands in 2020 were of African descent, and roughly 85 percent of those individuals were affiliated with a longstanding Christian denomination or with a newer sectarian offshoot.[1]

Legacies of slavery and colonialism, together with present-day challenges of globalization, leave the Caribbean's inhabitants wrestling with systemic poverty as the region's most pressing social and theological problem.[2] In 2015, Caribbean Development Bank President William Warren Smith declared that 21 percent of the Caribbean's population lived below the poverty line.[3] Since that year (as before it), African-descendant populations in the region have continued to face difficulties in accessing quality and affordable healthcare, among other life necessities. Local public medical and health infrastructures are weak, and budgets are strained.

When COVID-19 hit the Caribbean in early 2020, neither governments nor citizens could afford to engage in massive financial outlays. Tourism was a major component of the regional economy, and meeting ongoing costs of protecting local populations while expanding tourism-dependent economies was fraught with danger. A lack of economic diversification produced much health inequality in the Caribbean between and within states. Moreover, people in the region tended to approach healthcare using a biomedical paradigm. In my judgment, they needed to view healthcare

DOI: 10.4324/9781003214281-19

from a social perspective and thereby help raise the low status of public health and health promotion. Additionally, given that most black people in the Caribbean in 2021 are of African descent, the Christian Church in the region should engage creatively and constructively to respect black lives and bodies as physical, social, cultural, economic, political, and spiritual beings.[4]

## COVID-19 and Caribbean Social Vulnerabilities

Even before the COVID outbreak of late 2019 to early 2020, the Caribbean was one of the most indebted regions in the world. As stated above, Caribbean economies depended heavily on tourism. In Jamaica, for example, that industry was the country's largest. Twenty-five percent of the labor force worked in tourism, a sector that accounted for 30 percent of gross domestic product (GDP) and 50 percent of foreign exchange earnings.[5] Throughout the Caribbean, 2.4 million people worked in tourism, an industry responsible for more than $62 billion, roughly 16 percent, of GDP.[6]

After Caribbean officials announced the first case of COVID in the region toward the end of February 2020, they immediately closed national borders and enforced lockdowns, realizing they did not have the resources to manage a major hit from the pandemic. Officials focused on precautionary measures such as social distancing, mask-wearing, mandatory quarantines, curfews, and restricting travelers arriving from countries with high or rising numbers of infected people, including China and the United States. The trebling of unemployment figures and the halving of government revenues were direct consequences of border closings and lockdowns. The subsequent global pandemic worsened local Caribbean economies, with some places experiencing as much as a 23 percent drop in revenues or in exports on account of death, unemployment, and related occurrences in metropoles such as London, England, Montreal, Canada, New York City, New York, and Washington, DC.[7]

In September 2007, more than a decade before Chinese officials released information about twenty-seven cases of viral pneumonia that turned out to be to COVID,[8] Jamaican financial analyst and journalist Ralston Hyman identified challenges to economic growth and transformation in the Caribbean.[9] He declared, "The growth and development of many small Caribbean states are being negatively impacted by their onerous debt burdens, which ... prevent them from spending on infrastructure development and the provision of basic social services which are necessary to attract investments and improve their absorptive capacities."[10] Those problems remained in March 2020 when the World Health Organization pronounced COVID as a pandemic.[11] Speaking in June as the pandemic spread across the world, Barbados Prime Minister and Caribbean Community Chair (CARICOM) Mia Amor Mottley called for expanded discussions through a global leadership initiative whose members could create a vulnerability

*Table 16.1*  COVID-19 in Selected Caribbean Countries, June 2020 and September 2021[22]

| Country | June 2020 | | September 2021 | |
| --- | --- | --- | --- | --- |
| | *Cases* | *Deaths* | *Cases* | *Deaths* |
| Cuba | 2,340 | 86 | 689,674 | 5,703 |
| Haiti | 5,847 | 104 | 20,977 | 586 |
| Jamaica | 696 | 10 | 71,344 | 1,619 |
| Saint Lucia | 19 | 0 | 9,149 | 116 |
| Barbados | 97 | 7 | 5,349 | 51 |
| Trinidad and Tobago | 126 | 8 | 45,714 | 1,330 |
| Guyana | 230 | 12 | 26,611 | 647 |
| Totals | 9,355 | 227 | 868,818 | 10,052 |

index to determine how small island developing states (SIDS) could gain equitable access to fair allocation of international development funds: "Our small states have been suffering from high debt and low growth for decades, and we believe that there should be mature and relevant conversations for middle income, small island developing states across the globe as it relates to our debt obligations in the midst of this pandemic."[12]

Extreme vulnerability to climate change, natural disaster, and an assortment of other events that can impact temperature or weather conditions is another significant matter that SIDS face.[13] For example, when a hurricane strikes the Caribbean, force winds can wipe out the entire GDP of a SID. Often, the poorest people in that state suffer the most hardship. The need to build fiscal resilience and to invest in disaster preparedness are critical for reducing the large human and economic costs that climate changes, natural disasters, and related events can cause.[14]

In May 2020, as the COVID pandemic expanded, University of the West Indies Pro Vice-chancellor Clive Landis announced: "The English-speaking Caribbean has achieved containment of COVID."[15] Curves seemed to be flattening in much of the Dutch and French Caribbean as well. Data from June 2020 tended to bear out those assessments (Table 16.1). One year later, in contrast, COVID figures showed a growing number of cases and deaths, as governments reopened borders and economies.[16]

## The Christian Church in the Caribbean

With regard to Caribbean religiosity, another central aspect of this essay, all major world belief systems are present in the region. Several hybrids consisting of "elements of African and European beliefs and practices, and, in some cases, parts of American Indian and South Asian religious traditions" also are present in the Caribbean.[17] However, Christianity is predominant.[18]

The Caribbean Conference of Churches (CCC) and the Evangelical Association of the Caribbean (EAC), are the two major regional bodies for Christianity. Founded in 1973 and aligned with the World Council of Churches, the CCC is the ecumenical organization for the Caribbean.[19] By 2021, thirty-three member denominations existed in thirty-four territories from Cuna in the North to Suriname in the South.[20] The second major regional body, the EAC, originated in 1977 and is a network of eleven national evangelical associations that are aligned with the World Evangelical Alliance.[21] The CCC and the EAC do not collaborate formally, but both organizations are experiencing institutional and structural challenges that impede their abilities to create policies and deliver services such as COVID-19 assistance.

As primary institutions within Caribbean contexts, churches have performed pivotal roles in the COVID containment objectives of governments. When state officials locked down borders and instituted social, or physical, distancing, most Christian church leaders closed sanctuaries immediately. There was a small amount of church-based resistance to those occurrences, but congregations ultimately coalesced around individual denominational structures (versus looking to regional ecumenical bodies) to formulate responses that would not violate the law. For instance, the CCC has been receptive to vaccines produced in Europe and in North America, especially the United States. Accordingly, CCC leaders have encouraged ordinary members to comply with their respective national government vaccination policies. Leaders also have been involved in facilitating vaccination programs and have participated in international prayers of intercession for people affected by COVID.[23]

In addition to the CCC, Seventh-Day Adventist and Church of Christ denominations in the Caribbean posted COVID advisories to their websites. There also were cross-denominational initiatives in the region, albeit on a limited scale. One example will suffice: the United Theological College of the West Indies, an ecumenical institution based in Kingston, Jamaica, provided pastoral training wherein ministers of the New Testament Church of God (a member of the EAC) from various Caribbean territories learned how to deal with psychological effects of COVID. Though notable initiatives, individual churches with developed social ministries or pre-existing social initiatives have been best prepared to support their congregational members and local communities during the pandemic. Several have engaged in distributing food. Others have assigned health visitors to assist elderly people. All have adhered to government regulations regarding social distancing and appropriate sanitizing.

Many church leaders in the Caribbean decided independently how their denominationalists would operate during shutdowns. As demonstrated above, ministerial affairs continued, with ecclesiastical officers creating ways to interpret and to incorporate COVID prevention protocols on interpersonal levels. A majority of churches moved worship services, prayer meetings, and biblical studies online, using a variety of internet-based conferencing platforms. Churches streamed services using products such as Zoom, Skype, Microsoft Teams, Facebook, YouTube, posting live, or recorded videos on websites when possible.[24]

With restrictions on congregations gathering at physical places of worship, the digital divide and electronic poverty have become extraordinarily apparent during the COVID pandemic. Access to wireless services has not been widespread, as smart phones, tablets, and other mobile computers have been limited. The United Nations Educational, Scientific, and Cultural Organization noted that school "closures have left seven million learners and over 90[,]000 teachers across 23 countries and territories in the Caribbean sub-region grappling with a new reality of distance-learning" during the pandemic.[25] Of no surprise, well-off communities have fared better than poor communities.

In September 2020, the Organisation for Economic Co-Operation and Development Centre, the United Nations Economic Commission for Latin America and the Caribbean, the Development Bank of Latin America, and the European Union produced a report that noted disparities in internet usage between rich and poor sectors of the Caribbean. According to the report, 75 percent of the former population used internet and 37 percent of the latter did so.[26]

I witnessed the disparity on which the Organisation for Economic Co-Operation and Development Centre and its partners reported amid the COVID pandemic in 2020. Among the congregants I pastored in Saint Michael, Barbados, five children from one family had a single tablet to use with their online school lessons. To make matters worse, all lessons took place at the same periods each day. Compounding those problems, the parents of the children were able to pay for only three hours of internet service per day. Of course, COVID did not create the difficulty that family had accessing a quality education, but COVID made doing so more difficult.

The preceding paragraph warrants qualification: while basic literacy rates in Latin America and the Caribbean often have been higher than global averages in recent years, a point that authors Akanksha Sharma and Barbara Arese Lucini made in 2015, there remained "a gap in digital literacy and skills" during that year (2015).[27] "Insufficient infrastructure and teaching support for digital education," Sharma and Lucini explained, prevented "many mobile users from exploring the benefits of the internet."[28]

The two-pronged exclusion in both physical and digital worlds about which Sharma and Lucini wrote in 2015 remains in 2021, affecting ecclesiastical as well as academic work. For instance, the exclusion reduces the capacities of some churches to engage in pastoral ministries to their parishioners and to raise money for their service ministries. With the continued extension of national lockdowns and limits on how many persons can congregate at weddings, funerals, christenings, and other events, several independent churches have begun to agitate for the relaxation or the removal of COVID-19 restrictions.

## Church Responses to Medical and Economic
## Challenges of the COVID-19 Pandemic

As mentioned above, national leaders in Caribbean were able to stem the first tide of COVID in 2020 by imposing curfews, instituting lockdowns, and closing borders, among other means. The subsequent tide in 2021 has presented additional health and economic challenges to which widespread vaccination programs comprise one resolution. Regional policies began with vaccinating frontline workers such as those in the healthcare system. Next, aged and ill people with conditions that make them more suscepti-ble to COVID than healthier people received vaccines. Caribbean churches also have assisted the COVID containment process. For instance, numerous pastors have found ways to communicate with their congregants by using technology in innovate ways to hold services and perform other ministe-rial functions. Pastors also have encouraged congregants to consider gov-ernment policies and procedures regarding COVID vaccinations, thereby rebutting the idea that a vaccine was "the mark of the beast mentioned in Revelations."[29]

Not unlike evangelicals throughout the world, many in the Caribbean have questions vaccinations. While vaccines being marks of beasts perhaps rep-resent fringe thoughts, evangelicals more critically question ethical matters regarding vaccine development, testing, distribution, and implication for human life. While access to traditional media such as television and radio broadcasts are limited in many parts of the Caribbean, churchgoers have uti-lized social media when available to investigate conspiracy theories, to have debates about, and to perform other responsible duties regarding COVID and vaccinations. The African Methodist Episcopal Zion Church, the Pentecostal Assemblies of the West Indies, The Church of the Nazarene, and the EAC have facilitated discussions between medical practitioners and their parish-ioners to neutralize some of the negative attitudes toward vaccinations.[30]

Whereas many churchgoers support vaccines, getting requisite dosages has been difficult for Caribbean masses. Governments have not been able to purchase adequately from the vaccines pillar of the Coalition for Epidemic Preparedness Innovations and its partnering organizations' Access to the COVID-19 Tools Accelerator, or COVAX, program, nor have govern-ment secured enough vaccines through bilateral agreements with Indian, Chinese, European, or American governments, independent providers, or other legitimate means.[31] Based on a report the Pan American Health Organization released in January 2021, roughly one-tenth of the Caribbean population of more than over 653 million people had received a dosage of vaccine.[32] One in ten, the organization proclaimed, was "nowhere near the at least 500 million people [who needed to be immunized] in the Americas region to control the spread and achieve 'herd immunity.'"[33]

Some Cubans medical health officials are trying to do their parts to help people have access to vaccines and to reach the herd immunity about which the Pan American Health Organization reported in January 2021. As of mid-June, there were five emergency trials underway in Cuba, with certain Cubans working to immunize at least 2.2. million Cubans in the capital city of Havana by the end of the July. Regrettably, neither local ecumenical and evangelical church leaders nor regional governmental leaders in the Caribbean said much publicly about the trials in Cuba. Their collective silence reflected a lack of rigorous political or prophetic engagement in the face of COVID, one of the greatest health and economic challenges people in the Caribbean have faced in years. I believe having systematic and open discussions about vaccines is an important step in curtailing the pandemic. Such discussions are particularly vital in the Caribbean, where millions of people begged for vaccines by the time employees of the public health ministry in Cuba expanded vaccination trials in June as a coronavirus variant called delta spread across rapidly the region and the world.[34]

In addition to difficulties associated with obtaining sufficient vaccines, people in the Caribbean face mammoth fiscal hurdles that ultimately might cost more lives than COVID, delta, or some other variant. Having to divert funds from other hard pressed development sectors into health and medical provisions has come at great costs. The region has had marked success averting mass death and flattening the infection curve, but how government leaders will manage economies in the future is unknown. Tourism is a principal economic driver, and some global industry leaders predict it will take as many as five years for air travel to return to levels approaching the early months of 2020.[35]

As tourism revenues in the Caribbean dropped from the outset of 2020 through the middle of 2021, national debts rose. Trinidad and Tobago Prime Minister and CARICOM Chairman Keith Rowley address economic problems the "perilous pandemic [COVID]" caused during an intersessional virtual meeting of a conference for CARICOM government heads.[36] The pandemic, a writer covering the meeting reported, "had disrupted every segment of society as the Region continued to deal with traditional threats to development such as climate change, external economic shocks, blacklisting and de-risking of financial institutions."[37] Rowley, the writer continued, told meeting delegates that COVID highlighted vulnerabilities in the Caribbean and in other SIDS.[38] Before closing, Rowley advocated "for vulnerability indices that took into account the impact climate change, natural disasters and global pandemic had on their development. 'This will permit Small Island Developing States access to much needed concessional financing to aid our recovery and build our resilience,'" he declared.[39]

## Conclusion

The matters I discuss in this essay will have implications for Christian churches in the Caribbean as well as for governments in the region. In my judgment, the COVID pandemic has spotlighted a lack of theological urgency by Christian communities. There has been a proliferation of items I call bless-me sermons, enrich-me-quickly choruses, and feel-good prayers; however, there has not been much theological engagement about the qualities of life among the Caribbean masses. Church conferences, conventions, and crusades are held with a blatant refusal to address urgent regional problems. Matters ranging from international debt forgiveness, overdependence on tourism, lack of regional food security, inadequate health provisions, climate change, disgruntled youth, and growing crime seldom are on the agendas of church councils. I therefore call for a paradigm shift in Caribbean theology. The new approach should be grounded in an indigenous Caribbean sociocultural landscape whose primary aim is the radical transformation and liberation of Caribbean society for the betterment of Caribbean people.

It is my hope that learning from congregational experiences with and responses to the COVID pandemic will encourage greater regional coordination between churches in community related efforts and initiatives, especially on the part of local denominations and congregations whose members prefer to operate independently. The strengthening of regional bodies such as the CCC and the EAC will facilitate enhanced data collection, pastoral and lay training, and more effective coordinating of programs to address regional and international challenges, especially in a highly vulnerable region such as the Caribbean.

## Notes

1  Gordon-Conwell Center for the Study of Global Christianity, *Christianity in Its Global Context, 1970–2020: Society, Religion, and Mission* (South Hamilton, MA: Gordon-Conwell Center for the Study of Global Christianity, 2013), 9, 15, 54–57, 77, 78; "Population of Caribbean (2019 and Historical)," *Worldometer*, https://www.worldometers.info/world-population/caribbean-population/.
2  Glenn A. Bowen, "The Challenges of Poverty and Social Welfare in the Caribbean," *International Journal of Social Welfare* 16 (April 2007): 150–58.
3  "Poverty Grows as Caribbean Countries Face Economic Challenges—CDB President," *Jamaica Observer*, July 2, 2015, http://www.jamaicaobserver.com/news/Poverty-grows-as-Caribbean-countries-face-economic-challenges-CDB-president_19158281.
4  Regarding Caribbean governments not prioritizing social disparities in healthcare, see Patrick Cloos, "Health Inequalities in the Caribbean: Increasing Opportunities and Resources," *Global Health Promotion* 17 (March 2010): 73–76.
5  Joseph Kiprop, "The Biggest Industries in Jamaica," *World Atlas Economics*, May 16, 2018, https://www.worldatlas.com/articles/the-biggest-industries-in-jamaica.html.
6  Daphne Ewing-Chow, "The Environmental Impact of Caribbean Tourism Undermines Its Economic Benefit," *Forbes*, November 26, 2019, https://www.forbes.com/sites/daphneewingchow/2019/11/26/the-carbon-footprint-of-caribbean-tourism-undermines-its-economic-benefit/#5510d7da3cb5.
7  Maricruz Arteaga Garavito et al., *The Consequences of COVID-19 on Livelihoods in Barbados: Results of a Telephone Survey* (Washington, DC: Inter-American Development Bank, 2020), 5, 8, 10, 11; Sergio Ley López and

Salvador Suárez Zaizar, *Dealmaking with China amid Global Economic Uncertainty: Opportunities, Risks, and Recommendations for Latin America and the Caribbean* (Washington, DC: Atlantic Council, 2020), 2.

8  Zhangkai J. Cheng and Jing Shan, "2019 Novel Coronavirus: Where We Are and What We Know," *PubMed.gov*, February 18, 2020, https://dx.doi.org/10.1007%2Fs15010-020-01401-y.

9  Ralston Hyman, "The Impact of High Debt Burdens on Small Caribbean States," September 29, 2007, https://michelerobinson.net/yahoo_site_admin/assets/docs/The_Impact_of_debt_on_Small_Caribbean_States.13884815.pdf.

10  Hyman, "Impact of High Debt Burdens," 2.

11  "WHO Director-General's Opening Remarks at the Media Briefing on COVID-19," *World Health Organization*, March 11, 2020, https://www.who.int/director-general/speeches/detail/who-director-general-s-opening-remarks-at-the-media-briefing-on-covid-19. March 11, 2020.

12  Caribbean Media Corporation, "Mottley Repeats Call for Global Leadership Initiative," *Nation News*, June 3, 2020, https://www.nationnews.com/nationnews/news/245915/mottley-repeats-global-leadership-initiative.

13  Daphne Ewing-Chow, 2020, "Exploring the Unique Impact of Coronavirus on Small Island Developing States," *Forbes*, March 31, 2020, https://www.forbes.com/sites/daphneewingchow/2020/03/31/exploring-the-unique-impact-of-coronavirus-on-small-island-developing-states/#57d9617e2e17. In addition to serving as pro vice-chancellor at the University of the West Indies, Clive Landis headed its COVID-19 taskforce.

14  "The World Bank in the Caribbean: Overview," June 8, 2020, https://www.worldbank.org/en/country/caribbean/overview.

15  Tara Donaldson, "Caribbean Islands Will Begin Reopening to Americans in June," *Condé Nast Traveler*, May 28, 2020, https://www.cntraveler.com/story/caribbean-islands-will-begin-reopening-to-americans-in-june.

16  World Health Organization, "Coronavirus Disease (COVID-19) Situation Report."

17  George Eaton Simpson, "Caribbean Religions: Afro-Caribbean Religions," in *Encyclopedia of Religion*, ed. Mircea Eliade (New York, NY: Macmillan, 1987), 3:90–98 (quotation on 90).

18  Gordon-Conwell Center for the Study of Global Christianity, *Christianity in Its Global Context*, 9, 15, 54–57, 77, 78.

19  Caribbean Conference of Churches, "About CCC: Introduction," n.d., https://www.ccc-caribe.org/eng/intro.htm (hereafter cited as CCC); "Caribbean Conference of Churches," *World Council of Churches*, n.d., https://www.oikoumene.org/organization/caribbean-conference-of-churches.

20  "Caribbean Conference of Churches"; CCC, "About CCC."

21  Evangelical Association of the Caribbean, "History," n.d., https://www.caribbeanea.org/about-us/history/. Pentecostals and Full Gospel adherents belong to the Evangelical Association of the Caribbean.

22  World Health Organization, "Coronavirus Disease (COVID-19) Situation Report—162," June 3, 2021, https://www.who.int/docs/default-source/coronaviruse/20200630-covid-19-sitrep-162.pdf?sfvrsn=e00a5466_2; Reuters, "COVID-19 Tracker: Latin America and the Caribbean," September 7, 2021, https://graphics.reuters.com/world-coronavirus-tracker-and-maps/regions/latin-america-and-the-caribbean/.

23  Fred Hassell, "World Council of Churches Pray for End of Covid-19 Pandemic," *Royal Gazette*, April 3, 2021, https://www.royalgazette.com/religion/lifestyle/article/20210403/world-council-of-churches-pray-for-end-of-covid-19-pandemic/.

24  Jo Ella Holman, "Caribbean Churches Respond in This Time of COVID-19," *Presbyterian Mission*, June 1, 2020, https://www.presbyterianmission.org/ministries/missionconnections/letter/caribbean-churches-respond-in-this-time-of-covid-19/.

25  United Nations Educational, Scientific and Cultural Organisation Cluster Office for the Caribbean, "Education Response to COVID-19 in the Caribbean," January 3, 2020, https://en.unesco.org/caribbean-education-response.

26  Development Bank of Latin America, "Latin America and the Caribbean: Digital Transformation Key to Recovery and Building Back Better, Says New Report," September 24, 2020, https://www.caf.com/en/currently/news/2020/09/latin-america-and-the-caribbean-digital-transformation-key-to-recovery-and-building-back-better-says-new-report/, citing Organisation for Economic Co-Operation and Development Centre et al., *Latin American Economic Outlook 2020: Digital Transformation for Building Back Better* (Paros, France: OECD Publishing, 2020), 32.

27  Akanksha Sharma and Barbara Arese Lucini, *Connected Society: Digital Inclusion in Latin America and the Caribbean* (London: Global System for Mobile Communications, 2015), 3.

28  Sharma and Lucini, *Connected Society*, 3.

29  Clinton Chisholm, "No Sense in COVID-19 Vaccine being Mark of the Beast," *Jamaica Observer*, May 3, 2021, https://301-joweb.newscyclecloud.com/letters/no-sense-in-covid-19-vaccine-being-mark-of-the-beast_220563?profile=1449.

30  Hassell, "World Council of Churches."

31  World Health Organization, "COVAX," n.d., https://www.who.int/initiatives/act-accelerator/covax.

32  Pan American Health Organization, "Countries in the Americas Notified of First COVID-19 Vaccine Allocations through COVAX," January 31, 2021, https://www.paho.org/en/news/31-1-2021-countries-americas-notified-first-covid-19-vaccine-allocations-through-covax (hereafter cited as PAHO).

33  Jacqueline Charles et al., "'Shocking imbalance': Latin America's Poorest Shut Out of Vaccine Access as COVID Surges," *Miami Herald*, May 17, 2021, https://www.miamiherald.com/news/nation-world/world/americas/haiti/article251071689.html (quotation); PAHO, "Countries in the Americas Notified."

34  "Cuba Expands Emergency COVID-19 Vaccination in Havana," *Xinhua*, http://www.xinhuanet.com/english/2021-06/15/c_1310007823.htm.

35  Sarah Khan, "The Era of Peak Travel is Over," *Vox*, April 22, 2020, https://www.vox.com/the-highlight/2020/4/16/21216676/coronavirus-covid-19-travel-vacation-tourism-overtourism.

36  Michelle Nurse, "Pandemic Underscores Importance of Regionalism, Multilateralism, South-South Cooperation—CARICOM Chair," CARICOM Today, February 27, 2021, https://today.caricom.org/2021/02/24/pandemic-underscores-importance-of-regionalism-multilateralism-south-south-cooperation-caricom-chair/

37  Nurse, "Pandemic Underscores Importance."

38  Nurse, "Pandemic Underscores Importance."

39  Nurse, "Pandemic Underscores Importance."

# 17 Black Majority Church Responses to Black Health Urgencies in the United Kingdom

*Natasha Callender and Alton P. Bell*

## Introduction

Within the United Kingdom (UK), one of the most significant global health urgencies of the twenty-first century, COVID-19, has disproportionately affected black communities. Though one of the smallest minority ethnic groups in the UK, comprising 1.9 million of 63.2 million people in the country, black people have some of the highest rates of COVID-related deaths. That fact highlights troubling connections between socioeconomic and structural inequalities and poor health in black communities.[1]

A 2020 report on disparities in risks and outcomes from COVID drafted by Public Health England (PHE) indicated "people of Black, Asian and other minority ethnic groups may be more exposed to COVID-19, and therefore are more likely to be diagnosed. This could be the result of factors associated with ethnicity such as occupation, population density, use of public transport, household composition and housing conditions."[2] We believe long-standing social disadvantages underpinned by structural inequalities help explain health disparities in black communities.

Even though many researchers in the UK do not track indices of racial or ethnic inequality very accurately, that one in five children in black households live in poverty is a reasonable estimation, as black people often live in deprived areas and earn comparatively low pay.[3] A 2012 study demonstrated that black people of African Caribbean origin were up to three times more likely to develop Type 2 diabetes than white people of European origin.[4] A more recent survey, conducted in 2020 by the UK Office of National Statistics, found that 67.5 percent of 1,730 adult black respondents were overweight or obese; that percentage was the highest of any ethnic group the office surveyed (see Table 17.1).[5] Such comorbidities pose great risks of poor outcomes among black people who acquire COVID.[6]

In terms of the scale of impact of health urgencies, human immunodeficiency virus (HIV) and acquired immunodeficiency syndrome (AIDS) have been most devastating to black communities. In 2012, for example, black people made up 1.8 percent of the population in the UK but 34 percent of diagnosed HIV cases.[7] The prevalence of mental health conditions—for example,

DOI: 10.4324/9781003214281-20

Table 17.1 Percentage of Overweight or Obese Adults, 2019/2020[1]

| Ethnicity | Percentage | Number of respondents |
|---|---|---|
| All | 62.8 | 149,476 |
| Asian | 59.7 | 5,781 |
| Black | 67.5 | 1,730 |
| Chinese | 32.2 | 837 |
| Mixed | 59.6 | 1,755 |
| White British | 63.7 | 127,113 |
| White other | 58 | 8,281 |
| Other | 61.2 | 1,118 |

anxiety, depression, and psychiatric conditions such as schizophrenia—is another notable health urgency among black people in the UK. The association of racial discrimination with increased "weathering," or the difference between biological age and chronological age, is one explanation for such prevalence.[8] Racial discrimination is another. Scholars have shown that experiencing it can result in negative emotions that affect psychological well-being adversely, yielding "symptoms of distress and increasing the risk of discrete psychiatric disorders" and bad physical conditions.[9]

Negative emotions can cause biological dysregulation, thereby contributing to "indicators of subclinical disease and chronic physical illness. Coping with negative emotional states can also lead to increases in risky health behaviors, including declines in the utilization of and engagement with health care services."[10] As a 2018 report noted, black women were "most likely to have experienced a common mental disorder such as anxiety or depression in the last week," and black men were "most likely to have experienced a psychotic disorder in the past year. [Collectively, black adults] were more likely than adults in other ethnic groups to have been sectioned under the Mental Health Act."[11]

Black health vulnerabilities among socially disadvantaged groups have required the nation's black majority churches (BMC) to adopt innovative methods of pastoral care, physical health and well-being support. Although documentation of BMC support of black health communities is somewhat lacking, case reports of BMC work with local authorities, health agencies, and the voluntary sector organizations in addressing black health urgencies during the recent pandemic are notable, as discussed here.[12]

## Black Majority Churches: Backstories, Resources, and Responses to Health Needs

Black health vulnerabilities among socially disadvantaged groups have required BMC in the UK to adopt innovative methods of pastoral care, physical health, and well-being support. Although there is a dearth of information about such assistance, thousands of BMC have worked with local authorities, health agencies, and the volunteers to address black health urgencies for decades. Their collaborations during the COVID-19 pandemic are especially notable, and a few backstories to the modern-day presence of black people in the UK helps one understand the need for such collaborations.[13]

In 1948, a ship called the *MV Empire Windrush* docked in Tilbury with 492 British subjects, mainly from Jamaica.[14] The British government intended to use them to help rebuild the post-World War II economy, and their arrival coincided with the National Health Service (NHS), an agency the government created to provide universal access to healthcare.[15] Decades later, in 2012, the NHS published a constitution that reinforced many aspects of an equality act British officials ratified in 2010.[16] Key protections included universal healthcare access to all citizens irrespective of gender, race, disability, age, sexual orientation, religious belief, maternity or pregnancy, and marital or civil partnership status.[17] Present black health disparities in the UK, however, are at odds with notions of health equity promised in the NHS Constitution. Moreover, the disparities have existed since Caribbean immigrants aboard the *Empire Windrush* arrived in 1948.

Racial discrimination is a primary reason for decades of black health disparities in the UK. During the 1950s and 1960s, living conditions were unfavorable for the black Caribbean-born population because racism had a negative effect on employment, housing, religious observance, and many other elements of society.[18] Most black Caribbean people who immigrated to the UK were Christian, and many were Anglican, Methodist, Baptist, or Seventh Day Adventist who found churches monochromatic and unwelcoming.[19] The combination of social and religious discrimination led to the rapid growth of BMCs, with Pentecostal and Holiness churches gaining particular strength in the conurbations where Caribbean immigrants settled.[20] Similar trends arose among West Africans who arrived in the UK during the 1970s.[21]

By 2007, according to one estimation, there were as many as 500,000 committed black Christians in the UK.[22] Many attended independent or standalone BMCs, so an accurate number is difficult to calculate.[23] The demise of the African Caribbean Evangelical Alliance in 2010 worsened matters.[24] Fortunately, members of the National Churches Leaders Forum in London and the Council of Black Led (later Majority) Churches in the West Midlands helped fill the void.[25]

Although several historic churches and parachurch organizations have employed social justice relationship managers during the twenty-first century, many independent churches have not integrated well into their communities and therefore have been unaware of potential support available from local authorities and third sector organizations to advance public health initiatives.[26] For example, governmental agencies such as PHE have recognized the need to empower communities to screen for and potentially prevent HIV/AIDS, thereby improving public health. Some agency resources have benefited faith communities in particular. Catholics for AIDS Prevention and Support obtained funding from PHE to produce a 2017 video series called *Positive Faith*.[27] During the same year, PHE published *Guide to Healthy Living: Mosques* to promote the prevention of modifiable risk factors (e.g. obesity, high cholesterol) and to better long-term condition management.[28] The National AIDS Trust worked with a variety of organizations, to include BMCs and other faith-based entities, to reduce the stigmatizing of those with HIV or AIDS, to curb the spread of the diseases, and to promote healthy lifestyles in general.[29]

As stated above, there are mental health needs among African-Caribbean populations in the UK that BMCs can do more to address. Faith leaders can perform major roles in raising awareness about mental health. For example, they can help provide services to those in need, but fears and stigmas in black communities toward mental health often discourage individuals from accessing the services. Of equal significance as those occurrences, many BMCs have not approached mental health needs with the same degree of urgency as BMCs have approached physical health needs. Oftentimes, a lack of awareness or adequate training about mental health warnings is a key reasons BMCs prioritize physical health. Unbeknownst to many members, mental health can affect physical health.[30]

There are notable exceptions to the general rule above regarding mental health providers training BMC leaders. For instance, a mental health charity in London trained 100 leaders from across four boroughs over a three-year period, utilizing a ten-week course on spirituality and mental health developed.[31] In addition to that project, researchers and BMCs in the UK have joined forces to develop "'dementia-friendly,' community hubs."[32] Those kinds of collaborations between BMCs and local mental health services are not widespread in the UK, however, and need better publication and replication. Given that BMCs provide places of trusted peer and community support, the organizations are positioned to guide balanced theological and healthy living discourses and programs.

## Conclusion

Among the responses of BMCs, the National Church Leaders Forum produced a ten-point plan focused on short-term solutions and strategic asks to better resource BMCs whose members seek to assist with health urgencies.[33] Several BMCs and affiliated organizations provided structured well-being support campaigns to distribute personal protective equipment to essential workers or held seminars on health promotion and long-term condition management.[34] Black majority churches likewise provided online health workshops and seminars that professionals led.

In light of ongoing black health urgencies in the UK, the COVID-19 pandemic has made clear, we call for a national BMC registry to increase visibility, identify needs, and promote collaboration. We also encourage BMCs to work with voluntary organizations, local authorities, and health services to create interventions for church leaders to better support the well-being of BMC members; accelerate the training of health champions who, in turn, can advocate and provide long-term care for serious health conditions such as cardiovascular disease and diabetes; and, among other initiatives, expand empirical research exploring impact of racism on health outcomes.

## Notes

1 Population data are from 2011, the year of the most recent official decennial census available to the public. The 2021 census will not be available until 2022. See Aaron O'Neill, "United Kingdom—Ethnicity," *Statista*, April 15, 2021, https://www.statista.com/statistics/270386/ethnicity-in-the-united-kingdom/#:~:text=Black%20British%20citizens%2C%20with%20African,of%20the%20total%20UK%20population; Abdul Razaq et al., "BAME Covid-19 Deaths—What Do We Know? Rapid Data and Evidence Review," *Centre for Evidence-Based Medicine*, May 5, 2020, https://www.cebm.net/covid-19/bame-covid-19-deaths-what-do-we-know-rapid-data-evidence-review/; and Public Health England, *Beyond the Data: Understanding the Impact of COVID-19 on BAME Communities* (London: Public Health England, 2020), 5 (hereafter cited as PHE); and PHE, *Disparities in the Risk and Outcomes of COVID-19* (London: Public Health England, 2020), 4–8.
2 PHE, *Beyond the Data*, 6.
3 For general household data as of 2018 about black, white, and other people in the UK, see Cabinet Office, *Race Disparity Audit: Summary Findings from the Ethnicity Facts and Figures Website*, rev. ed. (London: Crown, 2018).
4 Therese Tillin et al., "Southall and Brent REvisited: Cohort Profile of SABRE, a UK Population-Based Comparison of Cardiovascular Disease and Diabetes in People of European, Indian Asian and African Caribbean Origins," *International Journal of Epidemiology* 21 (February 2012): 33–42.
5 Active Live Adults Survey, "Overweight Adults," *Gov.UK*, June 25, 2021, https://www.ethnicity-facts-figures.service.gov.uk/health/diet-and-exercise/overweight-adults/latest (hereafter cited as ALAS).
6 Jim McManus, "Positive Faith—A HIV Resource with a Difference," November 12, 2017, https://publichealthmatters.blog.gov.uk/2017/11/12/positive-faith-a-hiv-resource-with-a-difference/.
7 National AIDS Trust, *HIV and Black African Communities in the UK* (London: National AIDS Trust, 2014), 1, 4, 5.
8 Sarah Forrester, "Racial Differences in Weathering and Its Associations with Psychosocial Stress: The CARDIA Study," *Population Health* 7 (April 2019): 1–8.
9 David A. Williams and Brigette A. Davis, "Understanding How Discrimination Can Affect Health," *Health Services Research* 54 (December 2019): 1375, citing Rodney Clark et al., "Racism as a Stressor for African Americans: A Biopsychosocial Model," *American Psychologist* 54 (October 1999): 805–16.
10 Williams and Davis, "Understanding How Discrimination Can Affect Health," 1375.
11 Cabinet Office, *Race Disparity Audit*, 12. See also Mental Health Act 1983, https://www.legislation.gov.uk/ukpga/1983/20/contents; Mental Health Act 2007, https://www.legislation.gov.uk/ukpga/2007/12/contents; and Mental Health (Scotland) Act 2015, https://www.legislation.gov.uk/asp/2015/9/contents/enacted.
12 Maiden, op. cit.

13 See John Maiden, "'Race', Black Majority Churches, and the Rise of Ecumenical Multiculturalism in the 1970s," *Twentieth Century British History* 30 (July 2019): 531–56; and Cassandra J. St. Vil, "Training Up the Child: Youth Participation and Cultural Pride in Black Majority Churches in Britain, PhD diss., Howard University, 2009, v, 11–12.

14 See, for example, Karen Bonner, "Windrush and the NHS—An Entwined History," June 22, 2020, National Health Service, https://www.england. nhs.uk/blog/windrush-and-the-nhs-an-entwined-history/ (employing *HMT Empire Windrush*, one of several alternative handles for the ship).

15 Bonner, "Windrush and the NHS."

16 NHS Constitution for England, March 8, 2012, https://www.gov.uk/ government/publications/the-nhs-constitution-for-england.

17 NHS Constitution for England;

18 See Joe Aldred and Keno Ogbo, eds., *The Black Church in the Twenty-First Century* (London: Darton, Longman and Todd, 2010); Maiden, "Race"; and Israel Oluwole Olofinjana, "The History of Black Majority Churches in London," 2010, http://www.open.ac.uk/arts/research/religion-in-london/sites/ www.open.ac.uk.arts.research.religion-in-london/files/files/ecms/arts-rl-pr/ web-content/Black-Majority-Churches-in-London.pdf.

19 See Joe Aldred and Keno Ogbo, eds., *The Black Church in the Twenty-First Century* (London: Darton, Longman and Todd, 2010); John Maiden, "'Race', Black Majority Churches, and the Rise of Ecumenical Multiculturalism in the 1970s," *Twentieth Century British History* 30 (July 2019): 531–56; and Israel Oluwole Olofinjana, "The History of Black Majority Churches in London," 2010, http://www.open.ac.uk/arts/research/religion-in-london/sites/www.open. ac.uk.arts.research.religion-in-london/files/files/ecms/arts-rl-pr/web-content/ Black-Majority-Churches-in-London.pdf.

20 Olofinjana, "History of Black Majority Churches."

21 Olofinjana, "History of Black Majority Churches."

22 Joe Aldred, "Are Black Churches Contributing to Cohesion or Polarising Christians and Other Faith Groups?," *Churches Together in England*, June 15, 2007, https://www.cte.org.uk/Groups/236173/Home/Resources/Pentecostal_ and_Multicultural/Reports_Papers_Videos/Black_Church_in/Black_ Church_in.aspx.

23 See *What the London Church Census Reveals: London's Churches are Growing!* (London: London City Commission, 2012), 1–17; and Andrew Rogers, "How are Black Majority Churches Growing in the UK? A London Borough Case Study," December 28, 2016, https://blogs.lse.ac.uk/religionglobalsociety/2016/12/how-are-black-majority-churches-growing-in-the-uk-a-london-borough-case-study/.

24 "The African Caribbean Evangelical Alliance," *Charity Commission for England and Wales*, n.d., https://register-of-charities.charitycommission.gov.uk/ charity-search/-/charity-details/802887/linked-or-removed-charity-overview.

25 "The Council of Black Led Churches," *Local Prayers*, n.d., https://www. localprayers.com/GB/Birmingham/225287840845157/Council-of-Black-Led-Churches; "Council of Black Majority Churches," Open Charities, n.d., http://opencharities.org/charities/1121312; "The National Church Leaders Forum (NCLF)—a Black Christian Voice," n.d., https://nclf.org.uk/ nclf-steering-group-members/;

26 Leslie Fesenmyer, "African-Initiated Pentecostal Churches are on the Rise in the UK—What Role Do They Seek to Play in Wider Society?," November 23, 2016, https://blogs.lse.ac.uk/religionglobalsociety/2016/11/ african-initiated-pentecostal-churches-are-on-the-rise-in-the-uk-what-role-do-they-seek-to-play-in-wider-society/.

27 Positive Faith, "Church, Community and HIV," 2017, http://www.positive-faith.net/church-community-and-hiv.html.

28 Public Health England, *Guide to Healthy Living: Mosques* (London: Public Health England, 2017).

29 National AIDS Trust, *HIV and Black African Communities*; National AIDS Trust, *HIV and Finance: Exploring Access to Financial Services for People Living with HIV in the UK* (London: National AIDS Trust, 2017); National AIDS Trust, *HIV Support Services—The State of the Nations: Executive Summary* (London: National AIDS Trust, 2017).

30 Rachel-Rose Burrell, "The Black Majority Church: Exploring the Impact of Faith and a Faith Community on Mental Health and Well-Being," PhD diss., Middlesex University, 2019.

31 National Health Service Southwark Clinical Commissioning Group, *Working with Black Majority Churches (BMCs) to Improve the Mental Health and Well-being of Southwark People* (London: National Health Service, 2013).

32 University of Manchester, "Enabling Caribbean People to Live Well with Dementia: Development 'Dementia-Friendly', Community Hubs with Black Majority Churches," n.d., https://www.research.manchester.ac.uk/portal/en/projects/enabling-caribbean-people-to-live-well-with-dementia-development-dementiafriendly-community-hubs-with-black-majority-churches(7c-c7e3b2-06c3-466e-8feb-aaa41b9bed9a).html.

33 "NCLF Ten-Point Plan for Churches Post COVID-19 Lockdown," *Churches Together in England*, n.d., https://www.cte.org.uk/Articles/579375/Home/News/Latest_news/NCLF_ten_point.aspx.

34 Ade Amooba and R. David Muir, "Submissions to Statutory Reviews of the Impact of COVID-19 on BAME Communities," *National Church Leaders Forum*, https://nclf.org.uk/.

# 18 COVID-19, Cultural Competency, and Church Responsiveness in Nigeria

*Justina A. Ogodo, Martha Folashade Atanda, A. Christson Adedoyin, Sabrina A. Carter, and Jamar Thrasher*

## Introduction

The COVID-19 pandemic created much hardship for many Nigerians, particularly those in rural communities whose members value face-to-face interaction and where empathy and trust are measured through language and cultural contexts such as religion.[1] In northern Nigeria, a faith-based nonprofit organization called the Zion World Prayer and Missions (ZWPM) leveraged its cultural competency and responsiveness in rural communities of the Muslim-dominated region. During the pandemic, the ZWPM and similar organizations helped rural populations survive by formulating educated religious and secular responses to prevent COVID transmission.[2] This essay presents social and historical contexts of Nigeria to demonstrate how the ZWPM effectively engaged with under-resourced rural communities during the pandemic.

## Nigeria in Historical Perspective

Nigeria, the most populous country in Africa, lies in the sub-Saharan area and has about 219 million people, 250 ethnic groups, as well as 500 languages and dialects.[3] The country is partitioned into six geopolitical zones—North West, North Central, North East, South, South West, and South East—that represent the country's cultural, historical, and ethnic lines.[4] While Nigeria's existence dates to antiquity, its modern history begins with the British government's amalgamation of the border Northern and Southern regions, not zones, in 1914. Not only were those areas distinctly different linguistically, religiously, and politically but the areas also remain distinct a century later, as both regions strive for dominance. The North is predominantly Islamic, with a marginalized fraction practicing Christianity, whereas the South was home to several traditional religions before the advent of Christianity, which southerners embraced ardently.[5] According to 2020 estimates from the Pew Research Center, Muslims represented 51.1 percent of the Nigerian population and Christians 46.9.[6]

DOI: 10.4324/9781003214281-21

Regardless of the regions or the zones where Nigerians reside or the religious beliefs to which they adhere, most face challenges. For example, beyond the business capital, Lagos, and the federal capital territory, Abuja, many rural communities exist without basic amenities, including pipe-borne water, paved roads, functioning healthcare systems, and access to technology. According to National Bureau of Statistics data, about 82.9 million Nigerians lived under the poverty line set at 137,430 nairas ($381.75) per year, and 27.1 percent—a number that included many college graduates—were unemployed.[7] The absence of basic human needs notwithstanding, the rift between the North and the South has morphed with the insurgency of several militant groups, including Fulani herdsmen and the Boko-Haram (translated "Western education is forbidden").[8] Those groups have launched systematic attacks on individuals, communities, and even the Nigerian federal government, which Northern leaders control. Such egregious attacks continue daily without recourse from government officials, some of whom have openly supported the obliteration of southerners because of their predominant faith, Christianity.[9] The COVID-19 pandemic has expanded internal upheavals, human calamities, and property losses.

## COVID-19 and Nigerian Government Response

Nigeria's Federal Ministry of Health reported the first case of COVID-19 in Nigeria on February 27, 2020: An Italian businessman from Milan was infected.[10] When the World Health Organization declared COVID a global pandemic on March 11,[11] the Nigerian federal government established a presidential task force to spearhead the state fight against the pandemic.[12] As with former Ebola outbreaks that caused many African countries to invest in national public health institutes, the Nigeria Centre for Disease Control bolstered its support for training, emergency response preparedness, and public health messaging to deal with COVID.[13]

The Nigerian federal government's COVID readiness effort commenced before the first reported case. As Epidemiologist Chikwe Ihekweazu noted on January 2020, the Public Health Institute supported laboratories increasing testing and training in all thirty-six states by December 2019.[14] The existing systems would enable prevention, early detection, and prompt response to infectious disease.[15] Government officials imposed restrictive orders on gatherings and travels, and they mandated preventive measures such as social distancing and wearing a face mask in public.[16] Despite those initiatives, Nigeria recorded 29,789 confirmed COVID cases and 669 deaths by early July, according to the World Health Organization.[17] In brief, Nigeria had one of the highest infection rates in Africa, ranking next only to South Africa, reputed as the epicenter of the outbreak in Africa, with 215,855 and 3,502 deaths.[18]

The Nigerian federal government's presidential task force and its Centre for Disease Control provided information about COVID to citizens in 2020, but some communications did not reach the hinterlands where rural communities were severely under resourced, particularly with regard to formal education. Citizens in those places struggled more than those in urban communities because of multifaceted obstacles. A lack of functioning infrastructure, a flawed or non-existing healthcare system, lack of electricity, and an unreliable communications apparatuses were illustrative. Moreover, because of a general public distrust of the government, the onus fell on churches and other private organizations and philanthropists to combat the COVID pandemic at the grassroots levels.[19]

### Church Responses to COVID-19: Zion World Prayer and Missions as a Case Study

Nigerian church responses to COVID were not epochal. During the Ebola and the human immunodeficiency virus/acquired immunodeficiency syndrome (HIV/AIDS) epidemics, among other perilous times, churchgoers provided health education, participated in case findings and monitoring activities, influenced behavioral change, and communicated with quarantined people via text messaging. Members of the Redeemed Christian Church of God were microcosms. In addition to caring for Nigerians infected with HIV/AIDS and preventing the spread of the disease in their country, they used the international platform of the denomination to promote HIV/AIDS awareness to people across the globe.[20]

Many faith-based institutions in Nigeria have assumed comparable roles during the COVID pandemic. They have donated money and equipment to public health facilities, converted church-owned health centers and related facilities into isolation centers, and provided food and other in-kind resources to alleviate the impact of lockdowns, shutdowns, stay-at-home orders, and similar protective measures.[21] Faith-based institutions also have disseminated information about preventive protocols, provided psychosocial support, and modeled positive health behaviors and spiritual practices such as praying and fasting. Financial institutions and private citizens (e.g., philanthropists) have performed similar roles. Despite such laudable work, many Nigerian Christians have minimized potential dangers of COVID because they believed God can protect them from the virus; therefore, they have disregard government mandates to limit the sizes of in-person services, to cancel events, or to take similar precautions during the pandemic.[22]

The ZWPM has worked hard to ensure public safety in Nigeria during the COVID pandemic.[23] An indigenous organization founded by Martins Atanda in 1995, the ZWPM has been at the forefront in assisting minority Christian populations in rural, low resourced, and Muslim-dominated areas in North West Nigeria. The ZWPM anchors its vision in Matthew 9:36–38, which describes how Jesus showed compassion for the multitudes who were fainting and prayed for laborers in the field ripe for harvest.[24]

The ZWPM's holistic mission also is rooted in the call for the churchgoing community to be the "salt of the earth" and the "light of the world."[25]

Scholars Diana Garland and Gaynor Yancey suggest Christians should respond to God's word by addressing their neighbors' needs.[26] The King's Assembly, the church arm of ZWPM, provides such care for its estimated 450-member congregation, 95 percent of whom belong to minority groups in Sokoto City, the predominantly Muslim city where the church is situated.[27] The ZWPM collaborates with Zethar Al-Umma Foundation and other local, national, and worldwide nonprofit organizations to fund COVID initiatives in thirty-three villages across northern Nigeria as well as in twenty-eight other villages and towns in twenty more African countries.[28] Without disregarding scientific explanations for the occurrence of disease, including COVID, the ZWPM believes in the "hermeneutic of spiritual power" to combat illness.[29] For example, sermonizing, praying, fasting, encouraging, and dispelling fears are spiritual warfare against COVID, especially for church members, first responders, and frontline workers.

### Cultural Competency

Given cultural differences within the ZWPM membership as well as within the various rural communities the organization serves, cultural competency plays a crucial role in effective service. Cultural competency is the ability to center and respond to societal backgrounds and related differences of people to meet their needs.[30] To be culturally competent is to recognize the role of traditional beliefs, mores, norms, and similar items that govern decision-making processes in a targeted group.[31] Cultural competency is acquired over time through interactions and immersions with people who ordinarily distrust outsiders.[32]

The ZWPM's commitment to cultural competency and existing relationships has allowed the organization to communicate well with the rural communities it serves during the COVID-19 pandemic. Consequently, the ZWPM has been able to convey preventive care strategies because the organization has people with diverse ethnic and cultural backgrounds in its membership. The ZWMP, moreover, prioritizes no local cultural belief and adheres to three additional elements of cultural competency: active listening, empathy, and effective engagement.[33]

### Active Listening

Active listening is relational and requires being open and curious about others' experiences and perspectives while focusing on commonalities and differences. Face-to-face interactions, listening for meaning, and understanding to build trust are paramount activities. The ZWPM leaders' appreciation of scripture informs their choices and actions; however, in their work with rural communities, leaders also seek to understand local cultural practices by listening to indigenous stories. During the COVID pandemic, ZWPM leaders have used those stories, among other means, to identify and to meet the physical needs of indigenes. Lessons about proper handwashing and nutrition; providing face masks, food, and financial assistance; and building water purification and human waste disposal systems are representative acts.

### *Empathy*

The ZWPM trains its leaders to respect cultural differences when making decisions. Immersing themselves in the communities, they serve helps achieve that goal. Compassion is foremost. The ZWPM encourages its urban members—particularly, professionals and students—to be compassionate when leaving the comforts of their homes to help in rural communities where residents lack sufficient food, shelter, water, health services, income, education, and other basic sustainability items. The ZWPM also encourages urban members to identify with the culture of rural communities by eating local foods and by endorsing cultural dressings when appropriate.[34]

The COVID-19 pandemic has presented a real challenge to the ZWPM. For starters, many rural dwellers initially did not believe COVID existed. Hence, providing accurate information to them was crucial. The ZWPM taught preventative health by promoting immune-boosting foods and herbs, an act that reflected compassion and cultural competency because many rural communities were accustomed to preventing ailments with herbs. Furthermore, the ZWPM used ginger, garlic, pawpaw leaves, lemon, and other nutritious foods and herbs found locally to improve diets and thereby aid in COVID prevention. Those whom the ZWPM served received the information well.

### *Effective Engagement*

Forging mutually beneficial and nonjudgmental relationships are core elements of effective engagement. The ZWPM has done since 1995 by allowing individual ethnic groups to choose their modes of service. For example, before the COVID pandemic, the ZWPM established partnerships with indigenous, international faith-based, humanitarian, government, and other organizations whose members respected outside perspectives. The ZWPM also developed literacy and skill-building initiatives for women that included soap making, sewing, and knitting. The other ZWPM members, and organizational partners likewise funded and constructed handwashing stations using locally sourced materials to make soap available to those who otherwise would not have it readily.

The ZWPM has continued to forge similar relationships during the COVID pandemic. A leadership institute trains participants for public sector positions and challenges them to interact with the government. Via the King's Assembly and collaborations with humanitarian organizations such as the Zethar Al-Umma Foundation, the ZWPM has distributed face masks to churches and to individual community members throughout several villages. Though many people the ZWPM and its partners serve have limited internet access, the ZWPM's internet-based radio broadcasts, messaging applications, Facebook posts, and other devices play complementary roles in how ZWPM engages more than 2,500 people on regular bases. The ZWPM also uses technology to host Zoom meetings featuring medical professionals who educate rural communities about COVID updates and preventive measures, among other things. Regardless of religion or tribe, people benefit from such services.

## Conclusion

Despite notable successes for more than a quarter century, the ZWPM continues to face multiple challenges. Limited technology is foremost. As shown in the preceding paragraph, the ZWPM utilizes available resources as well as it can; however, unstable internet networks and a dearth of internet-compliant devices in rural communities have adverse effects on the disseminating of information throughout many villages. In addition to those problems, many residents do not have much access to formal education. Low literacy rates decrease the benefit of written materials. Persistent poverty and infrastructure underdevelopment are reflected in the scarce supply of food, clean water, and healthcare services in the areas the ZWPM serves. Those factors deepen the well of challenges the ZWPM must tackle, but threats of violence are the most challenging. Nevertheless, the ZWPM is dedicated to assisting people in underserved areas throughout North West Nigeria.

The work of the ZWPM during the COVID-19 pandemic is especially noteworthy. On May 7, 2020, the World Health Organization estimated Africa would suffer between 83,000 and 190,000 COVID-related deaths if the pandemic continued to spread unabated.[35] Many of those deaths would occur in Nigeria because it is the most populous country on the continent. As of June 26, 2021, however, Nigerian officials had recorded only 2,119 confirmed deaths.[36] That number is questionable because of low or no testing capacity in many places, but the general ability of Nigerians to have comparatively few verified deaths associated with COVID without access to sufficient healthcare systems and related services is remarkable.[37]

The ZWPM has an even more distinct COVID narrative than the national Nigerian story. The ZWPM has operated in an orthodoxy grounded in Christian scripture while also engaging in orthopraxis to curb the effects of COVID. Nigerian officials announced the first case in February 2020. As of June 2021, the ZWPM had not recorded any active case or death among its members or networks.

# Notes

1  Martin Atanda, "Key Help for Eliminating Rural Poverty and Helping Inform Rural Poor about COVID-19," (presentation during a Geneva Institute of Leadership and Public Policy videoconference, June 2–3, 2020).

2  Adebola Adegboyega et al., "Social Distance Impact on Church Gatherings: Socio-Behavioral Implications," *Journal of Human Behavior in the Social Environment* 31 (2021): 221–34.

3  Central Intelligence Agency, "Explore All Countries—Nigeria," *World Fact Book*, July 20, 2021, https://www.cia.gov/the-world-factbook/countries/nigeria/.

4  Endurance A. Ophori et al., "Current Trends of Immunization in Nigeria: Prospect and Challenges," *Tropical Medicine and Health* 42 (April 2014): 67–75.

5  John Gramlich, "Fast Facts about Nigeria and Its Immigrants as U.S. Travel Ban Expands," *Pew Research Center*, May 31, 2020, https://www.pewresearch. org/fact-tank/2020/02/03/fast-facts-about-nigeria-and-its-immigrants-as-u-s-travel-ban-expands/. In addition to the South, Nigerians in Middle West also adhered to traditional religious beliefs prior to embracing Christianity.

6  Pew-Templeton Global Religious Futures Project, "Nigeria—Religious Demography: Affiliation," n.d., http://www.globalreligiousfutures.org/countries/nigeria#/?affiliations_religion_id=0&affiliations_year=2020&region_name=All%20Countries&restrictions_year=2016.

7  National Bureau of Statistics, "2019 Poverty and Inequality in Nigeria: Executive Summary" (Abuja, Nigeria: National Bureau of Statistics, 2020), 1–25, esp. 5–6; National Bureau of Statistics, "Labor Force Statistics: Unemployment and Underemployment Report: Abridged Labour Force Survey Under COVID-19" (Abuja, Nigeria: National Bureau of Statistics, 2020), 1–90, esp. 2.

8  As Daniel E. Agbiboa recounted in 2014, the term *Boko Haram* "is derived from a combination of the Hausa word, boko (book), and the Arabic word, haram (forbidden). Put together, Boko Haram means 'Western education is forbidden.'" Agbiboa, "Peace at Daggers Drawn? Boko Haram and the State of Emergency in Nigeria," *Studies in Conflict and Terrorism* 37 (January 2014): 54.

9  Agbiboa, "Peace at Daggers Drawn," 41–67.

10  Osagie Ehanire, "First Case of Coronavirus Disease Confirmed in Nigeria," *Nigeria Centre for Disease Control*, February 28, 2020, https://www.ncdc.gov. ng/news/227/first-case-of-corona-virus-disease-confirmed-in-nigeria.

11  "WHO Director-General's Opening Remarks at the Media Briefing on COVID-19," *World Health Organization*, March 11, 2020, https://www.who.int/ director-general/speeches/detail/who-director-general-s-opening-remarks-at-the-media-briefing-on-covid-19. March 11, 2020.

12  Information about the Federal Government of Nigeria Presidential Task Force on COVID-19 can be found at https://statehouse.gov.ng/covid19/.

13  Chikwe Ihekweazu, "Steps Nigeria Is Taking to Prepare for Cases of Coronavirus," *Conversation*, January 28, 2020, https://theconversation.com/ steps-nigeria-is-taking-to-prepare-for-cases-of-coronavirus-130704.

14  Ihekweazu, "Steps."

15  Ihekweazu, "Steps."

16  Ebere Roseann Agusi et al., "The COVID-19 Pandemic and Social Distancing in Nigeria: Ignorance or Defiance," *Pan African Medical Journal* 35, supplement 2 (May 28, 2020): 1–3.

17  World Health Organization Regional Office for Africa, *COVID-19 Situation Update for the WHO African Region 8 July 2020: External Situation Report 19* (Brazzaville, Republic of Congo: World Health Organization, 2020), 2, 4 (hereafter cited as WHOROA).

18  WHOROA, *COVID-19 Situation Update*, 2, 4, 6.

19  Christian C. Ezeibe et al., "Political Distrust and the Spread of COVID-19 in Nigeria," *Global Public Health* 15 (December 2020): 1753–66.

20  Afe Adogame, "HIV/AIDS Support and African Pentecostalism: The Case of the Redeemed Christian Church of GOD (RCCG)," *Journal of Health Psychology* 12 (May 2007): 475–84; Ezeibe et al., "Political Distrust." Katherine Marshall, "Roles of Religious Actors in the West African Ebola Response," *Development in Practice* 27 (July 2017): 622–33, https://doi.org/10.1080/096145 24.2017.1327573; Wafaa M. El-Sadr and Jessica Justman, "Africa in the Path of Covid-19," *New England Journal of Medicine* 383, no. 3 (July 16, 2020): e11 (1–2), https://doi.org/10.1056/nejmp2008193.

21  Jesusegun Alagbe, "COVID-19: Winners Chapel Donates Ambulance, Ventilators, Others to FCT," *Punch*, April 4, 2020, https://punchng. com/covid-19-winners-chapel-donates-ambulance-ventilators-others-to-fct/; Gabriel Ewepu, "COVID-19: Dunamis Church Donates Medical Equipment to FCTA," *Vanguard*, March 26, 2020, https://www.vanguardngr.com/2020/03/ covid-19-dunamis-church-donates-medical-equipment-to-fcta/; Sam Eyoboka, "COVID-19: Adeboye, Oyedepo Donate Medical Supplies to Lagos, Ogun," *Vanguard*, April 1, 2020, https://www.vanguardngr.com/2020/04/ covid-19-adeboye-oyedepo-donate-medical-supplies-to-lagos-ogun/.

22  Oluwasegun Peter Aluko, "COVID-19 Pandemic in Nigeria: The Response of the Christian Church," *African Journal of Biology and Medical Research* 3 (2020): 111–25, https://abjournals.org/ajbmr/wp-content/uploads/sites/17/ journal/published_paper/volume-3/issue-2/AJBMR_YEEOATTF.pdf; and Ps. 91:10 KJV.

23  Martha Atanda, wife of Zion World Prayer and Missions' founder, Martins Atanda, studied the organization's response to COVID-19 as part of her capstone project in completion of a master of social work degree at the Diana R. Garland School of Social Work. Martha was a Global Mission Leadership Initiative fellow.

24  Matt. 9:36–38 King James Version (hereafter cited as KJV).

25  Matt. 5:13–16 KJV.

26  Diana R. Garland and Gaynor I. Yancey, *Congregational Social Work: Christian Perspectives* (Botsford, CT: North American Association of Christians in Social Work, 2014).

27  For information about the King's Assembly, visit https://www.thekingsassembly.org/.

28  The Zethar Al-Umma Foundation and King's Assembly are offshoots of ZWPM. The foundation is a humanitarian organization, and its homepage is http://www.zetharalumma.org/about.php.

29  Adogame, "HIV/AIDS Support and African Pentecostalism," 478 (an understanding premised on Matthews 17:21 and on Ephesians 6:10).

30  Geneva Gay, *Culturally Responsive Teaching: Theory, Research, and Practice*, 2nd ed. (New York: Teachers College Press, 2010); Leyla Feize and John Gonzalez, "A Model of Cultural Competency in Social Work as Seen through the Lens of Self-Awareness," *Social Work Education* 37 (June 2018): 472–89; Susan Mlcek, "Are We Doing Enough to Develop Cross-Cultural Competencies for Social Work?," *British Journal of Social Work* 44 (October 2014): 1984–2003.

31  Gay, *Culturally Responsive Teaching*; Feize and John Gonzalez, "Model of Cultural Competency."

32  Feize and Gonzalez, "Model of Cultural Competency"; United States Department of Education International Affairs Office, "Global and Cultural Competency," n.d., https://sites.ed.gov/international/global-and-cultural-competency/.

33 Maria Rosario T. de Guzman et al., *Cultural Competence: An Important Skill Set for the 21st Century* (Lincoln: University of Nebraska-Lincoln, 2016); and Josepha Campinha-Bacote, "The Process of Cultural Competence in the Delivery of Healthcare Services: A Model of Care," *Journal of Transcultural Nursing* 13 (July 2002): 181–84.

34 The United Nations adopted seventeen sustainable development goals (https://www.undp.org/sustainable-development-goals) in 2015. The goals included adequate food, shelter, water, health services, and other items referenced in the main text.

35 WHOROA, "New WHO Estimates: Up to 190 000 People Could Die of COVID-19 in Africa If Not Controlled," May 7, 2020, https://www.afro.who.int/news/new-who-estimates-190-000-people-could-die-covid-19-africa-if-not-controlled; and World Health Organization, "COVID-19 Weekly Epidemiological Update," May 25, 2021, https://apps.who.int/iris/bitstream/handle/10665/341525/CoV-weekly-sitrep25May21-eng.pdf?sequence=1&isAllowed=y (indicating the cumulative death tool in Africa was 85,964 as of May 23, a 2 percent increase from May 16).

36 Nigeria Centre for Disease Control, "COVID-19 NIGERIA," June 26, 2021, https://covid19.ncdc.gov.ng/.

37 Erigene Rutayisire et al., "What Works and What Does Not Work in Response to COVID-19 Prevention and Control in Africa," *International Journal of Infectious Diseases* 97 (August 2020): 267–69.

# Part III

# Public Education and Policy Considerations

# 19 The Black Church, Public Policy, and the Challenge of Health Equity

*Quardricos B. Driskell*

## Introduction

In a seminal 1899 social study titled *The Philadelphia Negro*, the pioneering African American scholar William E.B. Du Bois observed the most difficult problem regarding black health in the United States was the general attitude of white people.[1] According to Du Bois, a professor of economics and history at Atlanta University in Georgia, there were "few other cases in the history of civilized peoples where human suffering has been viewed with such peculiar indifference."[2] Sixty-seven years later, in 1966, the Rev. Martin L. King Jr. delivered a speech during a convention of the Medical Committee on Human Rights. King, an Atlanta native who had become a civil rights icon, echoed Du Bois. "Of all the forms of inequality," King proclaimed, "injustice in health care is the most shocking and inhuman."[3]

During the 1980s, decades after DuBois's and King's deaths, US Health and Human Services Secretary Margaret M. Heckler commissioned a task force to examine the overall health of black people and other social (racial, ethnic) minorities. Published in 1985 and 1986, the eight-volume report of the task force's thirty-eight primary and alternate members noted vast differences in health outcomes between the country's minority and majority, or white, populations. For example, the report indicated that homicide and accidents, infant mortality, heart disease, and stroke contributed the most significant numbers of excess death among black people younger than forty-five. Heart disease, stroke, and cancer were key causes of excess death in black people up to age seventy.[4]

In 2002, Congress commissioned a report titled *Unequal Treatment: Confronting Racial and Ethnic Disparities in Health Care*.[5] The committee responsible for the report declared, "Racial and ethnic minorities tend to receive a lower quality of healthcare than non-minorities, even when access-related factors, such as patients' insurance status and income, are controlled. The sources of these disparities are complex, are rooted in historical and contemporary inequities, and involve many participants at several levels, including health systems, their administrative and bureaucratic processes, utilization managers, health care professionals, and patients."[6] In 2015,

DOI: 10.4324/9781003214281-23

Robin L. Kelly, a congresswoman representing Chicago and other areas comprising the second district of Illinois as well as the chair of the Congressional Black Caucus Health Braintrust, authored a report about American healthcare to which thirty medical professionals, politicians, and other informed individuals contributed.[7] Drawing similar conclusions to the Heckler task force and the committee whose members penned *Unequal Treatment*, Kelly and her colleagues determined that grave racial/ethnic disparities continued to exist in healthcare despite improvements to access, increased research funding, and expanded insurance for underserved populations.[8]

The novel coronavirus, or COVID-19, began exacerbating preexisting inequalities from late 2019 into early 2020. Since then, numerous studies have shown that, despite significant advances in civil rights, race remains an important factor in determining whether an individual receives high-quality care, a principal factor in healthcare outcomes. In the United States, for instance, deaths due to severe acute respiratory syndrome coronavirus 2, or SARS-CoV-2, the virus that causes the COVID disease, are disproportionately high among African Americans compared with the general population. Factors contributing to that occurrence include structural, systemic determinants of health such as housing, underemployment, and climate. African Americans also are more likely to work in the service industry or to have diabetes, high blood pressure, or respiratory conditions. Predominately black neighborhoods are more likely to be exposed to pollutants and toxins, and there are racial/ethnic biases in medical treatment. I propose there needs to be a renewed focus on healthcare delivery for African Americans to ensure that adequate service is not a byproduct of privilege and that black churches can help ensure health equity.

### Bridging the Gap: Historical Healthcare Problems and Black Church Solutions

The history of the American healthcare system is fraught with racism, and only by acknowledging the effects of such racism can one work toward transformative change. Medical research activities such as the Tuskegee Study of Untreated Syphilis in the Negro Male, a government program in which physicians allowed black men to die from syphilis, a treatable condition, support my position. Begun in earnest in October 1932 and scheduled to last six months, the Tuskegee Experiment, as the study is known, continued for forty years, taking the lives of nearly 200 men during that period.[9]

The regrettable experience of Henrietta Lacks, a black woman born Loretta Pleasant in Roanoke, Virginia, is another well-known case of institutional racism in healthcare. In February 1951, medical staff at The Johns Hopkins Hospital in Baltimore, Maryland, diagnosed Lacks with cervical cancer. Her treatment was unsuccessful, and she died in October. For decades after that, white scientists and pharmaceutical companies used her cancer cells for many medical breakthroughs, including cancer and acquired immunodeficiency syndrome. Neither Lacks while living nor her survivors consented to such use.[10]

The abovementioned ordeals involving the unwitting Tuskegee men and Lacks are microcosms of other documented examples of biased, brutal, and unethical medical practices and programs in the United States. Consequently, numerous African Americans mistrust the healthcare system.[11] While certain officials have attempted to make amends for past injustices, Americans continue to grapple with racial/ethnic injustice. The COVID-19 pandemic highlights this fact. Black, Latino, and Native American people are more likely to get coronavirus, be hospitalized, and die than white people.[12] Furthermore, practically segregated hospitals, health clinics, and other medical facilities that care for high levels of racial/ethnic minorities continue to experience significant financial constraints.[13]

Each one of the inequalities I reference above is a major contributor to healthcare disparity in the United States. As regard COVID, a 2020 study about research and clinical trials found that black Americans were under-represented in both areas despite COVID affected them disproportionately when compared with white Americans.[14] While some people blame the gap on black mistrust of the healthcare system, Halo T. Borno, one of the physicians who conducted the study, said under recruitment was "the primary problem.... I think if we invest in engaging with the communities we want to see enrolled in our clinical trials, then trust won't be the barrier."[15]

Individual versus collective access to healthcare is a familiar conversation among physicians, researchers, politicians, lawmakers, patients, and other concerned parties in the United States. Oftentimes, when policymakers and researchers analyze data, they focus on individual-level factors. Thinking tends to be that if black, Latino, Native American, and other racial/ethnic minorities are more likely to have diabetes, high blood pressure, respiratory conditions, and other health concerns than white people, those likelihoods explain why the health outcomes of social minorities are worse than the majority. However, as a group of physicians, researchers, and writers affiliated with a nonprofit medical network called Sutter Health pointed out in 2020, nonwhite Americans without underlying chronic conditions still have adverse health outcomes at greater rates than white Americans.[16]

In relation to COVID-19, food availability and work environment are central factors in good health outcomes. People who are food insecure are represented disproportionately across the whole range of chronic conditions when compared with people who are food secure. If one lacks sufficient access to affordable and proper nutrition, one tends to develop a chronic disease sooner than someone with a nutritious diet. On balance, a higher percentage of white people in the United States are food secure than nonwhite people. Additionally, a lower percentage of white people than nonwhite people works in service industries or in frontline occupations such as groceries, retail stores, and custodial services that exposes one constantly with someone else who possibly is infected with COVID.[17]

Because of a long and storied history of influence and power despite decades of ill-treatment and racism to its congregants, the Black Church remains a pillar of African-descended communities in the United States. Black churches have promoted healthy living among other social contributions and helped offer disease prevention services, both formal and informal. Churchgoers have perpetuated and expanded their charitable services up through the early twenty-first century.[18]

As in previous eras of American history, black churches can assist in situations of a public health crisis. Congregants can serve as advocates and communicators of scientifically based public health messages, and they can educate individuals and communities about disease prevention, treatment, and other wellness matters, including promotion of healthy physical, mental, and emotional practices such as increased physical activity and greater fruit and vegetable intake. Moreover, adequately educated or trained congregants can work with local clinics, health departments, hospitals, and related entities to provide needed services such as cancer screenings and mammograms as well as more recent and procedures like COVID-19 checks. This assortment of services is an essential way church of virtually any size or socioeconomic status can contribute to black well-being. All the same, given the history of racism in the country, developing such partnerships can be a delicate process requiring significant investments of time, trust among multiple parties, and systematic planning.

Project CHURCH (Creating a Higher Understanding of Cancer Research and Community Health) exemplifies the type of collaboration that can be extremely useful to bettering African American health.[19] The University of Texas MD Anderson Cancer Center and several African American congregations in the Houston area formed Project CHURCH in 2008 to understand disparities in cancer prevention risk factors and to engage African Americans as partners in the research process.[20] Lorna H. McNeill, professor and chair of the Department of Health Disparities at the university cancer center, has been a critical participant in the development of Project CHURCH.[21] Selecting African Americans as the focus of the endeavor was sensible, she notes, because "their high cancer incidence and mortality rates, as well as their relative population size" in Houston and neighboring localities, make African Americans a prime community to research and help.[22]

Project CHURCH has proven successful and productive. By 2017, McNeill and others affiliated with the project had published approximately twenty scientific articles about cancer risks among African Americans. Simultaneously, she and her associates sponsored myriad activities with more than eighty churches in and around Houston. Throughout, McNeill and her colleagues worked hard to gain the confidence of the congregants with whom they worked. As McNeill and several other Project CHURCH participants remarked in 2018, establishing trust is vital for any individual or group of individuals seeking to engage racially and ethnically diverse communities in beneficial research initiatives.[23]

Project CHURCH is an exemplar of local collaborative cancer research and treatment among public institutions and private citizens. Additionally, the Prostate Health Education Network, founded in 2003, represents a comparably valuable endeavor on a larger scale. The network is a leading patient education and advocacy charitable organization for men living with prostate cancer, particularly black men, and their families. Volunteers, partners, and others involved with the organization began partnering with churches in 2009 through an annual Father's Day rally meant to support survivors and caretakers through praying, fellowship, and education about prostate cancer. From then until 2020 the network collaborated with more than 1,000 churches throughout the country. The organization expanded its partnership initiatives with black churches through educational symposiums, social media, television programs, and other creative efforts to educate and to mobilize African Americans in the fight against prostate cancer.[24]

There are several advocacy fronts for black churches. First, black churches should spark local, state, and federal actions on health disparities by partnering with organizations that advocate for health equity. In so doing, churches can find spaces within civil society institutions where the battle over health equity ideas does not descend into a meaningless debate but proper policy solutions. Second, churches should advocate for legislative protection and improvement of Medicare and Medicaid (e.g., adding dental and vision benefits for adults) as well as the Patient Protection and Affordable Care Act that President Barack Obama signed into law in 2013. Third, churches should pressure lawmakers to increase funding for pivotal programs and partnerships that strive to close health gaps among racial and ethnic groups nationwide, such as the Ryan White HIV/AIDS program, National Institutes of Health, and Healthy Start Initiative. Four, churches should press lawmakers on every level to pass black maternal care, mental health, and substance abuse legislation. Fifth, churches should engage with persons across the Black Atlantic in meaningful and mutual ways that help address disparities abroad and domestically.

## Conclusion

For me, a crucial question is this: Can black churches in the United States design and foster comprehensive faith responses to health equity and justice concerns effectively centered in both theological and public policy imperatives? I think churches not only can but also must engage policymakers, public health professionals, scientific researchers, practicing clinicians, and other parties to assist in bridging the wide gap between rich and poor citizens. Together, they should retool health strategy to achieve parity. The same idea applies to black churches, which need to take more active roles in matters regarding prevention, education, and advocacy relating to combatting chronic conditions and managing health disparities.

Essential targets of policy advocacy should include the Health Equity and Accountability Act of 2020, a signature measure of the Congressional Black Caucus, the Congressional Hispanic Caucus, and the Congressional Asian and Pacific American Caucus.[25] The Maternal Care Access and Reducing Emergencies Act, which Kamala Harris of California introduced into the US Senate in 2018 and reintroduced in 2019, is another significant piece of legislation.[26] It seeks to create a $25 million program to "address racial bias in maternal health care [and] allocate $125 million to identify high-risk pregnancies, and provide mothers with the culturally competent care and resources they need" to survive the birthing process.[27] Congresswoman Robin Kelly introduced the Mothers and Offspring Mortality and Morbidity Awareness Act and reintroduced it in 2019 to improve federal efforts to prevent maternal mortality, especially among black women, is another piece of legislation I think black churches should champion.[28] With respect to existing laws I believe worthy of Black Church support, the Action for Dental Health Act that Congressman Kelly introduced in 2017 and that President Donald J. Trump signed into law in 2018 is an exemplar.[29] It focuses on improving "essential oral health care for low-income and other underserved individuals by breaking down barriers" to such care.[30]

African-descended masses in the US cannot sit idly while lawmakers, insurance companies, physicians, and other providers make significant healthcare decisions. Resolving disparities is a moral and an ethical issue in which representatives of every sector of American society should participate. How black churches respond to disparity and to allied healthcare urgencies will shape how future generations view the churches. Therefore, present-day churchgoers should remain engaged and provide leadership in achieving health equity throughout the country.

## Notes

1 See W.E. Burghardt Du Bois, "The Health of Negroes," chap. 10 in *The Phila-delphia Negro: A Social Study* (Philadelphia, PN: University of Pennsylvania, 1899), 147–63, esp. 163.
2 Du Bois, "Health of Negroes," 163.
3 Martin Luther King Jr., as quoted in, among sources, John Dittmer, *The Good Doctors: The Medical Committee for Human Rights and the Struggle for Social Justice in Health Care*, updated ed. (Jackson: University of Mississippi Press, 2017), xi (employing inhumane rather than human, as have many people, even though Chicagoan physician Quentin Young recalled King using inhuman; Young served as chairman of the Medical Committee for Human Rights when King delivered the 1966 speech, which no one seems to have recorded in its entirety via audio, video, or transcription).
4 United States Department of Health and Human Services, *Report of the Secretary's Task Force on Black and Minority Health*, 8 vols. (Washington: US Department of Health and Human Services, 1985–1986) (hereafter cited as DHHS, *Secretary's Task Force Report*).

5 Committee on Understanding and Eliminating Racial and Ethnic Disparities in Health Care, *Unequal Treatment: Confronting Racial and Ethnic Disparities in Health Care*, Brian D. Smedley, Adrienne Y. Stith, and Alan R. Nelson, eds. (Washington: National Academies Press, 2002) (hereafter cited as CUEREDHC).

6 CUEREDHC, *Unequal Treatment*, 1.

7 Robin L. Kelly, *2015 Kelly Report: Health Disparities in America* (Chicago: Robin L. Kelly, 2015).

8 Kelly, *2015 Kelly Report*.

9 United States Centers for Disease Control and Prevention, "U.S. Public Health Service Syphilis Study at Tuskegee," April 22, 2021, https://www.cdc.gov/tuskegee/index.html.

10 "The Legacy the Henrietta Lacks," n.d., *Johns Hopkins Medicine*, https://www.hopkinsmedicine.org/henriettalacks/frequently-asked-questions.html.

11 Katrina Armstrong et al., "Racial/Ethnic Differences in Physician Distrust in the United States," *American Journal of Public Health* 97 (July 2007): 1283–89.

12 National Public Radio, Robert Wood Johnson Foundation, and Harvard T.H. Chan School of Public Health, *The Impact of Coronavirus on Households, by Race/Ethnicity* ([N.P.]: National Public Radio, Robert Wood Johnson Foundation, and Harvard T.H. Chan School of Public Health, 2020).

13 David A. Asch and Rachel M. Werner, "Segregated Hospitals Are Killing Black People. Data from the Pandemic Proves It," *Washington Post*, June 18, 2021, https://www.washingtonpost.com/opinions/2021/06/18/segregated-hospitals-are-killing-black-people-data-pandemic-proves-it/, citing David A. Asch et al., "Patient and Hospital Factors Associated with Differences in Mortality Rates among Black and White US Medicare Beneficiaries Hospitalized with COVID-19 Infection," *JAMA: Journal of the American Medical Association* 4 (June 17, 2021), 1–11, doi:10.1001/jamanetworkopen.2021.12842.

14 Hala T. Borno, Sylvia Zhang, and Scarlett Gomez, "COVID-19 Disparities: An Urgent Call for Race Reporting and Representation in Clinical Research," *Contemporary Clinical Trials Communications* 19 (September 2020): 1–4, https://doi.org/10.1016/j.conctc.2020.100630.

15 "Black and Latino Americans Underrepresented in COVID-19 Vaccine Trials, Despite Being Hit the Hardest," September 11, 2020, https://www.cbsnews.com/news/covid-19-vaccine-trials-minorities-recruitment/.

16 Kristen M. Azar et al., "Disparities in Outcomes among COVID-19 Patients in a Large Health Care System in California," *Health Affairs* 39 (July 2020): 1253–62.

17 Sandra R. Hernández and Kara Carter, "COVID-19: A Perfect Storm of Health Care Inequality," April 10, 2020, https://www.chcf.org/blog/covid-19-perfect-storm-health-care-inequality/.

18 Rayford W. Logan, *The Negro in American Life and Thought: The Nadir, 1877–1901* (New York, NY: Dial Press, 1954).

19 See Clayton Boldt, "Preaching Better Health," *University of Texas MC Anderson Cancer Center*, spring 2017, https://www.mdanderson.org/publications/conquest/preaching-better-health.h37-1591413.html; and Lorna H. McNeill et al., "Engaging Black Churches to Address Cancer Health Disparities: Project CHURCH," *Frontiers in Public Health* 6 (July 2018): 1–11.

20 Boldt, "Preaching Better Health."

21 McNeill et al., "Engaging Black Churches," 3.

22 Boldt, "Preaching Better Health."

23 Boldt, "Preaching Better Health"; McNeill et al., "Engaging Black Churches," 2.

24 Additional information about the Prostate Health Education Network is located at http://prostatehealthed.org/page.php?id=26.

25  Health Equity and Accountability Act, H.R. 6637, 116th Cong. (2020).
26  Maternal Care Access and Reducing Emergencies Act, S. 3363, 115th Cong. (2018); Maternal Care Access and Reducing Emergencies Act, S. 1600, 116th Cong. (2019).
27  "Harris Reintroduces Legislation Addressing Black Maternal Morality Crisis," May 22, 2019, https://www.harris.senate.gov/news/press-releases/harris-reintroduces-legislation-addressing-black-maternal-mortality-crisis. As of July 28, 2021, the legislation remained in the US Senate Health, Education, Labor, and Pensions Committee.
28  Mothers and Offspring Mortality and Morbidity Awareness Act, H.R. 5977, 115th Cong. (2018) (hereafter cited as MOMMA's Act); MOMMA's Act, H.R. 1897, 116th Cong. (2019). The death rate of 43.5 per 1,00,000 live births among black women in 2018 and 2019 was significantly higher than the 12.7 deaths per 1,00,000 among white women and the 14.5 deaths per 1,00,000 among other ethnicities.
29  Action for Dental Health Act, H.R. 2422, 115th Cong. (2017); Pub. L. 115–302, December 11, 2018, 132 Stat. 4369.
30  Action for Dental Health Act.

# 20 Black Mental Health Challenges and Responses by Britain's Black Majority Churches

*Babatunde Adedibu*

## Introduction

Because Britain is a melting pot culturally and ethnically, the country is a hotbed of religious pluralism. Black majority churches (BMCs), some of the fastest growing Christian formations in Britain, have been quite creative in meeting the religious needs of their members; however, BMCs have been less attentive to health needs, especially mental conditions.[1] That omission is serious, as much scientific research and scholarly writing have revealed disproportionate mental health challenges among black African and Caribbean men compared with white European men in Britain.[2] For example, in 2011 the Department of Health in the United Kingdom projected the probability of psychosis in black Caribbean groups to be approximately seven times higher than white groups.[3] The 2014 Adult Psychiatric Morbidity Survey found that black men were 3.2 percent more likely than men in other ethnic groups to experience psychotic disorders.[4] As of 2018, criminal justice were in the UK were four times more likely to utilize the 1983 Mental Health Act, as amended in 2007, to direct African and Caribbean people to mental health services as a function of detention.[5] Such racial/ethnic disparities, which continue to exist throughout Britain, have contributed to the poor mental health status of black, African, and minority ethnic populations.[6]

Ethnicity and race are emotive and complex factors requiring attention when analyzing mental health landscapes within British society, especially disparities. In addition to being more likely than white Britons to develop mental health conditions, BME Britons are less likely to receive care for mental conditions, according to scholars such as Anjum Memon.[7] I contend that British social and political institutions have been critical to mental health challenges experienced by BME populations, especially black populations, and that churches and other religious institutions have performed important roles in responding to the needs of those populations, including during the COVID-19 pandemic.

DOI: 10.4324/9781003214281-24

## Mapping Dynamics of BME Mental
## Health Challenges in Britain

Inequalities that BME populations in Britain have faced during the twenty-first century necessitate pushing mental health challenges of ethnic minorities to the fore of policy formulation.[8] In 2009, the National Health Services Information Centre for Health and Social Care published results from a 2007 household survey that found the "age standardised prevalence of psychotic disorder was significantly higher among black men (3.1%) than men from other ethnic groups (0.2% of white men, no cases observed among men in the South Asian or 'other' ethnic group)."[9] A 2014 academic book indicated that, regardless of gender or sex, black Britons of Caribbean origin had higher rates of depression and schizophrenia than other ethnic groups and that all BME groups were overrepresented in mental health inpatient settings.[10]

Researchers and authors have identified several factors that contribute to mental health disparities in the UK. Economic inequality is one factor. In 2013, according to one study, 37 percent of the BME population was statutorily homeless,[11] as per the 1996 Housing Act.[12] From October 2019, not long before Chinese officials publicized the first known cases of COVID-19, through September 2020, amid the pandemic, 29 percent of BME people in the UK aged sixteen to twenty-four was unemployed.[13]

Inadequate information, understanding, and empathy account for some BME mental health disparities in the UK: Numerous service providers are unfamiliar with general BME social, cultural, and linguistic norms.[14] Additionally, many BME people stigmatize mental health conditions and shun available services. Yet again, inadequacy is a part of the issue: BME families, members of religious communities, and other individuals do not realize or wish to admit the importance of mental healthcare, including getting help from professionals when necessary.[15] Despite such challenges, greater inclusion of BME people in mental health services is possible, and BMC have created blueprints that other people can follow.

## Actual and Potential BMC Responses
## to Mental Health Challenges

The proliferation of BMCs across the UK has changed the country's religious landscape. Caribbean Pentecostal denominations began the groundswell during the late 1940s and into the 1950s after British officials used a vessel called the *MV Empire Windrush* to relocate hundreds of subjects from the Caribbean to Britain to help build up the national economy after World War II.[16] Often treated disrespectfully by white citizens, including churchgoers, the subjects created autonomous institutions in the years following their 1948 arrival in Britain.[17] The BMC was a foremost institution among the so-called Windrush generation.[18] Later, Caribbean-born Britons created African Indigenous, Pentecostal, and Neo-Pentecostal denominations, which flourished in Britain and elsewhere in the UK by the end of the century.[19] Given their numbers, I describe such BMCs as "migrant sanctuaries."[20]

In general, BMCs in the UK have been less responsive to the mental health needs of congregants than to their religious needs. However, among the BMCs that members of the Windrush generation established, responsiveness has been greater than among African Indigenous, Pentecostal, and Neo-Pentecostal churches that subsequent generations of Caribbean-born people founded in the UK. That God's centrality to all aspects of life should prevent believers from falling into anxiety, depression, and related conditions is one reason for the difficulty. In sum, if one is aligned properly with God, one can avoid mental health challenges, as only imbalances such as sinfulness and wrongdoing—for example, living above one's means, thereby leading to financial difficulties and stress—cause such challenges. Therefore, interventions such as continuous prayer is the approach many MBCs take to restore the balance of spirit and mind. Regrettably, the spiritualization of mental illness has led to several cases of psychological, physical, sexual, and emotional abuse in both children and adults, and a few cases of witchcraft accusations and exorcist practices that have resulted in scandal.[21]

When BMC leaders believe the causative factors of mental health conditions to primarily be spiritual, I contend that belief often prevents them from recognizing other factors. In my judgment, their singular approach to causation is a sign of a flawed theological presupposition or scriptural exegesis due to insufficient religious training. That dynamic, I argue further, perpetuates approaches to mental health that keep the same BMC leaders from advising mentally ill parishioners to seek professional psychiatric assistance.

Revisiting public policy and criminal justice, I think BMCs in Britain can do better jobs advocating for racially inclusive employment policies in prison mental health services than BMCs do presently. Leading and ordinary BMC members also can promote the integration of holistic care delivery schemes that emphasize cultural sensitivity. Encouraging black people to pursue careers in law enforcement, government, and comparably important decision-making positions is yet another scheme BMCs can adopt. Redeemed Christian Church of God minister Agu Irukwu has led the charge for such endeavors. For example, in 2020 Irukwu, senior pastor of the Jesus House in London and a prominent leader of an interdenominational organization known as Churches Together in England, urged black people "to take very seriously the call to serve in the police, in local and central government, in politics, in the education system, and in the judiciary.... Our faith enjoins us to stand against injustice, sometimes at great cost."[22] Noting the systemic racism, the ethnic bias, and other injustices that pervaded many British institutions, Irukwu said godly people needed to identify and, moreover, work to eradicate the bias that countless officials had spoken about ending but whose deeds had not matched their words.[23]

If BMCs wish to address adequately the inequalities about which Irukwu spoke in 2020, members perhaps should consider answering a past call from black executives in the National Church Leaders Forum and establish a public policy think tank to facilitate research-based engagement of the British government. In 2015, the forum issued a report criticizing the government for the disproportionate imprisonment of black people. The report also urged the government to develop schemes to reduce the numbers of black inmates in British prisons and to address mental health concerns. Such initiatives are especially relevant during the COVID-19 pandemic, which has devastated black communities throughout the world.[24]

## BMCs and COVID-19

Despite shortcomings, BMCs provide a sense of community for adherents through religious ritual, worship, and Bible study, thereby facilitating well-being, hope, and optimism. Those acts help decrease incidences of loneliness, depression, and other conditions the COVID-10 pandemic has exacerbated. According to 2020 data from Public Health England, for the typical black, African, or minority ethnic person in Britain aged twenty to sixty-four, the risk of a test-confirmed COVID-19 infection was 56 percent higher than the same risk for a white Briton and 69 percent higher for someone sixty-five or older.[25] Financial insecurity, family dysfunction, employment loss, and reduced access to healthcare are associated risk factors that worsen mental health challenges, which have increased during the COVID pandemic.[26]

Additional occurrences that can affect mental health adversely include a loss of social connections due to stay-at-home orders, lockdowns, shutdowns, and related preventive measures. To lessen the impact of such restrictions, BMCs have utilized various technologies and social media platforms to provide a sense of community for their congregants. By shifting pastoral praxis from open, or public, physical gatherings to communicating via text messages, telephone calls, electronic mails, videoconferences, and similar methods. Such virtual connections facilitated the good mental and physical conditions that in-person services often aided prior to the pandemic. That religious churchgoing can affect well-being positively is not an anecdotal belief. Authors have written that regular attendance can increase life expectancy by up to fourteen years.[27]

Utilizing technology is important to counterbalancing a host of negative effects of the COVID-19 pandemic; however, vaccinations are invaluable counterbalances. In the UK, BMC leaders have been involved in major public education and endorsement efforts to assuage church and broader community members fears of possible bad side effects of vaccines. In February 2021, for example, Pastor Agu Irukwu of the Jesus House in London spoke for numerous other leading BMC members when he declared: "Our message is to encourage our congregations to take the vaccines, and to provide information that answers the many legitimate questions raised."[28] Culturally competent and hence sensitive to local norms, Irukwu said his fellow BMC leaders and he would bring "experts—a large proportion from within the communities, people they trust, people they know—to address concerns and answer questions."[29] In addition to the foregoing endeavors, Irukwu and his Jesus House congregation has joined with other mainline BMC congregants to make equip their sanctuaries to become COVID vaccination hubs.

## Conclusion

Systemic inequalities in mental healthcare and in social conditions contributing to mental health vulnerabilities have had significant adverse impacts on BME populations. Although BMCs have provided supportive communities for their constituencies, there has been a lack of proactive and pragmatic engagement by BMC leaders on public policies related to systemic inequalities in Britain. Specifically, there is a need for much greater BMC attention to the lack of cultural sensitivity within British mental healthcare and the degree to which cultural and structural biases and inequities have limited access by blacks in particular to mental healthcare. BMCs must reposition their energies and resources as demonstration of their concern for the holistic health of their adherents and for that of black persons in general.

## Notes

1 In this essay, I use the term *black* to identify someone of African or Caribbean ancestry, as viewed through a Pentecostal prism. For more on such usage, see J.D. Aldred, *Respect: Understanding Caribbean British Christianity* (Peterborough: Epworth, 2005); Joe Aldred and Keno Ogbo, eds., *The Black Church in the 21st* Century (London: Darton, Longman and Todd, 2010); Mark Sturge, *See What the Lord Has Done! An Exploration of Black Christian Faith in Britain* (Milton Keynes: Scripture Union, 2005); and Arlington Trotman, "Black, Black-Led or What?," in *Let's Praise Him: An African Caribbean Perspective on Worship*, ed. Joel Edwards, 12–35 (London: Kingsway, 1992).

2 See, among other studies, Paul Fearon et al., "Incidence of Schizophrenia and Other Psychoses in Ethnic Minority Groups: Results from the MRC AESOP Study," *Psychological Medicine* 36 (November 2006): 1541–50; and Sally McManus, Paul Bebbington, and Traolach Brugha, eds., *Mental Health and Wellbeing in England: Adult Psychiatric Morbidity Survey 2014* (Leeds: NHS Digital, 2016).

3 United Kingdom Department of Health and Social Care, "No Health Without Mental Health: A Cross-Government Mental Health Outcomes Strategy for People of All Ages: Analysis of the Impact on Equality (AIE)," (London: Department of Health and Social Care, 2011), 1–49, esp. 29.

4 McManus, Bebbington, and Brugha, *Mental Health and Wellbeing in England*, 132 (finding that psychotic disorder "did not vary significantly in rate between ethnic groups among women"), 140, 147.

5  NHS Digital, "Mental Health Act Statistics, Annual Figures 2017–18," October 9, 2018, https://digital.nhs.uk/data-and-information/publications/statistical/mental-health-act-statistics-annual-figures/2017-18-annual-figures. See also Carl Baker, *Mental Health Statistics for England: Prevalence, Services and Funding* (London: House of Commons Library, 2020); Mental Health Act 1983, https://www.legislation.gov.uk/ukpga/1983/20/contents; and Mental Health Act 2007, https://www.legislation.gov.uk/ukpga/2007/12/contents.

6  Frank Keating and David Robertson, "Fear, Black People and Mental Illness: A Vicious Circle?," *Health and Social Care in the Community* 12 (September 2004): 439–47; Caroline Lawlor et al., "Ethnic Variations in Pathways to Acute Care and Compulsory Detention for Women Experiencing a Mental Health Crisis," *International Journal of Social Psychiatry* 58 (January 2012): 3–15.

7  Anjum Memon et al., "Perceived Barriers to Accessing Mental Health Services among Black and Minority Ethnic (BME) Communities: A Qualitative Study in Southeast England," British Medical Journal Open 2 (2016): 2, doi: 10.1136/bmjopen-2016-012337.

8  Commission for Healthcare Audit and Inspection, *Count Me In: Results of a National Census of Inpatients in Mental Health Hospitals and Facilities in England and Wales November 2005* (London: Commission for Healthcare Audit and Inspection, 2005); Commission for Healthcare Audit and Inspection, *Count Me In: Results of the 2006 National Census of Inpatients in Mental Health and Learning Disability Services in England and Wales* (London: Commission for Healthcare Audit and Inspection, 2007) (hereafter cited as *2006 Count Me In*).

9  Sally McManus et al., eds, *Adult Psychiatric Morbidity in England, 2007: Results of a Household Survey* (Leeds: National Health Services Information Centre for Health and Social Care, 2009), 89.

10  Anne Rogers and David Pilgrim, *A Sociology of Mental Health and Illness*, 5th ed. (Maidenhead: Open University Press/McGraw-Hill, 2014).

11  Institute of Race Relations, "Inequality, Housing and Employment Statistics," 2020, https://irr.org.uk/research/statistics/poverty/.

12  Housing Act 1996, part 7: homelessness, https://www.legislation.gov.uk/ukpga/1996/52/part/VII/enacted.

13  Brigid Francis-Devine, "Unemployment by Ethnic Background" (briefing paper 6385, House of Commons Library—UK Parliament, June 1, 2021), 1–5, esp. 4.

14  Marija Kovandžić et al., "Access to Primary Mental Health Care for Hard-to-Reach Groups: From 'Silent Suffering' to 'Making It Work,'" *Social Science and Medicine* (March 2011): 763–72, esp. 767, 771.

15  Lee Knifton et al., "Community Conversation: Addressing Mental Health Stigma with Ethnic Minority Communities," *Social Psychiatry Epidemiology* 45 (2010): 497–504.

16  On June 22, 1948, the *MV Empire Windrush* docked in Tilbury, England, with more than 500 people, mostly Jamaican, from the Caribbean. They experienced categorical racism and social depravation. Many were Anglicans, but white Anglicans prohibited them from worshipping alongside white church-goers. Therefore, the immigrants formed autonomous churches such as the New Testament Church of God and The Church of God of Prophecy. For further study, see Babatunde Aderemi Adedibu, "African and Caribbean Pentecostalism in Britain," chap. 2 in *Pentecostals and Charismatics in Britain: An Anthology*, ed. Joe Aldred, 19–33 (London: SCM Press, 2019); and Adedibu, *Coat of Many Colours: The Origin, Growth, Distinctiveness and Contributions of Black Majority Churches to British Christianity* (Blackpool, England: Wisdom Summit, 2012).

17  Babatunde Adedibu, "Migration, Identity, and Marginalization: The Case of Britain's Black Majority Churches," *Journal of Africana Religions* 2 (2014): 110–17; Adedibu, *Coat of Many Colours.*

18  Adedibu, "Migration, Identity, and Marginalization"; Adedibu, *Coat of Many Colours.*

19  Adedibu, "African and Caribbean Pentecostalism in Britain"; Adedibu, "Migration, Identity, and Marginalization."

20  Babatunde Adedibu, "Reverse Mission or Migrant Sanctuaries? Migration, Symbolic Mapping, and Missionary Challenges of Britain's Black Majority Churches," *Pneuma: The Journal of the Society for Pentecostal Studies* 35 (2013): 405–23.

21  Eleanor Stobart, *Child Abuse Linked to Accusations of "Possession" and "Witchcraft"* (Nottingham: Department of Education and Skills, 2006).

22  Harriet Sherwood, "UK Institutions Need More Black People, Says Pentecostal Church Leader," *Guardian*, June 10, 2020, https://www.the-guardian.com/world/2020/jun/10/uk-institutions-need-more-black-people-says-pentecostal-church-leader.

23  Sherwood, "UK Institutions Need More Black People."

24  National Church Leaders Forum, *Black Church Political Mobilisation—A Manifesto for Action* (London: National Church Leaders Forum, 2015); Tim Wyatt, "Black Majority Churches Slam 'British Rule,'" *Church Times*, February 27, 2015, https://www.churchtimes.co.uk/articles/2015/27-february/news/uk/black-majority-churches-slam-british-rule.

25  Peter Kenway and Jabeer Butt, "Evidence in Action: A Review of the Report by Public Health England into Disparities in Risks and Outcomes of COVID-19 between Ethnic Groups and by Level of Deprivation" (briefing paper, New Policy Institute and the Race Equality Foundation, June 2020), 5; Eugenio Proto and Climent Quintana-Domeque, "COVID-19 and Mental Health Deterioration by Ethnicity and Gender in the UK," *PLOS One* 16 (January 6, 2021): 2, https://doi.org/10.1371/journal.pone.0244419.

26  Proto and Quintana-Domeque, "COVID-19 and Mental Health Deterioration," 2.

27  Alex Bunn and David Randall, "Health Benefits of Christian Faith" (Christian Medical Fellowship files, no. 44, Easter 2011), http://admin.cmf.org.uk/pdf/cmffiles/44_faith_benefits.pdf. See also, among numerous other contemporary works, Andrew Sims, *Is Faith Delusion? Why Religion is Good for Your Health* (London: Continuum, 2009).

28  Harriet Sherwood, "UK Faith Leaders Join to Counter Fears Over Vaccine in BAME Communities," *Guardian*, February 7, 2021, https://www.theguardian.com/society/2021/feb/07/faith-leaders-join-to-counter-fears-over-vaccine-among-bame-communities.

29  Sherwood, "UK Faith Leaders Join."

# 21 Cultural and Religious Influences on Genetic Interventions in Sub-Saharan Africa

*Murugi Kagotho and Njeri Kagotho*

> Genetic advances will only be acceptable if their application is carried out ethically, with due regard to autonomy, justice, education and the beliefs and resources of each nation and community.
>
> —World Health Organization (2000)

## Introduction

In the months following the first diagnosed cases of COVID-19, the Tanzanian government, among others in Africa, called for national days of prayer, fasting, and reflection seeking divine protection from the virus.[1] Those acts reflected the deep religiosity and spirituality in sub-Saharan Africa,[2] though ecclesiastical beliefs and scientific advances coexist. In matters of health, the relationship between church and scientific institutions is complex. While religious, spiritual, and other cultural gatekeepers work in close collaboration with the scientific community, there are cases where a clash of worldviews have created a public rebuff of medical advancements, research studies, and public health literacy campaigns.[3]

Sub-Saharan Africans (SSA) bear an inordinately large burden in the form of disease and healthcare disparity, and that burden has increased during the COVID-19 pandemic.[4] Biomedical technologies, including genetic and genomic advancements, hold tremendous promise for tackling such hardships. Across the region, research initiatives are advancing genetic and genomic research, which now includes collaborations to curtail COVID, a disease that has exhibited patient variations based on host genetic factors such as an individual's blood group (e.g., A, B, AB, O).[5]

Sub-Saharan spirituality, cultural taboos and social norms are especially salient in health decision-making. As we prepare for the rapid genetic and genomic response needed to deal effectively with SARS-CoV-2, the virus that causes COVID disease, we pause to examine factors that can impact the uptake of those interventions—specifically, dilemmas that might arise when genetic-genomic interventions offer a perspective contrary to religious, spiritual, and other customary dictates. This essay

DOI: 10.4324/9781003214281-25

contextualizes that possibility by drawing lessons from genetic conditions such as sickle cell disease, concluding that, to realize the promise of genetic and genomic health interventions, stakeholders should consider a multi-pronged approach in which researchers leverage informal institutions by weaving genetic-genomic technologies into religious, spiritual, and cultural philosophies.[6]

In sub-Saharan Africa, Judeo-Christianity and Islam are the two largest belief systems based on numbers of adherents. Though on the decline, African traditional religions remain central to regional culture. Expressed through taboos, social norms, and customary laws, indigenous religious traditions—which are unique to each ethnic group and adjudicated by each group's cultural gatekeepers—are experiential in nature and share common beliefs that supernatural beings and spirits perform significant roles in daily life.[7] Judeo-Christianity, Islam, and other religions coexist alongside traditional systems of faith, and it is not uncommon for individuals to amalgamate traditions when making life decisions.[8] For instance, both organized and traditional religions frame people's understanding of and interactions with genetic information and therapies.[9]

Many people use the terms *genetics* and *genomics* interchangeably; however, genetics, the study of heredity, focuses on the functioning of a single gene, whereas genomics refers to the study of the entire genome, particularly how genes interact with other genes and the individual's environment.[10] Oftentimes, much uneasiness accompanies researching and manipulating human genetics, as doing so warrants profound social and ethical consideration. Religion ascribes indelible rights to a God or to multiple gods, and countless people consider usurping those rights through genetic manipulation to be a direct violation of humanity's relationship with God or gods. In collectivist, culture, that violation has wide-reaching implications, as members of the culture believe the violation will lead to social imbalance and discord. By remaining engaged in biomedical debates, religious, spiritual, and cultural gatekeepers seek to protect community interests by establishing boundaries around a society whose members might otherwise feel compelled to adapt unchartered scientific advances.[11]

## Genetic and Genomic Studies in SSA

A review of medical and public health literature from sub-Saharan African reveals a growing body of work on genetic research and intervention to address genetic disorders such as sickle cell disease (a heritable group of disorders that affects the normal functioning of red blood cells and has a high morbidity and mortality rate).[12] According to one 2012 study, Africa accounted for approximately 233,750 (85 percent) of the 270,000 children born with sickle disease.[13] While exact mortality rates were not known, another study estimated 50 to 90 percent of sub-Saharan children with the disorder died in early childhood.[14]

Most Western countries had eliminated child mortality owing to the disease by 2012, and young patients tended to experience fine qualities of life.[15] Many of those countries achieved success through multidisciplinary interventions that included prenatal diagnosis and genetic counselling. For example, invasive and noninvasive in-vitro tests screened for genetic and related abnormalities, thereby helping physicians, mothers, fathers, and other concerned parties make informed clinical decisions about reproductive health.[16] While some religious people in the West and elsewhere in the world opposed prenatal testing, especially in cases involving pregnancy termination, other religious people had more permissible attitudes toward testing—but still rejected termination.[17]

In considering genetic-genomic technologies and global religions, many denominations demand that science acknowledge the sanctity of life, which, according to many denominational dogmas, begins at conception and emanates from a preeminent life giver—for example, a God.[18] Judeo-Christianity decrees "thou shalt not kill."[19] In Islam, Allah "created death and life."[20] In African traditional religions, the concept of family includes the unborn; therefore, the value that adherents place on life in-utero is at odds with genetic counseling and other interventions that might lead to pregnancy termination.[21]

Health literacy (i.e., the ability to obtain and comprehend information well enough to make logical decisions) is a central part of the religion versus science debate.[22] Genomic literacy, a subset of health literacy, is key in the use of genetic interventions starting from diagnosis, prevention, interventions, and therapy.[23] A considerable amount of scholarship examines what we consider to be ideology informed by the ascription of disease to supernatural forces and to misinformed sociocultural beliefs.[24] For example, religious or spiritual connotations attached to the collecting of blood, saliva, hair, or some other specimen necessary for genetic testing might result in one being reticent about participating in a genetic intervention.[25]

Guided by patriarchal structures and social hierarchies, many people in sub-Saharan Africa have gender blamed, stigmatized, and hence discriminated against women who suffer with hereditary or genetic conditions such as sickle cell disease or who give birth to children with such conditions; and that discrimination has created additional barriers to accessing care or to adhering to care plans.[26] In a 2011 study about sickle cell disease on the Kenyan coast, a group of scholars that included Vicki M. Marsh found that mothers were likely to bear the brunt of blame for hereditary diseases even when conditions were not evident in maternal lines.[27] While not unique to reproductive health or to Africa, gender blaming is pervasive across the African continent. Even when a hereditary diagnosis is not a primary cause of stigmatization, the diagnosis can reinforce a negative label associated with a condition.[28]

Communalism is another driver of stigmatization in Africa. In many societies, informal communal norms prioritize group welfare over individual interest. Because family is the core unit where decisions that affect individual are first canvassed,[29] hereditary diagnoses that carries social stigmas can have devastating consequences on entire families, as opposed to a single member (e.g., mother, diagnosed child), further decreasing the willingness of a family member or members to engage in care. Accordingly, any researcher who investigates such matters should consider ethical factors that extend beyond an individual subject, or medical patient, and consider research implications on whole families and communities.[30]

A financial demand associated with the management, or the treatment of a hereditary condition can further compound alienation or outright exclusion from community life. An individual with a modicum of fiscal autonomy is not as likely to experience social stigma when diagnosed with a genetic condition than someone who is less well-off monetarily.[31] Moreover, because Africa has the lowest global gross domestic product in the world, the intersection of stigma and poverty often presents a moral, an ethical, or a pecuniary dilemma medical technology is used to diagnose a hereditary condition: one might lose a social network, and the cost of a potential treatment might be prohibitively high.[32] Considering those possibilities, we cannot understate the significance that cultural gatekeepers can perform in demystifying hereditary conditions and scientifically based treatments, as they broker relationships between researchers and communities, helping to ensure strategies align with local norms and mores.[33]

## Moving Forward

We believe increased community participation is imperative if professional and lay investigators are to diversify global genomic research to include data on African genetic ancestry, of which there is a great deficit. Ancestry is known to impact disease outcomes and the ways individuals respond to medical therapies, including vaccines.[34] As regard SARS-CoV-2, the official name of COVID-19, we propose understanding the link between human genetic variations, susceptibility, and resistance will be key to controlling the disease.[35] Scientists are looking at symptomatic and asymptomatic individuals to determine genetic protective and risk factors associated with COVID resistance.[36] However, most genetic databanks consist primarily of information about people of European descent; African and other ancestry groups are greatly underrepresented even though Africa has the most genetically diverse people in the world.[37] Together with ineffective genomic-based surveillances, insufficient genetic databases have major implications in determining vaccine equivalency across racial and ethnic groups.

Exploring genetic variation in Africa doubtless will be beneficial to COVID research; however, improving research capacity throughout the continent is another important endeavor. Africans face significant barriers in bridging global research gaps and translating genetic-genomic interventions into practical healthcare settings. Resource limitations, research costs, and delayed knowledge transfers are foremost barriers.[38] Sub-Saharan Africa is a case in point. The use of genomic surveillance techniques such as genome sequencing to track COVID mutations in the region have been modest at best. Fortunately, by July 2021, amid the pandemic, notable attempts were underway to better guide public health responses.[39]

Infrastructure and technological lessons learned from past pandemics position sub-Saharan Africa well for undertaking viral genomic sequencing.[40] Key public and private sector actors include the Africa Centres for Disease Control and Prevention and a continent-wide body the centers formed in February 2020 called the Africa Taskforce for Novel Coronavirus.[41] Such groups are laying the foundation for an integrated scientific model that includes monetary investments to advance genomic sequencing, coordinating intracontinental data and technology sharing. Already efforts to standardize protocols to facilitate coordination between institutional laboratories and individual scientists to help advance understanding about COVID are ongoing.[42]

In addition to scientific challenges and advancements, the COVID pandemic has shown a light on political issues in sub-Saharan Africa. Numerous politicians and policymakers seem to be unfamiliar with genomics, as demonstrated by meager budgetary allocations for viral genomic research. While faith leaders and cultural gatekeepers might not hold sway in matters relating to public resource allocation, their individual and collective impact on the uptake of research can bolster social participation and help scientists, physicians, and other stakeholders realize the full potential of pertinent technologies.

At the community level, low health literacy rates in sub-Saharan Africa have proven to be major barriers to genomic research during the COVID pandemic. People's reservations about participating in genomic studies have had a negative impact on attempts to obtain samples needed to sequence COVID.[43] By forming more transparent partnerships with cultural gatekeepers, we believe scientists and other individuals who wish to conduct further research on COVID are likely to get more local buy-in for new and usually unfamiliar technologies. Lessons from researchers engaged in sickle cell disease interventions suggest that informed consent practices are potential tools to facilitate transparency. Practices tailored to specific local contexts, or communities, might empower potential participants to understand the benefits and the drawbacks of research studies and biomedical interventions.[44]

In relation to genetic-genomic research, we think it should engage African worldviews and sociocultural values, including faith dictates. While religious and spiritual beliefs, norms and mores, and various taboos can contradict the science that informs health behavior and health services, collaborations with community gatekeepers can help mediate religious and secular relationships.[45] For instance, many sub-Saharan societies are grappling with scientific directives related to COVID that, when viewed through a cultural lens, are anathema. Government regulations have altered religious dying and death rituals, to include viewing, washing, burying, and other ministrations on the deceased. Some people in the region have accepted regulations, albeit reluctantly in many cases, while other people have staged violent public events to oppose regulations.[46]

If intolerable socially, a COVID intervention is likely to face much opposition in a sub-Saharan community. Meaningful engagement with cultural gatekeepers who hold significant sway with other indigenes will help facilitate peaceful engagement.[47] About this matter, too, we cannot overstate the role of spiritual leaders in helping disseminate health information and engender adherence to government regulations. In a 2020 study of more than 400 religious leaders and traditional healers in Ethiopia conducted approximately three months after the federal ministry confirmed the first COVID case in the country, a set of researchers found that most of the leaders and healers they studied were highly knowledgeable about the prevention and the early detection of COVID but oftentimes did not distance physically, avoid mass gatherings, or wear masks, among other acts.[48] Because those surveyed represented individuals who had a duty to help care for the health and the safety of others, such findings were and remain disquieting.

## Conclusion

Genetic and genomic research and practice hold great promise in global health disparities. Success in sub-Saharan Africa, as well as elsewhere in other regions of the continent, depends in part on how well scientists, physicians, government officials, cultural gatekeepers, and other decision-makers approach not only scientific matters but also social constructs such as religion and spirituality. Owing to cultural sensitivity, acceptance of genomic research regarding the prevention, control, or elimination of existing, emerging, and reemerging infections such as Lassa fever, Ebola, and COVID as it increases in Africa as of July 2021. However, continuing to bridge genetic and genomic gaps to advance the study of African genes in relation to emergent diseases will require sustained buy-in from local communities, improved infrastructures, and greater access to technologies.[49]

## Notes

1 Syriacus Buguzi, "Covid-19: Counting the Cost of Denial in Tanzania," *British Medical Journal Online* 373 (April 27, 2021): 1–2, doi: 10.1136/bmj.n1052.
2 Pew Forum on Religion and Public Life, *Tolerance and Tension: Islam and Christianity in Sub-Saharan Africa* (Washington, DC: Pew Research Center, 2010).
3 John B. Blevins, Mohamed F. Jalloh, and David A. Robinson, "Faith and Global Health Practice in Ebola and HIV Emergencies," *American Journal of Public Health* 109 (March 2019): 379–84; Angellar Manguvo and Benford Mafuvadze, "The Impact of Traditional and Religious Practices on

the Spread of Ebola in West Africa: Time for a Strategic Shift," *Pan African Medical Journal* 22, supplement 1 (October 2015): 1–4; Fredrick Nzwili, "African Catholic Bishops Emphasize Hope amid COVID-19," *Catholic World Report*, April 15, 2020, https://www.catholicworldreport.com/2020/04/15/african-catholic-bishops-emphasize-hope-amid-covid-19/.

4   N.S. Munung, B.M. Mayosi, and J. de Vries, "Genomics Research in Africa and Its Impact on Global Health: Insights from African Researchers," *Global Health, Epidemiology and Genomics* 3 (June 8, 2018): 1–8.

5   H3Africa Consortium, "Enabling the Genomic Revolution in Africa," *Science* 344 (June 20, 2014): 1346–48; H3Africa Working Group, "Harnessing Genomic Technologies Toward Improving Health in Africa: Opportunities and Challenges," Emmanuel K. Peprah and Charles N. Rotimi, eds. (working paper, National Institutes of Health and the Wellcome Trust, January 2011); Severe Covid-19 GWAS Group, "Genomewide Association Study of Severe Covid-19 with Respiratory Failure," *New England Journal of Medicine* 383, no. 16 (October 15, 2020): 1522–34; Severe Covid-19 GWAS Group, "Genomewide Association Study of Severe Covid-19 with Respiratory Failure," *New England Journal of Medicine* 383, no. 16 (October 15, 2020): 1522–34.: Sofonias K Tessema et al., "Accelerating Genomics-Based Surveillance for COVID-19 Response in Africa," *Lancet Microbe* 1 (October 2020): e227–28.

6   Regarding Sub-Saharan Africa, spirituality, cultural taboos, social norms, and health decision making, see Njeri Kagotho, Alicia Bunger, and Kristen Wagner, "'They Make Money Off of Uso': A Phenomenological Analysis of Consumer Perceptions of Corruption in Kenya's HIV Response System," *BMC Health Services Research* 16 (September 2016): 1–11, doi: 10.1186/s12913-016-1721-y; and Vicki M. Marsh, Dorcas M. Kamuya, and Sassy S. Molyneux, "'All Her Children Are Born That Way': Gendered Experiences of Stigma in Families Affected by Sickle Cell Disorder in Rural Kenya," *Ethnicity and Health* 16 (August 2011): 343–59.

7   John S. Mbiti, *African Religions and Philosophy* (Garden City, NY: Doubleday, 1969).

8   Kasomo Daniel, "An Assessment of Religious Syncretism: A Case Study in Africa," *International Journal of Applied Sociology* 2 (2012): 10–15; Mbiti, *African Religions and Philosophy*.

9   Amina Abubakar et al., "Socio-Cultural Determinants of Health-Seeking Behaviour on the Kenyan Coast: A Qualitative Study," ed. Nicholas Jenkins, *PLOS One* 8, no. 11 (November 2013): e71998, doi: 10.1371/journal.pone.0071998; Joseph B. Fanning and Ellen Wright Clayton, "Religious and Spiritual Issues in Medical Genetics," *American Journal of Medical Genetics, Part C: Seminars in Medical Genetics* 151 (February 15, 2009), 1–5, doi: 10.1002/ajmg.c.30191.

10  National Human Genome Research Institute, "Genetics vs. Genomics Fact Sheet," September 7, 2018, https://www.genome.gov/about-genomics/fact-sheets/Genetics-vs-Genomics.

11  Evangelical Lutheran Church in America, *A Social Statement on Genetics, Faith and Responsibility* (Chicago: Evangelical Lutheran Church in America Office of the Presiding Bishop, 2011); Paulina O. Tindana et al., "Aligning Community Engagement with Traditional Authority Structures in Global Health Research: A Case Study from Northern Ghana," *American Journal of Public Health* 101 (October 2011): 1857–67.

12  Jemima A. Dennis-Antwi et al., "Relation Between Religious Perspectives and Views on Sickle Cell Disease Research and Associated Public Health Interventions in Ghana," *Journal of Genetic Counseling* 28, no. 1 (February

2019): 102–18; Vicki Marsh et al., "Consulting Communities on Feedback of Genetic Findings in International Health Research: Sharing Sickle Cell Disease and Carrier Information in Coastal Kenya," *BMC Medical Ethics* 14 (December 2013): 41; Lucky L. Mulumba and Lynda Wilson, "Sickle Cell Disease among Children in Africa: An Integrative Literature Review and Global Recommendations," *International Journal of Africa Nursing Sciences* 3 (September 2015): 56–64.

13  Banu Aygun and Isaac Odame, "A Global Perspective on Sickle Cell Disease," *Pediatric Blood and Cancer* 59 (August 2012): 386–90, esp. 386.

14  Scott D. Grosse et al., "Sickle Cell Disease in Africa: A Neglected Cause of Early Childhood Mortality," *American Journal of Preventive Medicine* 41, no. 6, supplement 4 (December 2011): S398–S405.

15  Sophie Lanzkron, C. Patrick Carroll, and Carlton Haywood Jr., "Mortality Rates and Age at Death from Sickle Cell Disease: U.S., 1979–2005," *Public Health Reports* 128, no. 2 (March–April 2013): 110–16.

16  Nagwa E. A. Gaboon et al., "Attitude toward Prenatal Testing and Termination of Pregnancy among Health Professionals and Medical Students in Saudi Arabia," *Journal of Pediatric Genetics* 6 (September 2017): 149–54.

17  Rebecca Rae Anderson, "Religious Traditions and Prenatal Genetic Counseling," *American Journal of Medical Genetics, Part C: Seminars in Medical Genetics* 151C (February 15, 2009): 52–61, doi: 10.1002/ajmg.c.30203; Chantelle Jennifer Scott, Merle Futter, and Ambroise Wonkam, "Prenatal Diagnosis and Termination of Pregnancy: Perspectives of South African Parents of Children with Down Syndrome," *Journal of Community Genetics* 4 (January 2013): 87–97.

18  Fanning and Clayton, "Religious and Spiritual Issues in Medical Genetics."

19  Exodus 20:13, King James Version Online.

20  Surah Al-Mulk 67:2, Qur'an.

21  Mbiti, *African Religions and Philosophy.*

22  Matombo Ondwela et al., "'I Visited a Traditional Healer Because I Felt I Wasn't Getting Any Better by Using Active Antiretroviral'. Understanding Cultural Imperatives in the Context of Adherence to Highly Active Antiretroviral Therapy," *Open Public Health Journal* 12 (August 2019): 315–20.

23  Gerald Mboowa and Ivan Sserwadda, "Role of Genomics Literacy in Reducing the Burden of Common Genetic Diseases in Africa," *Molecular Genetics and Genomic Medicine* 7 (July 2019): e00776, 1–8, doi: 10.1002/mgg3.776.

24  Owusu Boahen et al., "Community Perception and Beliefs about Blood Draw for Clinical Research in Ghana," *Transactions of the Royal Society of Tropical Medicine and Hygiene* 107 (April 2013): 261–65; Dennis-Antwi et al., "Relation Between Religious Perspectives and Views"; Amal Gedleh et al., "'Where Does It Come From?': Experiences among Survivors and Parents of Children with Retinoblastoma in Kenya," *Journal of Genetic Counseling* 27 (June 2018): 574–88; Marsh et al., "Consulting Communities."

25  Boahen et al., "Community Perception and Beliefs"; Eunice Kamaara, Camillia Kong, and Megan Campbell, "Prioritising African Perspectives in Psychiatric Genomics Research: Issues of Translation and Informed Consent," *Developing World Bioethics* 20 (September 2020): 139–49.

26  Jantina de Vries et al., "Investigating the Potential for Ethnic Group Harm in Collaborative Genomics Research in Africa: Is Ethnic Stigmatisation Likely?," *Social Science and Medicine* 75 (October 2012): 1400–407; Marlyn C. Faure et al., "Does Genetics Matter for Disease-Related Stigma? The Impact of Genetic Attribution on Stigma Associated with Rheumatic Heart Disease in the Western Cape, South Africa," *Social Science and Medicine* 243

(December 2019), 1–6, doi: 10.1016/j.socscimed.2019.112619; Gedleh et al., "Where Does It Come From?"; Marsh, Kamuya, and Molyneux, "All Her Children Are Born That Way"; Fasil Tekola et al., "Impact of Social Stigma on the Process of Obtaining Informed Consent for Genetic Research on Podoconiosis: A Qualitative Study," *BMC Medical Ethics* 10 (August 22, 2009): 1–10, doi: 10.1186/1472-6939-10-13.

27 Marsh, Kamuya, and Molyneux, "All Her Children Are Born That Way."
28 de Vries et al., "Investigating the Potential for Ethnic Group Harm"; Marsh, Kamuya, and Molyneux, "All Her Children Are Born That Way."
29 Hill et al., "Achieving Optimal Cancer Outcomes."
30 Tekola et al., "Impact of Social Stigma"; Fasil Tekola et al., "Tailoring Consent to Context: Designing an Appropriate Consent Process for a Biomedical Study in a Low Income Setting," *PLoS Neglected Tropical Diseases* 3 (July 2009): e482, 1–6.
31 Marsh et al., "Consulting Communities."
32 Rwamahe Rutakumwa et al., "What Constitutes Good Ethical Practice in Genomic Research in Africa? Perspectives of Participants in a Genomic Research Study in Uganda," *Global Bioethics* 31 (2020): 169–83.
33 Paulina Tindana et al., "Community Engagement Strategies for Genomic Studies in Africa: A Review of the Literature," *BMC Medical Ethics* 16 (April 2015): 1–12.
34 Jerome Amir Singh, "The Case for Why Africa Should Host COVID-19 Candidate Vaccine Trials," *Journal of Infectious Diseases* 222 (August 2020): 351–56.
35 Michael F. Murray et al., "COVID-19 Outcomes and the Human Genome," *Genetics in Medicine* 22 (July 2020): 1175–77.
36 Hugo Zeberg and Svante Pääbo, "A Genomic Region Associated with Protection against Severe COVID-19 is Inherited from Neandertals," *Proceedings of the National Academy of Sciences* 118, no. 9 (March 2, 2021), e2026309118, 1–5, https://doi.org/10.1073/pnas.2026309118; Severe Covid-19 GWAS Group, "Genomewide Association Study of Severe Covid-19 with Respiratory Failure," *New England Journal of Medicine* 383, no. 16 (October 15, 2020): 1522–34.
37 Sarah A. Tishkoff, "The Genetic Structure and History of Africans and African Americans," *Science* 22 (May 2009): 1034–44.
38 Konstantinos Mitropoulos et al., "Success Stories in Genomic Medicine from Resource-Limited Countries," *Human Genomics* 9 (June 18, 2015): 1–7, doi: 10.1186/s40246-015-0033-3.
39 Tessema et al., "Accelerating Genomics-Based Surveillance."
40 "Genomic Sequencing in Pandemics," *Lancet* 397 (February 6, 2021): 445, doi: 10.1016/S0140-6736(21)00257-9.
41 Africa Centres for Disease Control, "Africa CDC Establishes Continent-Wide Task Force to Respond to Global Coronavirus Epidemic," *Africa Union*, February 5, 2020, https://africacdc.org/news-item/africa-cdc-establishes-continent-wide-task-force-to-respond-to-global-coronavirus-epidemic/.
42 Tessema et al., "Accelerating Genomics-Based Surveillance."
43 Sara Jerving, "Strengthening Africa's Ability to 'Decode' the Coronavirus," *Devex*, May 28, 2020, https://www.devex.com/news/strengthening-africas-ability-to-decode-the-coronavirus-97319.
44 Daniel Asmelash et al., "Knowledge, Attitudes and Practices toward Prevention and Early Detection of COVID-19 and Associated Factors among Religious Clerics and Traditional Healers in Gondar Town, Northwest Ethiopia: A Community-Based Study," *Risk Management and Healthcare Policy* 13 (2020): 2239–50; J. De Vries et al., "Research on COVID-19 in South Africa: Guiding Principles for Informed Consent," *South African Medical Journal* 110 (July 2020): 635–39.

45 Blevins, Jalloh, and Robinson, "Faith and Global Health Practice in Ebola and HIV Emergencies"; Bankole Falade, "Religious and Traditional Belief Systems Coexist and Compete with Science for Cultural Authority in West Africa," *Cultures of Science* 2 (March 2019): 9–22; Bankole A. Falade and Lars Guenther, "Dissonance and Polyphasia as Strategies for Resolving the Potential Conflict Between Science and Religion among South Africans," *Minerva* 58 (September 2020): 459–80.

46 Anne Atieno, "Family in Shock as Musician's Body is Buried at Dawn," *Standard*, June 14, 2020, https://www.standardmedia.co.ke/nyanza/article/2001375037/two-musicians-two-contrasting-burials.

47 Gedleh et al., "Where Does It Come From?"; Kamaara, Kong, and Campbell, "Prioritising African Perspectives"; Vicki M. Marsh et al., "Experiences with Community Engagement and Informed Consent in a Genetic Cohort Study of Severe Childhood Diseases in Kenya," *BMC Medical Ethics* 11 (July 2010): 1–11; P. Tindana et al., "Developing the Science and Methods of Community Engagement for Genomic Research and Biobanking in Africa," *Global Health, Epidemiology and Genomics* 2 (2017): 1–5, doi: 10.1017/gheg.2017.9.

48 Asmelash et al., "Knowledge, Attitudes and Practices."

49 Seth C Inzaule et al., "Genomic-Informed Pathogen Surveillance in Africa: Opportunities and Challenges," *Lancet Infectious Diseases* 21 (February 12, 2021): 1–9, https://doi-org.libproxy.clemson.edu/10.1016/S1473-3099(20)30939-7.

# 22 Pastoral Care, the COVID-19 Pandemic, and Oppression in Port-au-Prince, Haiti

*B. Denise Hawkins and Ervin E. Dyer*

## Introduction

Amid summer days that blaze hotter than normal in Haiti's capital of Port-au-Prince, a small band of young adults in bright white and blue tee shirts ventures out from a church called Rendez-Vous in the Delmas section of the city. Sweat rolls down their foreheads, landing in the creases of the colorful cloth masks that cover their noses and mouths. The teens are on Pastor Julio Volcy's team.

Not unlike much of the rest of the world in the spring of 2020, Haiti found itself in the grip of a pandemic-fueled public health crisis, and Volcy called the youth to the frontline. His ministry needed to count on them more than ever before, as COVID-19 had hit Haiti. The national ministry of health reported the first confirmed cases of the highly contagious respiratory disease caused by SARS-CoV-2, a coronavirus, on March 19, 2020,[1] eight days after the World Health Organization proclaimed COVID a pandemic.[2] The Haitian government swiftly declared a state of emergency, closed borders, and shuttered schools for some 300,000 children.[3] The emergency declaration came a week before Rendez-Vous Church planned to celebrate its fourth anniversary. Government officials ordered Volcy's 2,800-member church (and many other establishments) to cease activities, as Port-au-Prince had become a center of the island nation's outbreak.

Despite growing numbers of COVID-19 cases by summer 2020, many Haitians in the capital and in rural communities outside the capital doubted COVID was a real threat. The government affirmed the presence of the coronavirus and alerted Haitians about the pandemic; however, because "there is no trust in the government, no matter what is said, they don't believe it," Volcy explained in June.[4] Some Haitians who understood the seriousness of COVID remained silent, Volcy continued, because they viewed the disease with fear and shame.[5] As loved ones became infected, the stigma associated with the coronavirus in Haiti kept many people from seeking medical care or from leaving their homes if they had symptoms such as a persistent cough, abdominal pain, or

DOI: 10.4324/9781003214281-26

fever. If there was a death, they attributed it to another illness or kept the burial a secret.

Despite such denials, Volcy said Haiti was expected to be under a third public health state of emergency until late July 2020. For a society where much of life depended on using public transportation and where people operate in close contact with others, the COVID lockdown devastated livelihoods. No longer did vendors sell fruits and vegetables, flip flops, and meats, among other items, in sprawling, congested, open-air markets, or while huddling by candlelight on the sides of dark roads. The COVID pandemic also caused more people to live hand to mouth. Others sank deeper into hunger, a phenomenon that began to surge in 2019. The burden of a deadly, global pandemic being layered on top of a hunger crisis would only add to the growing political instability and soaring inflation, which had already left close to four million people, nearly half the population, undernourished, food insecure and unable to afford even rice and beans (basic staples of the Haitian diet), according to reports that track global food crises.[6] For this reason and others, "an impending humanitarian crisis," loomed for the island nation, said Dr. Carissa F. Etienne, Director of the Pan American Health Organization.[7]

## The Pandemic's Burden on Health and Wellness

The toll and strain of COVID, an outsized contagious disease, were compounded in a nation already made fragile by a broad swath of health, education and other inequities. By January 2020, an estimated 6 million Haitians live below the poverty line, earning $2.41 a day.[8] As many as 2.5 million others lived on $1.12 a day.[9] More than a third of Haitians lacked access to clean drinking water, and two thirds had no sanitation.[10] The healthcare system was weak, and for those who could not afford to pay for healthcare, they received no service. That lack of access matters. Large numbers of Haitians suffer with chronic diseases like diabetes and hypertension, and their island has the highest rates of tuberculosis in the Americas.[11] To make matters worse, Haiti for decades before the COVID pandemic was burdened with human immunodeficiency virus/acquired immunodeficiency syndrome, the leading cause of death for adults and adolescents.[12]

Quality education is essential to breaking the cycle of poverty in Haiti, but, similar to healthcare, education is for those who can afford it. Every four out of five schools in the county are private, and there are few spaces available for children in the handful of free public schools. The COVID-19 pandemic deepened the crisis. Impoverished and unable to obtain adequate healthcare or education, millions of children born in Haiti are unlikely to realize their full potentials. According to the World Bank's 2019 Human Capital Index, Haitian adults were only 45 percent as productive as they could have been with sufficient money, healthcare, education, and related items.[13]

## Connecting to Public Health

Much of life in Haiti is characterized by oppressive economic classism and cultural rifts stemming from language and religious differences as well as colorism. Those schisms help perpetuate health inequities in Haiti. In brief, how one looks and where one lives often determines where one can go to school, find at job, access healthcare, or have food security.[14] Persistent and habitual stress associated with such oppression increases the risk for chronic conditions such as inflammatory and autoimmune disorders, heart disease, and diabetes. Each one of those social determinants of health makes someone more vulnerable to contracting COVID-19 than someone without one of the determinants.[15]

Once COVID arrived in Haiti, its inhabitants found themselves confronting deeply entrenched inequities within social and institutional life and the highly infectious virus. Volcy and the almost 3,000 members of the multisite Rendez-Vous Church expanded their ongoing efforts to provide education and health services to those the government failed to reach. At Rendez-Vous, a church whose membership constitute a mosaic of Haiti, Volcy uses the pillars of faith and service to encourage personal growth in young people and participation in community—what he calls "love in action."[16] If youth practice both acts, Volcy emphasizes, they can create change in a nation struggling with poverty, corruption, and inequality, three conditions that erode positive public health.

In battling COVID, Volcy has dispatched young people, many of whom are active participants or alumni of a mentoring and self-improvement program called Haiti Teen Challenge, to the same poor and densely packed neighborhoods they call home. Love in action means youth haul buckets of clear, clean water and bountiful supplies of soap for makeshift handwashing stations. Besides providing those items, Volcy instructs his team to show people how to properly wash their hands. The practice is part of a basic hygiene regiment, but is one that has taken on a greater urgency during the COVID pandemic.

In addition, Haiti Teen Challenge girls have sewn and distributed hundreds of colorful masks to residents across Port-au-Prince, among other places. Other youth have volunteered to feed people, thereby keeping them healthy, as many would go hungry without such supports. Restrictions on social gatherings have caused Volcy to repurpose Rendez-Vous Church's ministry teams. Members still pray together virtually or gather online for Bible study and to figure out additional ways to demonstrate love in action.

On the streets of Port-au-Prince, young congregants of Rendez-Vous Church have been visible signs of whole church's response to the COVID-19 pandemic and commitment to assisting people in need. Guest services and other church staff, program leaders, and members of the music ministry were among those who responded. With in-person worship suspended because of pandemic restrictions, their official jobs paused, but they took up new assignments and ministries that kept them on the payroll thanks to donations from church members and other Haitian supporters as well as from charitable people throughout the world. Youth and various other ministries at Rendez-Vous Church fetched medicine for homebound seniors and delivered parcels of rice, beans, dried fish, and other nonperishable staples. Ideally, those products would provide nutritious food for a six-member family for an entire month.

While fighting COVID, oppression, and corruption, the people with whom Volcy works have been mindful of the interconnectedness of nationwide vulnerabilities. Haiti is divided by haves and have-nots, with the latter outnumbering the former. Stressed by food insecurity, poverty, political, and other challenges, the have-nots often lash out against the haves by robbing, killing, and kidnapping. Such acts create constant unrest and unease in Haiti. But stressful conditions are not limited to have-nots. Volcy notes that such insecurity also impacts a person of means: "I have to think about where I go for a walk. It is a challenge because I have to think with every step how to avoid the possibility of being robbed because I could be identified as a person who has something."[17]

Volcy believes Haiti's public health can be improved through a practice of engaged spirituality. To build a healthy, safe, and unified society, he explains, people must stop seeing each other as enemies—as haves and have-nots. "You can't overcome evil with evil," Volcy contends: "You can only overcome evil by doing good. You can't battle oppression with oppression. Society needs to be made more equal and less corrupt to be healthy."[18]

Volcy starts with youth, teaching them to free their minds, as guided by Mark 9:23: "All things are possible for one who believes."[19] Teaching youth the principles of sacrifice and service to build a better Haiti is his goal: "I choose the young people—I know for a fact they are young, but they are learning and leading by example."[20] Volcy likewise believes youth are Haiti's destiny because they have more free time, more energy, and more access to technology than older Haitians. He insists, "To win them is to win the entire country. It's more than changing government leaders."[21]

Volcy's advice is sage. As of 2020, almost 65 percent of the Haitian population was under twenty-five years old. To change the youth, then, is to change the nation, Volcy professes. Enhancing educational opportunities constitute a significant part of that change. Formal learning will engender mindsets of integrity and help children formulate new ideas about proper society. "We have to do it," Volcy implores his fellow Haitian adults, as "someday [from younger generations] will come the next president of this country."[22]

## Conclusion

Julio Volcy is a caring and engaged pastor in Haiti who is devoted to combatting oppression in Port-au-Prince. Adequate public healthcare is a principal area of concern. For Volcy and like-minded individuals, successful healthcare reform can generate a new spirit of possibility. He wants the youth to follow a simple principle: "If I can do it for you, I will do it; and the same thing I want for me is what I want for you."[23] That principle underscores Volcy's belief that everyone has a role to play in creating a better Haitian society and eliminating systemic oppression. When those things happen, the threat to public health can be erased, which not only helps those who are impoverished but also every person in Haiti. "We have to provide an opportunity for everyone to thrive. And without eliminating oppression of their minds and spirits, which are at the root of so many evils in Haiti," Volcy declares, "we will never have a healthy society."[24]

## Notes

1 Sandra Lemaire and Matiado Vilme, "Haiti Confirms Its First Coronavirus Cases," *Voice of America*, March 20, 2020, https://www.voanews.com/science-health/coronavirus-outbreak/haiti-confirms-its-first-coronavirus-cases.

2 "WHO Director-General's Opening Remarks at the Media Briefing on COVID-19," *World Health Organization*, March 11, 2020, https://www.who.int/director-general/speeches/detail/who-director-general-s-opening-remarks-at-the-media-briefing-on-covid-19. March 11, 2020.

3 Jude Mary Cénat, "The Vulnerability of Low- and Middle-Income Countries Facing the COVID-19 Pandemic: The Case of Haiti," *Travel Medicine and Infectious Disease* 37 (September–October 2020), 101684, https://doi-org.libproxy.clemson.edu/10.1016/j.tmaid.2020.101684.

4 Julio Volcy, interview by B. Denise Hawkins and Ervin E. Dyer, June 25, 2020 (hereafter cited as Hawkins, Dyer, and Volcy Interview).

5 Hawkins, Dyer, and Volcy Interview, June 25, 2020.

6 Caitlin Hu, "Millions in Haiti Face Hunger in 2020," *CNN*, December 30, 2019, https://www.cnn.com/2019/12/30/world/haiti-hunger-doctors-intl/index.html; Food and Agricultural Organization of the United Nations et al., *The State of Food Security and Nutrition in the World 2019: Safeguarding against Economic Slowdowns and Downturns* (Rome, Italy: Food and Agricultural Organization of the United Nations, 2019), 60, 74–75, 87, 94, 149, 168, 177, 179, 213; United Nations World Food Programme, "Haiti," https://www.wfp.org/countries/haiti.

7 "Weekly Press Briefing on COVID-19: Director's Opening Remarks, May 5, 2020," *Pan American Health Organization*, https://www.paho.org/en/documents/weekly-press-briefing-covid-19-directors-opening-remarks-may-5-2020.

8 Opportunity International Canada, "Where We Work: Haiti," 2021, https://www.opportunityinternational.ca/what-we-do/where-we-work/haiti; United States Department of State, "2020 Investment Climate Statements: Haiti," https://www.state.gov/reports/2020-investment-climate-statements/haiti/.

9 Joseph Maria, "Haiti's COVID-19 Response," *Borgen*, September 10, 2020, https://www.borgenmagazine.com/haitis-covid-19-relief-response/.

10 "Haiti Reaches One-Year Free of Cholera," *Pan American Health Organization*, January 23, 2020, https://www.paho.org/en/news/23-1-2020-haiti-reaches-one-year-free-cholera.

11 United States Centers for Disease Control and Prevention, "One Year Later: Haiti Public Health System Rebounds with Help from US, Other Partners," July 1, 2020, https://www.cdc.gov/globalhealth/countries/haiti/stories/haiti_public_health_system.html.

12 UNAIDS, "Haiti," 2020, https://www.unaids.org/en/regionscountries/countries/haiti.

13 "World Bank to Strengthen Human Capital and Climate Resilience in Haiti," *World Bank*, May 17, 2019, https://www.worldbank.org/en/news/press-release/2019/05/17/world-bank-to-strengthen-human-capital-and-climate-resilience-in-haiti.

14 United States Department of Health and Human Services Office of Disease Prevention and Health Promotion, "Social Determinants of Health," *Healthy People.gov*, June 23, 2021, https: www.healthypeople.gov/2020. See also Laurent Dubois, *Haiti: The Aftershocks of History* (2012; repr., New York, NY: Picador, 2013), 6–7, 360–70.

15 United States Centers for Disease Control, "People with Certain Medical Conditions," May 13, 2021, https://www.cdc.gov/coronavirus/2019-ncov/need-extra-precautions/people-with-medical-conditions.html?CDC_AA_refVal=https%3A%2F%2Fwww.cdc.gov%2Fcoronavirus%2F2019-ncov%2F-need-extra-precautions%2Fgroups-at-higher-risk.html

16 Hawkins, Dyer, and Volcy Interviews, October 15–16, 2017, November 22–27, 2019, and June 25, 2020.

17 Hawkins, Dyer, and Volcy Interview, June 25, 2020.

18 Hawkins, Dyer, and Volcy Interview, June 25, 2020

19 Mark 9:23, King James Version.

20 Hawkins, Dyer, and Volcy Interview, June 25, 2020.

21 Hawkins, Dyer, and Volcy Interview, June 25, 2020.

22 Hawkins, Dyer, and Volcy Interview, June 25, 2020.

23 Hawkins, Dyer, and Volcy Interview, June 25, 2020.

24 Hawkins, Dyer, and Volcy Interview, June 25, 2020.

# 23 Black Women's Reproductive Health, Justice, and COVID-19 Complications in the United States

*Bernetta D. Welch*

## Introduction

For women of color, contending as they have with systemic racism, social injustice, and the right to control their own bodies, ensuring reproductive justice has been an urgent need for generations. Certain predominantly white initiatives have addressed reproductive justice in general but often have not dealt with particularities related to race, ethnicity, or class. Consequently, gross maleficence on the part of medical professionals and racism-laced care delivery systems remain. Such malfeasance includes sterilizing women of color without their knowledge or consent, imposing stricter sentences on pregnant women of color who have drugs in their systems while giving birth than on white women in similar conditions, more judicial impositions of contraceptive measures on black women than their white counterparts in exchange for lighter sentences, and making abortions more accessible for affluent white women than for poorer white women and women of color.

Such acts violate biomedical ethics, a healthcare construct grounded in four basic moral principles: Respect for autonomy, beneficence, nonmaleficence, and justice.[1] While a relatively new discipline, biomedical ethics developed as an outgrowth of neglected areas of the Hippocratic tradition. The aforementioned principles are ethical norms that form the rules and obligations of how medical professionals in the context of healthcare should treat patients, distribute resources and information, and make decisions regarding the care of their patients.[2]

Respect for autonomy is the recognition of the rights of individuals to make choices based on personal values and beliefs, providing the individual has the mental capacity to do so.[3] Regarding women, their decision to give birth or not give birth constitutes an autonomous act. Nonmaleficence delineates several rules, including not causing unnecessary pain, incapacitating, or offending as well as not depriving others of the life necessities. Nonmaleficence also means equal treatment without regard to sex, religion, race, nationality, gender, or ethnicity and prohibits the threat of a punitive act or action (e.g., family division, unfair

DOI: 10.4324/9781003214281-27

removal of a child). Nonmaleficence furthermore obligates one to neither withhold nor withdraw beneficial treatment if a patient likely will recover and live a full life.[4]

Beneficence, a more affirmative principle of rights and protections than nonmaleficence, is concerned with an obligation to act for the benefit of others. Given that physicians often are in authoritative positions to determine patients' interests, beneficence mandates that, whenever possible, patients are active in decision-making processes.[5] As regards justice, the principle prevents unfair or wrongful acts such as denying needed resources or lawful protections or receiving social benefits on the basis of an undeserved advantage.[6] In some instances, self-made choices by women of color seem to have been excluded from legal protections; instead, their choices have been subjected to much interference and obstruction.[7]

This essay explores the principles of healthcare ethics as aids to the reproductive justice movement in the United States that various women of color launched during the mid-1990s. They responded to persistent race-based health disparities., especially among black women. The essay also explores ways public resources, including resources emanating from black religious life, should be mobilized and leveraged to ensure collective reproductive justice for women of color. The essay also examines how the COVID-19 pandemic has affected reproductive health among women of color. Research indicates women of color suffer higher rates of prenatal stress, anxiety, and depression than white women and that such conditions can have long-term effects on mothers and their children.[8]

## Reproductive Health, Reproductive Rights, and Reproductive Justice

The global reproductive justice movement emerged against a backdrop of predominantly white reproductive rights activism focused largely on abortion rights and contraceptive choice. In the United States, the women of color who helped launch the movement recognized their white mainly economically well-off white contemporaries did not advocate for many needs in communities of color. The American reproductive justice movement thus broadened the abortion debate, creating a mechanism to address unfair polices and legal interpretations that placed limits on the reproductive freedoms of women of color. Movement organizers stressed the need to make decisions to have children or not have children in safe environments.[9]

Regarding the international context of the reproduction justice movement, the year 1994 is pivotal. While preparing to attend the International Conference on Population and Development in Cairo, Egypt, a set of black women used the term *reproductive justice* to emphasize the idea that an individual's right to plan a family was central to global development. Members of the group named themselves Women of African Descent for

Reproductive Justice and started a campaign (later movement) rooted in three core principles. One, every woman had the right to decide if or when she would have a baby as well any other condition regarding childbirth. Two, a woman could prevent or terminate a pregnancy. Finally, a woman should be able to parent a child with necessary social support in a safe environment and a healthy community without fear of violence from another individual or government.[10]

Since 1994, numerous women of color have expanded the framework the Women of African Descent for Reproductive Justice created to include economic injustice, welfare reform, prisoner's rights, environmental justice, immigration, and drug policy in addition to reproductive choice.[11] Linda Ross, an African American author, activist, and cofounder of a Southern-based national organization called Sister Song (or SisterSong),[12] often discusses "reproductive oppression," or systematic population control via the regulating of women's bodies.[13] As she and her colleague, scholar Ricker Solinger, explained in 2017, reproductive justice combines social and reproductive rights and then centers that combination as a human right.[14]

"Convention on the Prevention and Punishment for the Crime of Genocide," a document the United Nations General Assembly ratified on December 9, 1948, is of utmost importance to the human rights element of the reproductive justice movement.[15] According to the document, "imposing measures intended to prevent births within [a] group, and forcibly transferring children of the group to another group," was a genocidal act.[16] That definition matched the experiences of countless African American women who suffered sterilization without consent, who lost children to an unfair foster care system, or whose pregnancies officials criminalized. Such reproductive control fostered reproductive oppression, which often resulted in detrimental outcomes for affected women and other loved ones.

The reproductive justice movement has proceeded along three major service delivery trajectories: health, rights, and justice.[17] Reproductive health addresses the improvement and the expansion of services (e.g., information, research, data) pursuant to developing prevention mechanisms that are culturally sensitive to women of color.[18] Reproductive rights form the basis of the delivery model embodying legal and other advocacy services. The model functions to safeguard existing constitutional protections that are not applied sufficiently to reproductive matters. By my estimation, incarcerated women, women clients of social assistance programs, and women and girls of color in poor communities who are without recourse in fighting structural and institutional racism concerning their bodies are most vulnerable to reproductive rights abuses.[19] The third trajectory, justice, takes the form of movement-building by women concerned with the intersectionality of reproductive rights, environmental and sociocultural issues, economics, and politics.[20]

## Impacts of COVID-19 on Women of Color
## and Federal Legislation

According to Diana Bianchi, a medical geneticist and neonatologist who directs the Eunice Kennedy Shriver National Institute of Child Health and Human Development, the COVID-19 pandemic has resulted in further endangerment of maternal health. Increased incidents of infant mortality, complications related to high blood pressure, postpartum hemorrhaging, and premature delivery are illustrative. As far as race/ethnicity are concerned, disparities have long been evident in pregnancy outcomes. For instance, black women have endured higher pre-term birth rates and maternal morbidity than their white counterparts. My research shows that other historical indices of disparity (e.g., anxiety, depression, underemployment) often worsen the mental health of pregnant black women.[21]

In addition to the matters discussed above, widespread shifting to routine care using telehealth systems during the COVID pandemic has posed major risks to women of color and to other marginalized women in the United States. Sometimes, during telephone conferences, physicians or other caregivers do not pay as close attention to what those pregnant women say as the caregivers would during traditional in-person, or face-to-face, consultations. Additionally, caregivers might not take the concerns of pregnant women of color as seriously as they would if consultations were in person. Of equal significance as those two possibilities, some pregnant women of color are not positioned well to pick up on symptoms of prenatal complications that physicians and other caregivers might catch during traditional face-to-face visits. Restricting such visits also means fewer ultrasound tests, cervical checks, laboratory work, and opportunities for additional health screenings.[22] According to Michelle Williams, dean of faculty at the Harvard T.H. Chan School of Public Health, those and related matters lead to a "disproportionate burden of morbidity and mortality" in black, brown, and poor white communities.[23]

Changing policies that limit maternal support during labor and delivery constitute an additional reproductive concern during the COVID pandemic. Fear of spreading the disease has caused hospital administrators to eliminate doulas, family members, and other individuals from being present during deliveries and post-delivery stays. Angelina Aina, interim director for Black Mamas Matter Alliance, confirmed the stories of black maternal advocates who have separated mothers suspected of having COVID from their babies. That act interrupted the skin-to-skin, or bonding, period between mother and child. While prudent, as the life of both mother and baby are at risk if a mother is infected with COVID, hospital administrators have separated more black mothers and babies than their white counterparts. Furthermore, black women have expressed being pressured into having Caesarean sections to limit the length of their hospital stays, increasing risks, and complications during delivery.[24]

Despite an assortment of major challenges on which COVID has cast a bright light, black and other women of color have demonstrated much resilience. From April 17, 2020, to May 1, as the pandemic spread around the world, a group of medical researchers in the United States conducted a survey among 787 pregnant women.[25] Two hundred sixteen were black, non-Hispanic/Latina women who completed a twenty-one-item questionnaire covering five factors of resilience: Emotion regulation, supportive close relationships, non-hostile close relationships, and perceived neighborhood safety.[26] Results indicated high levels of resilience among the black women surveyed, as expressed in their abilities to push through anxieties and take care of personal and familial needs.[27]

Although resilience is critical to the health prospects of women of color, achieving changes and reforms to reproductive healthcare policies and practices is more important. Policymakers are considering changes to Medicaid coverage for postpartum mothers, increasing insurance services, training more black female doctors, and encouraging current healthcare providers to not only listen to but also heed the concerns of black women.[28] With respect to Medicaid, there has been a growing cry among Democrats in the United States House of Representatives to expand coverage for pregnant women and new mothers.[29] In November 2019, the majority in the House Energy and Commerce Committee approved two bipartisan bills to address maternal mortality by voice vote, but the bills have not come to the floor.[30] The bills authorize coverage under Medicaid and the Children's Health Insurance Program for one-year postpartum care, new funding for state programs that address maternal health, and coverage for midwifery.[31]

Several advocacy groups have led the charge for legislative reform. For example, members of the Black Mamas Maternal Association lobbied for passage of the Black Maternal Health Momnibus Act, a piece of legislation Congresswoman Lauren Underwood, a Democrat from Illinois, introduced into the US House of Representatives in March 2020 and reintroduced in February 2021.[32] The act focuses on increasing prenatal workforces, among other things. Additional policy initiatives the association supports include using doulas as support persons in delivery rooms and obtaining grants to fund a larger number of midwives and physician assistants. It is important to note, these bills have not yet been passed but are supported by 93 groups, including The American College of Obstetricians and Gynecologists.[33] A separate organization, the Black Maternal Health Association, wants to see the US Department of Health and Human Services award grants to improve maternal outcomes and reduce bias and discrimination in maternal care.[34]

Sister Song is yet another organization whose members have promoted action steps that provide means to mobilize resources to fight against reproductive punishment and other forms of oppression. Members understand the intersectional reproductive needs of women of color, the constitutional rights to have needs addressed, and the necessity of collaborating with other reproductive justice organizations to achieve common goals. Collaboration is particularly important for black women, whom white people, especially men, historically have refused to fully acknowledgment humanity and identity. Sister Song's concerns emanate not only from pro-choice and pro-life differences, but also from a broader range of matters bearing on family development, respect for a black woman's body, autonomy, and the demand for quality medical care.[35]

## Conclusion

The fight for reproductive justice is not a new struggle. For example, the dark history of forced sterilization without proper consent is one aspect that is centuries old. Today, black women lead the charge to address such injustice, but additional warriors are needed. Bioethicists, lawmakers and other public policymakers, and medical professionals are simply three groups whose members can diversify the aforementioned army of women battling to achieve reproductive justice. In so doing, they set an example for other faith soldiers who seek to leverage multifaceted resources to ensure the health and wellness of women.

## Notes

1　Tom L. Beauchamp and James F. Childress, *Principles of Biomedical Ethics*, 6th ed. New York, NY: Oxford University Press, 2009). Some scholars expand the list of biomedical ethics to as many as seven, adding health maximization, efficiency, and proportionality to nonmaleficence, beneficence, respect for autonomy, and justice. Peter Schröder-Bäck et al., "Teaching Seven Principles for Public Health Ethics: Towards a Curriculum for a Short Course on Ethics in Public Health Programmes," *BMC Medical Ethics* 15 (October 7, 2014): 1–10, http://www.biomedcentral.com/1472-6939/15/73.

2　Beauchamp and Childress, *Principles of Biomedical Ethics*, 1–14.

3　Beauchamp and Childress, *Principles of Biomedical Ethics*, 105.

4　Beauchamp and Childress, *Principles of Biomedical Ethics*, 149–53.

5　Beauchamp and Childress, *Principles of Biomedical Ethics*, 208.

6　Beauchamp and Childress, *Principles of Biomedical Ethics*, 241.

7　Dorothy Roberts, *Killing the Black Body: Race, Reproduction, and the Meaning of Liberty* (New York, NY: Pantheon Books, 1997), 294.

8　Raquel E. Gur et al., "The Disproportionate Burden of the COVID-19 Pandemic among Pregnant Black Women," *Psychiatric Research* 293 (November 2020): 1–8, doi: 10.1016/j.psychres.2020.113475.

9　Loretta J. Ross and Rickie Solinger, *Reproductive Justice: An Introduction* (Oakland, CA: University of California Press, 2017), 9. See also Rebecca J. Cook and Bernard M. Dickens, "From Reproductive Choice to Reproductive Justice," *International Journal of Gynecology and Obstetrics* 106 (August 2009): 106–9.

10　Zakiya Luna and Kristin Luker, "Reproductive Justice," *Annual Review of Law and Social Science* 9 (2013): 327–52; Ross and Solinger, *Reproductive Justice*, 9 (enumerating the trio of core principles).

11  Cook and Dickens, "From Reproductive Choice to Reproductive Justice."

12  For information about Sister Song, visit https://www.sistersong.net/.

13  Loretta Ross, "Understanding Reproductive Justice: Transforming the Pro-Choice Movement," *Off Our Backs* 36 (January 2006): 14.

14  Ross and Solinger, *Reproductive Justice*, 9.

15  United Nations General Assembly, "Convention on the Prevention and Punishment for the Crime of Genocide," December 9, 1948, https://web-cache.googleusercontent.com/search?q=cache: n-076PqZ0xEJ: https://www.un.org/en/genocideprevention/documents/atrocity-crimes/Doc.1_Convention%2520on%2520the%2520Prevention%2520and%2520Punishment%2520of%2520the%2520Crime%2520of%2520Genocide.pdf+&cd=1&hl=en&ct=clnk&gl=us (hereafter cited as UNGA, "Convention.").

16  UNGA, "Convention."

17  Ross, "Understanding Reproductive Justice.

18  Ross, "Understanding Reproductive Justice."

19  Luna and Luker, "Reproductive Justice."

20  Ross, "Understanding Reproductive Justice," 14–19.

21  Regarding infant mortality, high blood pressure, postpartum hemorrhaging, and premature delivery, among other matters I discuss in the main text, see Diana W. Bianchi and *Janine Clayton,* "A Mother's Day Message: Time for Action to Improve Maternal Health," *National Library of Medicine Musings from the Mezzanine,* May 12, 2021, https://nlmdirector.nlm.nih.gov/2021/05/12/a-mothers-day-message-time-for-action-to-improve-maternal-health/.

22  Eona Harrison and Ebonie Megibow, "Three Ways COVID-19 is Further Jeopardizing Black Women's Health," *Urban Wire,* July 30, 2020, https://www.urban.org/urban-wire/three-ways-covid-19-further-jeopardizing-black-maternal-health.

23  Sandhya Raman, "COVID-19 Amplifies Racial Disparities in Maternal Health," *Roll Call,* May 14, 2020, https://www.rollcall.com/2020/05/14/covid-19-amplifies-racial-disparities-in-maternal-health.

24  Raman, "COVID-19 Amplifies Racial Disparities."

25  Gur et al., "Disproportionate Burden," 2–3.

26  Gur et al., "Disproportionate Burden," 3.

27  Gur et al., "Disproportionate Burden."

28  Jamila Taylor et al., "Eliminating Racial Disparities in Maternal and Infant Mortality: A Comprehensive Policy Blueprint," *Center for American Progress,* May 2, 2019, https://www.americanprogress.org/issues/women/reports/2019/05/02/469186/eliminating-racial-disparities-maternal-infant-mortality/.

29  Raman, "COVID-19 Amplifies Racial Disparities."

30  Raman, "COVID-19 Amplifies Racial Disparities."

31  Raman, "COVID-19 Amplifies Racial Disparities."

32  Raman, "COVID-19 Amplifies Racial Disparities."

33  Raman, "COVID-19 Amplifies Racial Disparities."

34  Raman, "COVID-19 Amplifies Racial Disparities."

35  Regarding white Americans' historical denial of black women's humanity, see Roberts, *Killing the Black Body,* 302.

# 24 Film as a Pedagogical Tool for Trauma- and Resiliency-Informed Theology and Liturgy

*Phil Allen*

## Introduction

In 2020, I screened *Open Wounds: A Story of Racial Tragedy, Trauma, and Redemption*, a documentary short film about the 1953 murder of my grandfather, Nate Allen, in Georgetown, South Carolina. On his death certificate, officials stated he died from an accidental drowning. They ignored the bullet hole in the back of his head.[1]

After viewing the film during a virtual screening, Reena Evers-Everette, daughter of Medgar Evers, the NAACP field worker a violently racist white man shot and killed in 1963, responded through tears of pain as she recounted being a witness to her father's murder fifty-seven years earlier. She recognized the film as necessary work to tell the unspoken narrative of intergenerational trauma in the African American community, but it stimulated memory capsules her body had stored for decades. She could see and, moreover, feel her family's story in mine. No longer, Evers-Everette decided, would she sit in shadows; it was time to write her chapter in Evers family's long saga, a decision with potential to further her personal healing process. Such responses to *Open Wounds* have been commonplace at screenings. Viewers have exposed unattended traumas lingering beneath the surface of consciousness their bodies have hosted.[2]

The COVID-19 pandemic not only has provided context for the awareness of trauma but it also has been a catalyst for stimulating trauma, especially among African Americans. In May 2020, as the rapid spread of COVID in the United States slowed the pace of life almost to a halt for millions of people, several concerned citizens in Minneapolis, Minnesota, videotaped the brutally unnecessary police killing of George Floyd, an African American resident. After detaining Floyd for trying to use a twenty-dollar counterfeit bill—a minor legal violation—policeman thrust him to the ground and knelt hard on his neck for nine minutes and twenty-nine seconds until he died. That fatal act demonstrated the widespread racial/ethnic injustice that African Americans long knew existed but that innumerable others denied. Furthermore, videotaped victims became more than statistics; their recorded demises enabled viewers to connect names and faces. No longer

DOI: 10.4324/9781003214281-28

was it easy for many people to ignore racially/ethnically motivated violations, though some people continued to do so.[3]

The disproportionate number of African Americans who have become ill or died from complications associated with COVID-19 has prompted citizens to look at other racial/ethnic violations, to include inequities in the healthcare system, a matter I explore below. For African Americans themselves, however, the pandemic has triggered myriad emotions because not only has every day been a reminder of social inequity but also of isolation from community and interruptions of normal rhythms of life. All ancestry groups have experienced similar isolation and interruptions, but, because of the long history of racial/ethnic discrimination in the US, COVID-related hardships have been especially trying for African Americans. Vaccinations constitute a case in point. Because of the memory of the 1932 to 1972 syphilis experiment in Tuskegee, Alabama, among other public and private experimentations on black bodies, a considerable segment of the African American population has been leery of becoming vaccinated during the COVID pandemic.[4]

Clinical psychologist and trauma specialist Gladys K. Mwiti believes COVID has escalated mental health challenges and social breakdowns among vulnerable groups such as the depressed, poor, or unemployed as well as among people with histories of domestic violence and verbal abuse.[5] Her list of vulnerable people is not exhaustive. For example, frontline workers in occupations whom state and federal lawmakers deem essential—agriculture, child and healthcare, food production, retail, transportation—and incarcerated individuals are two additional groups who fit the vulnerable description, and people of color make up a sizeable portion of both groups.[6] Though numbers are inexact, much data confirm that African Americans, Latino Americans, and Asian Americans comprise a large segment of the essential workforce across the country.[7] Accordingly, they have greater exposure to COVID than people in nonessential occupations, especially white collar fields.

In relation to incarcerated populations, in 2019, the year for which the latest data from the National Prison Statistics program of the United States Bureau of Justice Statistics are available, African Americans and Latino Americans comprised 53 percent of the total prison population (but only 32 percent of the US population).[8] For many incarcerated individuals, the spread of COVID in facilities has deepened existing traumas. As several scholars have noted, emotional abuse such as youth abandonment is prevalent among imprisoned adults.[9] In one study, Nancy Wolff and Jing Shi reported 25 percent of incarcerated men were abandoned during their childhood or adolescent years.[10]

In this essay, which deals primarily with African Americans, I use film to show how intergenerational trauma can be a contributing factor in behavioral and physical health concerns. Regrettably, many individuals, especially clerics, have neglected to consider how such trauma might affect present behavior. I likewise demonstrate that film, as storytelling, is as a useful pedagogical tool to bring attention, as well as healing, to trauma. Specifically, film aids in developing trauma- and resiliency-informed theology and liturgy.

### Open Wounds

The film *Open Wounds* and the COVID-19 pandemic reveal the significance of three concepts: Intergenerational trauma, intergenerational resiliency, and redemptive potentiality. In my judgment, the open wounds of trauma concretize a statement James Baldwin made in 1961: "To be Black and conscious in America is to be in a constant state of rage."[11] Such rage also presents an opportunity to invite others to look more deeply into African American experiences to conceive a narrative of empathy and hopefulness.[12]

*Intergenerational Trauma.* The body is a storehouse for trauma. A community of bodies, even an intergenerational multigenerational community, expands into a compound for trauma that creates an infirmary of what I term dis-eased bodies. In his 2014 book, *The Body Keeps the Score*, Bessel A. van der Kolk asserted that one way "the memory of helplessness is stored is as muscle tension or feelings of disintegration in the affected body area."[13] As a body keeps score, it creates and then sustains a narrative about the person until something disrupts and replaces the narrative with something else that gives new life.[14]

As regards African Americans, I submit their collective narrative is uninterrupted because the toxicity of racial/ethnic stress (i.e., trauma) is chronic. The beliefs of family therapist Robin Karr-Morse, lawyer Meredith S. Wiley, and neurologist Robert Scaer are foundational.[15] In a 2012 book titled *Scared Sick*, Karr-Morse and Wiley built on the work of Scaer and confirmed that several traumatic diseases resulted from "chronic perceptions of helplessness and hopelessness added to toxic stress, leading to the overstimulation of the autonomic nervous system."[16] Continually stressed, the traumatized mind manifests as health issues over time, rendering one vulnerable to further trauma.[17] Psychotherapist Resmaa Menakem suggests the way many people respond to that cycle is an undiscerned part of their narrative that becomes intergenerational, or part of a seemingly familial cultural norm.[18] Those in his profession often refer to that process as traumatic retention: the ostensible norms informs the narrative that minds or bodies tell and that people believe from one generation to the next.[19]

*Intergenerational Resiliency.* Having resilience, or being elastic, essentially means possessing the ability to rebound, spring back, stretch, or withstand.[20] In relation to human life, a resilient person is one who endures a challenge, or trial, and recovers from it.[21] Writing about African Americans, Menakem affirms they "have proven very resilient, in part because, over generations, African Americans have developed a variety of body-centered responses to help settle their bodies and blunt the effects of racialized trauma. These include individual and collective humming, rocking, rhythmic clapping, drumming, singing, grounding touch, wailing circles, and call and response, to name just a few."[22]

In countless instances, stories of resistance that people tell invite others to see themselves in their own untold stories. Similar to many African American families, mine held on to my grandfather's killing in secrecy, likely to avoid revisiting trauma and thereby protecting future generations. If concealed, however, trauma goes undiagnosed, unnamed, and untreated. Likewise, in muting one's own narrative, one's resiliency is neither recognized nor honored.

*Redemptive Potential.* Healing can occur in the process of metabolizing trauma by remembering, naming, and telling a story. My father, in discussing his depression in recent years, shared with me that his therapist suggested his condition resulted from the deaths of his brother and mother only six months apart—in October 2015 and May 2016, respectively. I followed up by asking him if he believed he also was depressed because he never knew his father. He replied he was two years old when someone murdered his father. That fact was my point: he had been grieving his father's death all his life, never addressing the trauma in a healthy way. Instead, he displayed grief through anger, violence, and medicating with substance use. Our exchange was revelatory, and my father agreed to reflect further during his therapy sessions.

Healing occurred between my father and me in the midst of discussing his own father. While recalling stories that relatives and other persons told him about his father, he and I took comfort in how much we were like my grandfather. Our conversation created a new family narrative that I extended via my short film, *Open Wounds*.[23]

## The COVID-19 Pandemic, or Pause

Film is not a cure-all, or instant healer, for trauma; however, film can contribute to healing by providing opportunities for connecting trauma to its source, thereby facilitating a solution. Film reclaims the narrative, or historical account, for an individual or a group whom another more individual or group dominates or redacts. With regard to racial/ethnic minorities who have undergone traumatic experiences, film presents opportunities for others to enter into narratives with those who carry the trauma in their bodies. The COVID-19 pandemic, or pause, as I term the phenomenon, is an exemplar. Though traumatic, it has presented people with an opportunity to engage the narrative of discrimination. In the United States, where people of African descent have endured much injustice since enslavement, descendants of enslavers and others who have benefited from white privilege can help alleviate trauma by admitting and furthermore discussing the history of bias in the country in open and honest manners. Those courageous acts,

I believe, can assist in the closing of personal and communal wounds, which in turn will constitute a giant first step on the path of American healing.

African Americans are principal actors in both discrimination and COVID narratives. As several scholars have shown in recent decades, contemporary African American bodies store loads of historical trauma: from chattel slavery to Jim and Jane Crowism to unfair police and justice system cruelty that result in disproportionate levels of mass incarceration.[24] The COVID pandemic has made those loads heavier. As of March 7, 2021, almost a year after the World Health Organization designated COVID a pandemic,[25] black Americans have died from complications associated with the disease at a rate of 1.4 times more than white Americans, according to the COVID Tracking Project.[26]

While COVID has had a disproportionate impact on communities of color, particularly African Americans, the pandemic in my opinion has been advantageous in one regard: The forced Sabbath (i.e., compelled collective pause) of stay-at-home, lockdown, and shutdown orders has caused many other Americans to not only see but also feel the trauma that historically discriminatory racial/ethnic structure have forced on African Americans. For example, disparities between white and nonwhite students who have had access to the internet for remote learning during the pandemic is evidence of structural inequity, both economic and social.[27] The high percentage of nonwhite Americans who work as frontline workers in essential occupations, which typically are blue collar jobs, is further evidence of such inequity. As stated above, those laborers are more likely than those in nonessential occupations, especially white collar jobs, to test positive, become sick or, worse, die from COVID complications.[28]

The COVID pandemic has crystallized abstract notions of racism that countless members of dominant groups in the US—most notably, certain affluent white people—have not discerned. Fortunately, the slowed pace of many survivors, together with the hundreds of millions of lost lives, has resulted in shared empathies among people worldwide. The cluster of racially/ethnically motivated tragedies (e.g., the death of George Floyd) that have made national and international news have birthed multiracial/multiethnic global movements unlike the localized and predominantly African American protests that occurred after murders caught on video cameras before the pandemic. While some opponents of such movements have caused violence and bloodshed, I believe supporters of the movements should not retaliate in kind. Supporters should not frame their protests as stages of anger; instead, protests should be spaces for shared lament, empathy, hope, and healing. The COVID pandemic has presented similar opportunities for positive advancement.[29]

As stated earlier in this essay, black people in the United States carry generations of trauma; hence, their immune systems are comprised—metaphorically if not literally, acknowledged or unacknowledged. Because the damage COVID does to people extends beyond their immune systems,

COVID is an apt metaphor for the assortment of societal diseases biased white people have created to attack black people. As I see matters, the assault on blackness demands a response featuring newly oriented language, or theology, and practice, or liturgy, from caring individuals and groups, and the Black Church is positioned well to help fashion that response.[30]

## The Body Tells the Story

Storytelling is a tool that churchgoers can use to educate, provide space for lament and empathy, or build solidarity, among other things that help generate resilient language and practices in theology and liturgy. Film, in particular, provides an opportunity to tell a story vividly because film contains visual imagery. Seeing, not simply reading or hearing, the story facilitates understanding fully any underlying cause—in my instance, an act of bigotry that led to the death of my grandfather. As scholars like David R. Williams make plain, such traumatic acts can have serious adverse effects on the emotional, physical, and psychological health of individuals and families.[31]

The palliative element of storytelling is not a new concept, nor is it unique to African Americans. Oral traditions (e.g., passing down informative histories, sharing encouraging testimonies, singing songs that evoke individual, familial, or community memories) have been generational bridges and healing balms for many ethnic groups in the United States and abroad. However, because of decades of legal and extralegal devices that kept enslaved people of African descent from becoming literate before federal and state adoption of the Thirteenth Amendment to the US Constitution abolished racial/ethnic slavery in the country, orality has played an integral part in African American culture.[32]

Among other things, oral stories have preserved histories, testimonies, and cultural norms that have helped black people and black institutions such as The Church strengthen their resistance to unwelcome white assimilation processes. In the South Carolina Lowcountry, where my grandfather lived and died, Gullah, or Geechee, people have preserved their distinct culture longer than any other racial/ethnic group in the United States, and storytelling has been a crucial part of their heritage. In a similar vein, black churches throughout the South Carolina Lowcountry have told stories, given testimonies, sang songs, and performed other acts that have helped congregants understand God equally as well, if not better, than simply hearing lecture style sermons.[33]

Storytelling often inspires new language. As I say often, storytelling is the language of imagination, the language of poetry and improvisation versus the language prose and predictability. Even though historical storytelling needs to be accurate, a central feature of my short film, *Open Wounds*, the story a historian tells can offer or engender new insight. In the case of the Black Church, storytelling can result in new theology.[34] For example, the Eucharist, as a sacrament, is storytelling, poetry, a symbiosis of tragedy and beauty. The tragedy Jesus withstood enabled him to fulfill God's will, and beauty rests in the eternal implication of his faithfulness and resilience for humanity's benefit. Jesus's story enables followers to not only have faith in ultimate victory but also to cohere his narrative with their own. Viewed through that lens, the suffering of Christians connects with the suffering of their Christ, Jesus. A follower might lament, but a follower also can have faith that healing is possible. I convey a similar idea in my short film, *Open Wounds*, and other African American churchgoers can do the same in relation to COVID-19.[35]

## Conclusion

The COVID pandemic has functioned as the context for personal and collective awareness of undiscerned trauma. For me the pandemic, mask-wearing, and vaccines all are metaphors for identifying/naming and controlling/slowing down the spread of another disease, racial/ethnic injustice. The drama of the COVID pandemic, as tragic as it has turned out to be, also is an invitation to diagnose and, moreover, treat the discrimination that has ravaged the US since the early republic. As I make clear throughout this essay, the Black Church can help generate such healing, and film can help document that godly work.

## Notes

1 Phil Allen Jr., *Open Wounds: A Story of Racial Tragedy, Trauma, and Redemption* (Minneapolis, MN: Fortress Press, 2021). For more information about the Open Wounds Project and access to a short film, visit www.openwoundsdoc.com. Unless I note otherwise, each reference I make to *Open Wounds* is in regard to the film. *Open Wounds*, prod. Phil Allen, Jr., dir. L. Michael Lee (Los Angeles, CA: Twlve21 Media and Divyzed Media Group, 2019).

2 Medgar Evers, *The Autobiography of Medgar Evers: A Hero's Life and Legacy Revealed through His Writings, Letters, and Speeches*, Myrlie Evers-Williams and Manning Marable, eds. (New York, NY: Basic Books, 2006); Michael Vincent Williams, *Medgar Evers: Mississippi Martyr* (Fayetteville, NC: University of Arkansas Press, 2011).

3 The murders of Brunswick, Georgia, citizen Ahmaud Arbery in February 2020 and Breonna Taylor of Louisville, Kentucky, in March constitute a cluster of tragedies that embody the long history of contemporary anti-black violence and injustice at the hands of white police officers and ordinary citizens. According to one 2018 scholarly article, police officers killed "more than 300 black Americans—at least one quarter of them unarmed—each year in the USA. These events might have spillover effects of the mental health of people not directly affected." Jacob Bor et al., "Police Killings and Their Spillover Effects on the Mental Health of Black Americans: A Population-Based, Quasi-Experimental Study," *Lancet* 392 (June 28, 2018): 302.

4 Debbie Elliott, "In Tuskegee, Painful History Shadows Efforts to Vaccinate African Americans," *NPR*, February 16, 2021, https://www.npr.org/2021/02/16/967011614/in-tuskegee-painful-history-shadows-efforts-to-vaccinate-african-americans; Sabrina R. Liu and Sheila Modir, "The Outbreak

That Was Always Here: Racial Trauma in the Context of COVID-19 and Implications for Mental Health Providers," *Psychological Trauma: Theory, Research, Practice, and Policy* 12 (July 2020): 439–42; United States Centers for Disease Control and Prevention, "The Tuskegee Timeline," April 22, 2021, https://www.cdc.gov/tuskegee/timeline.htm. April Dembosky is one of many people who have proven African American vaccination concern is more multitudinous than the so-called Tuskegee Experiment and includes health safety and religious preference. Dembosky, "No, the Tuskegee Study Is Not the Top Reason Some Black Americans Question the COVID-19 Vaccine," *KQED*, February 25, 2021, https://www.kqed.org/news/11861810/no-the-tuskegee-study-is-not-the-top-reason-some-black-americans-question-the-covid-19-vaccine.

5   Gladys K. Mwiti, "Building Hope and Resilience in the COVID-19 Storm: Lament, Communities of Care and the New Normal," *Evangelical Focus Europe*, February 2, 2021, https://evangelicalfocus.com/lausanne-movement/9973/building-hope-and-resilence-in-the-covid-19-storm.

6   National Conference of State Legislatures, "COVID-19: Essential Workers in the States," January 11, 2021, https://www.ncsl.org/research/labor-and-employment/covid-19-essential-workers-in-the-states.aspx; United States Cybersecurity and Infrastructure Security Agency, "Identifying Critical Infrastructure during COVID-19," https://www.cisa.gov/identifying-critical-infrastructure-during-covid-19.

7   While white Americans make up the majority of frontline workers overall, people of color are overrepresented in many occupations. See Jocelyn Frye, "On the Frontlines at Work and at Home: The Disproportionate Economic Effects of the Coronavirus Pandemic on Women of Color," *Center for American Progress*, April 3, 2020, https://www.americanprogress.org/issues/women/reports/2020/04/23/483846/frontlines-work-home/; Sandra R. Hernández and Kara Carter, "COVID-19: A Perfect Storm of Health Care Inequality," *California Health Care Foundation*, April 10, 2020, https://www.chcf.org/blog/covid-19-perfect-storm-health-care-inequality/; Celine McNicholas and Margaret Poydock, "Who Are Essential Workers? A Comprehensive Look at Their Wages, Demographics, and Unionization Rates," *Economic Policy Institute*, May 19, 2020, https://www.epi.org/blog/who-are-essential-workers-a-comprehensive-look-at-their-wages-demographics-and-unionization-rates/; and Hye Jin Rho, Hayley Brown, and Shawn Fremstad, "A Basic Demographic Profile of Workers in Frontline Industries," *Center for Economic Policy and Research*, April 7, 2020, https://cepr.net/a-basic-demographic-profile-of-workers-in-frontline-industries/.

8   E. Ann Carson, *Prisons in 2019* (Washington: United States Department of Justice, 2020); John Gramlich, "The Gap Between the Number of Blacks and Whites is Shrinking," *Pew Research Center*, April 30, 2019, https://www.pewresearch.org/fact-tank/2019/04/30/shrinking-gap-between-number-of-blacks-and-whites-in-prison/.

9   Michelle A. McManus and Emma Ball, "COVID-19 Should Be Considered an Adverse Childhood Experience (ACE)," *Journal of Community Safety and Well-Being* 5 (December 2020): 164–67; Nancy Wolff and Jing Shi, "Childhood and Adult Trauma Experiences of Incarcerated Persons and Their Relationship to Adult Behavioral Health Problems and Treatment," *International Journal of Environmental Research and Public Health* 9 (May 2012): 1908–26.

10   Wolff and Shi, "Childhood and Adult Trauma Experiences," 1909.

11   James Baldwin et al., "The Negro in American Culture," *Cross Currents* 11 (summer 1961): 5. Baldwin made the statement originally in January 1961 during a moderated discussion at WBAI-FM radio station in New York City,

New York. Baldwin, Emile Capouya, Lorraine Hansberry, Langston Hughes, and Alfred Kazin were discussants. Nathan Hentoff, onetime editor of *Downbeat* magazine, was moderator.

12 Here I am using Soong-Chan Rah's definition for lament. "Lament in the Bible Is a Liturgical Response to the Reality of Suffering and Engages God in the Context of Pain and Trouble." *Prophetic Lament: A Call for Justice in Troubled Times* (Downers Grove, IL: InterVarsity Press, 2015), 21. "Hopefulness" is used to highlight within the black experience/narrative is seen in the improvisational, creative, and resilient traits of being African American.

13 Bessel A. van der Kolk, *The Body Keeps the Score: Brain, Mind, and Body in the Healing of Trauma* (New York, NY: Penguin Books, 2014), 265.

14 van der Kolk, *Body Keeps the Score*.

15 Robin Karr-Morse and Meredith S. Wiley, *Scared Sick: The Role of Childhood Trauma in Adult Disease* (New York, NY: Basic Books, 2012); Robert Scaer, *The Trauma Spectrum: Hidden Wounds and Human Resiliency* (New York, NY: W.W. Norton, 2005).

16 Karr-Morse and Wiley, *Scared Sick*, 43.

17 Karr-Morse and Wiley, *Scared Sick*, 43.

18 Resmaa Menakem, *My Grandmother's Hands: Racialized Trauma and the Pathway to Mending Our Hearts and Bodies* (Las Vegas: Central Recovery Press, 2017), 9.

19 Menakem, *My Grandmother's Hands,* 9.

20 "Resilience," *Online Etymology Dictionary*, n.d., https://www.etymonline.com/search?q=resilience.

21 Scaer, *Trauma Spectrum*.

22 Menakem, *My Grandmother's Hands*, 15.

23 *Open Wounds.*

24 Michelle Alexander, *The New Jim Crow: Mass Incarceration in the Age of Color Blindness*, 10th anniversary ed. (New York, NY: New Press, 2020); Douglas Blackmon, *Slavery by Another Name: The Re-Enslavement of Black Americans from the Civil War to World War II* (New York, NY: Doubleday, 2008); Joy DeGruy, *Post Traumatic Slave Syndrome: America's Legacy of Enduring Injury and Healing* (Portland, OR: Uptone Press, 2005).

25 "WHO Director-General's Opening Remarks at the Media Briefing on COVID-19," *World Health Organization*, March 11, 2020, https://www.who.int/director-general/speeches/detail/who-director-general-s-opening-remarks-at-the-media-briefing-on-covid-19. March 11, 2020.

26 COVID Tracking Project, "COVID-19 is Affecting Black, Indigenous, Latinx, and Other People of Color the Most," *COVID Racial Data Tracker*, March 7, 2021, https://covidtracking.com/race.

27 Sara Atske and Andrew Perrin, "Home Broadband Adoption, Computer Ownership Varies by Race, Ethnicity in the U.S.," *Pew Research Center*, July 16, 2021, https://www.pewresearch.org/fact-tank/2021/07/16/home-broadband-adoption-computer-ownership-vary-by-race-ethnicity-in-the-u-s/.

28 Leah Harris, "COVID-19's Devastation in Black Communities Began Long Ago," *Saint A.*, April 24, 2020, https://sainta.org/covid-19s-devastation-in-black-communities-began-long-ago/.

29 I employ the term *lament* similar to Soong-Chan Rah, who says it "is a liturgical response to the reality of suffering and engages God in the context of pain and trouble. The hope of lament is that God would respond to human suffering that is wholeheartedly communicated through lament. Unfortunately, lament is often missing from the narrative of the American church." Rah, *Prophetic Lament: A Call for Justice in Troubled Times* (Downers Grove, IL: InterVarsity Press, 2015), 21.

30  For a representative study about nonphysical effects of health issues, see Lisa M. Brown et al., "The Influence of Race on the Development of Acute Lung Injury in Trauma Patients," *American Journal of Surgery* 201 (April 2011): 486–91, esp. 488.

31  David R. Williams, Jourdyn A. Lawrence, and Brigette A. Davis, "Racism and Health: Evidence and Needed Research," *Annual Review of Public Health* 40 (2019): 106–7.

32  U.S. Const., amend. XIII.

33  Jason R. Young, *Rituals of Resistance: African Atlantic Religion in Kongo and the Lowcountry South in the Era of Slavery* (Baton Rouge, LA: Louisiana State University Press, 2007), 20.

34  *Open Wounds.*

35  *Open Wounds.*

# 25 Shifting the Tide Toward Health Equity

*Lydell C. Lettsome*

## Introduction

When many of my physician colleagues and I heard people use *we're all in this together* as a catchphrase for how American society would navigate a deadly pandemic, COVID-19, we had a fast comeback: *We may all be in this together, but we're not in the same boat.*

Those of us on the frontlines of healthcare and health access interpreted the togetherness platitude as a shallow response to the country's failure to create a healthcare system that welcomes all citizens. Essential workers, the working poor, and jobless always have been disproportionately affected by sickness, loss of life, and medical bankruptcy; indeed, the COVID-19 pandemic simply have laid bare the hard facts of how many Americans, particularly black Americans, are sailing in different boats—if they have a boat at all—than white Americans. In general, blacks have lived sicker and died younger than whites, but that gap has expanded during the pandemic.[1]

## Boats Adrift

In 2019, a year before the COVID pandemic, I started working with the New York Theological Seminary as a research professor. I anchored my work on the premise that many people of color were drowning in the rough seas, or biases, of American healthcare. I previously attended a lecture given by the Rev. Dr. Frederick D. Haynes III, senior pastor of Friendship-West Baptist Church, who contended black churches had become very good at fishing people of color out of rough waters. Nonetheless, he voiced a need for preventative work that kept people from falling into waters in the first place.

The Vanbert Health Equity Project (VHEP), a nonprofit composed of an eclectic group of people of faith who have agreed to look upstream for ideas that keep people on solid ground during healthcare storms, was borne out of my research on healthcare inequities. In my review of more than twenty articles, I identified disparities in several areas of healthcare. Neurological strokes,[2] medication use,[3] and hospice were representative subjects of my investigation.[4]

DOI: 10.4324/9781003214281-29

The organizers of VHEP believed many churches had excellent boats in the sense that, via health fairs, health ministries, or health activities, congregations provided a measure of healthcare access and stability to communities; however, most of those boats were adrift at sea with no safe harbor to dock. No matter how big or how opulent a boat might have been, it still could only carry a finite amount of resources. When it came to healthcare, for instance, fairs and screenings usually constituted the proverbial tip of the iceberg because healthy living was much bigger than a community education event or a screening.

Vanbert strives to connect churches with healthcare institutions and infrastructures in their local communities to improve delivery and to diminish disparities. For example, mobile mammograms and pap smears are not maximally impactful without proper gynecological and oncological follow up. Empowering a church to build a proactive relationship with community healthcare providers and payers is one way we at Vanbert get boats to safe harbors. We believe surviving the COVID-19 pandemic and future health storms depends not only on the boats in which people sail but also the types of harbors where boats dock.

## Captains and Harbors

As the leaders of trusted community institutions, clergy function as community captains and gatekeepers. Regardless of socioeconomic status, pastors, preachers, and other people of the cloth often are the most organized mouthpieces in communities of color. Hence, we at the VHEP explore with faith leaders the reasons the United States healthcare system is profit-driven rather than patient-centered. Foundationally, we know improving healthcare and making it more accessible and affordable for all citizens begins with equipping those on the margins of healthcare, especially people of color and poor people of every persuasion, to ask proper questions about a system, healthcare, that many individuals find intimidating.

The VHEP has targeted spiritual leaders because the organization believes they are reliable gatekeepers to communities of color. Therefore, they are potential champions of health who can add better value to the physical well-being of congregants and communities. The research the VHEP has conducted indicates people of color tend to resist pathways to equity because of mistrust of the healthcare system. The organization seeks to address that barrier to health equity by providing practical responses to longstanding disparities in healthcare access and health outcomes. To achieve that goal, the VHEP trains faith-based and other community leaders in the fine points of healthcare policy and practice, with a primary aim to empower spiritual leaders to become healthcare advocates for the communities where they minister or reside. By building their capacities to do outreach and advocacy, among other efforts, the healthcare expectations of those they serve often rise. With enhanced understanding, outcomes tend to improve.

Even though COVID-19 is not a primary initiative of the VHEP, the organization's work on the disease and vaccines to treat it had helped many pastors and communities navigate their ways through the pandemic. We ensure leaders are versed well in necessary clinical and socioeconomic strategies that are crucial to undoing some of healthcare inequities their communities face. To illustrate, in the area of hereditary cancer screening, the VHEP has shown spiritual leaders how tremendous disparities in cancer screenings among people of color and white people have led to higher morbidity rates among the former group. Afterward, the VHEP has empowered spiritual leaders with access to various self-screening tools, such as Myriad's *MyRisk* questionnaire, to share with their communities.[5]

While cancer is not always preventable, death because of cancer often is preventable. Since the human genome's mapping, the discovery and linkage of various genes to human cancers have grown exponentially. In general, black and other people of color get screened and tested at a significantly lower rates than white people. Hereditary cancer screening is a lifesaving treatment tool with tangible benefits. For example, many blacks dismiss breast cancer 1 and breast cancer 2 genes as genetic markers of breast cancer in whites and not blacks. As more black women get tested, the more they test positive for those genes.[6]

Scientific researchers have discovered at least ten additional genes with clinical links to breast cancer, and genes with clinical significance in more than seven other cancers.[7] Proper screening for such genes can save lives by identifying and treating at-risk patients before cancer manifests. Because African Americans remain disproportionately unaware of their cancer risks, the VHEP recently joined a collaboration with the Drew Theological School Religion and Global Health Forum to improve screening access for communities of color.[8] Something as simple as a family filling out a chart can save lives for generations.

The VHEP shares data regarding the effectiveness of self-screening tools in the hope that newfound awareness will raise healthcare expectations. Regrettably, studies have shown that, when it comes to hereditary cancer screenings, people of color cannot rely solely on their healthcare providers to screen them, even when screenings are clinically indicated. Because of those occurrences, the VHEP distributes hereditary cancer screening assessment sheets to educate patients about their risk factors before they see primary care doctors. Getting certain patients to trust medical advice or, in some cases, to become patients that receive advice is a different matter.[9]

Regardless of how some mistrust of the healthcare system is, COVID has confirmed the value of Black Church leaders being able to influence more ordinary members to comply with safety measures and accept vaccines. The significance of the leaders' willingness to encourage such potentially life-saving behavior is immeasurable. For months before and after the World Health Organization declared COVID a pandemic in March 2020, houses of worship were notorious for being hotspots of transmission as certain churchgoers doubled down on the notion that religious facilities were essential places where people could gather and hence exempt from government closing, lockdown, or shutdown orders.[10]

## Compasses, Captains, and Harbors

Scholars such as Jonathan M. Metzl and Helena Hansen have proven that structural and cultural competencies have provided much needed dialogue, research, and processes to reduce the way institutional systems, policies, and healthcare harm the patients those items are meant to assist.[11] In that way and others, healthcare is an interesting service industry whose ethics is particularly important because the final product also is the chief customer, a healthy patient. As both product and customer, a patient should know what is needed to become or to remain healthy. Although the VHEP is excited about the improvements in understanding that structural and cultural competencies bring to relationships and outcomes in healthcare, the organization remains concerned that such competencies leave too much control in the hands of vendors, meaning healthcare providers. Because we at the VHEP believe strongly that no one has more to lose or to gain in healthcare than a patient, we strive to empower each patient with whom we work to have the knowledge and other tools needed for healthy living.

While the healthcare industry is working on structural competency, we at the VHEP are working with churches to provide healthcare and healthy living competencies. For example, black Americans and poor people, among other marginalized groups, are less likely than affluent white people to get an electrocardiogram when they visit an emergency room with chest pain even though that process is a standard diagnostic for anyone who has such pain. Instead of hoping structural competency alone will be enough for emergency rooms clinicians who do not conduct themselves properly, the VHEP explores ways for African Americans themselves to know more about basic chest pain evaluation.[12] In addition, our hereditary cancer screening assessment sheets seek to educate patients about their risk factors before they see their primary care doctors.

## Physicians and Prophets

The COVID pandemic gave VHEP more opportunities with spiritual leaders seeking to guide their boats as the disease roughened waves, meaning caused illnesses or deaths. At the New York Theological Seminary, people often asked me to use my background in religion and medicine to give perspective to spiritual leaders regarding COVID, then various government responses, and finally vaccine use. Unlike the acquired immunodeficiency syndrome and opiate crises, houses of worship were on the frontlines of the COVID pandemic from the beginning, as congregants often fellowshipped in close quarters, even at megachurches. Moreover, physicians, scientists, and other usually informed people did not know much about COVID, especially how to treat it. Consequently, pastors and other church leaders had to contend with a disease without the benefit of secular (e.g., medical) strategies or insights.

Once researchers provided people around the world the science care givers needed to treat COVID, many of my fellow clinical colleagues and I frequently gave more counsel than scientific advice; we gave prophetic words of hope, especially to home congregations, pastors, and other people of faith who were willing to hear us. Several concerns were common. How bad is COVID, and what should I do to prevent it? Is the government prepared? Where can I find reliable help? Some pastors asked what they should tell or give to their congregants. Other pastors wanted to know how to minister or to worship safely. Almost every person with whom my colleagues and I communicated had questions about vaccines or the cost of healthcare if they became infected and did not have adequate healthcare coverage.

For decades, cost dominated public discourse about healthcare. Numerous physicians, hospital administrators, pharmaceutical company executives, and other people claimed matters of cost efficiency, morality, and compassion in the dispensing of care were wasteful or unrealistic. We at the VHEP believe the failure to prioritize reliable healthcare coverage over costs has led to avoidable premature deaths, untreated diseases, as well as the bankruptcies of families and healthcare entities. Such occurrences have continued to resonate during the COVID pandemic. When I speak with pastors, for instance, tremendous losses of life and pressing healthcare needs the pandemic has revealed had placed the desire for reliable healthcare coverage above many concerns about cost.

When the federal government authorized vaccines in December 2020, those items instantly became the waters I found myself trying to navigate.[13] By that month, politicians and clergy had taken over the discourse, and they pushed the science to the edges of public conscience. By July 2021, matters had not changed much: Many Americans' perceptions of vaccines were linked more to their political or religious views than to their understanding of the science about vaccines.[14] Further complicating matters with some of African Americans with I spoke, I had to encourage trust to people who had endured a long and dark history of neglect, deceit, or abuse from organized healthcare providers, including government sources.[15] Even through monitors and screens, I could see looks of concern, doubt, or fear as I spoke about the safety of the vaccines, a task that especially hard in January. As I championed vaccines, many major black preachers were telling their congregations to wait for more evidence of safety.

## Imagining Universally Safe Harbors

As I have spoken with pastors, other churchgoers, and other people about COVID, vaccines, healthcare costs, and related matters, I have imagined the United States having a health plan that is not linked to employment status, valid in each state, or accepted by every hospital, nursing home, and most clinicians. I also have imagined the country having a plan that covers mental health, dental care, and long-term care. In short, I have imagined universal healthcare.

Free care at the point of delivery based on an individual's need and not the ability to pay is a core principle of universal healthcare. That principle, not rationing care or providing low technology care, is a cornerstone of a universal system, which since World War I (1914–1918) has become the standard, not the anomaly, for healthcare in most industrialized countries. Norway instituted universal healthcare in 1914, two years before the war commenced.[16]

Of the many Americans who have contracted COVID-19 while being unemployed or without health insurance, some likely have desired universal healthcare. While the Patient Protection and Affordable Care Act that US President Barack Obama signed into law in 2010 has given insurance coverage to millions of Americans, expanded coverage for millions of others, and prevented health insurance companies from discriminating against individuals with preexisting health conditions, we who affiliate with the VHEP believe the law is not enough to erase thick health disparities.[17]

The preceding statement requires qualification. We at the VHEP understand constraints of the US healthcare system and therefore provides interventions that help people work through such constraints morally, ethnically, and legally. For example, screenings for obesity related disease and hereditary cancer are the two low-cost tactics the VHEP has chosen to implement to achieve high-impact health outcomes. Such screenings are significant given high rates of preventable diseases among African Americans and the great risk of dying from COVID-19 that obese people face.[18]

Obesity affects black Americans disproportionately to white Americans.[19] Not only does the condition hurts blacks' quality of life but it also shortens their life expectancy.[20] Obesity also fuels high cost, potentially deadly diseases such as diabetes, hypertension, sleep apnea, venous stasis and COVID.[21] Building on the efforts of former US First Lady Michelle Obama's "Let's Move" campaign, the VHEP connects target communities with nutritionists and physical therapists.[22] The VHEP also works with the African Methodist Episcopal International Health Commission on a religious initiative to reduce obesity among people of color, thereby increasing their chances to longer and healthier lives.[23]

On average, obese people die nine years sooner than non-obese people.[24] Obesity also causes those living with the condition to miss 56 percent more workdays than non-obese people miss.[25] The former individuals hence run the risk of experiencing losses to income and to quality of life that often come from steady paychecks. In 2015, for example, cancer cost Americans an estimated 8.7 million years in life lost and $94 billion in lost future earnings.[26] The work of the VHEP helps cut such losses, and we are confident our strategies and programming will allow faith-based organizations to continue their traditions of making significant community impact in financially responsible ways. We know such organizations, given for whom they care and serve in numerous other manners, are crucial to any strategy to lessening health disparities, especially disparities linked to race/ethnicity.

## Jesus as Model Caregiver and Captain

Health inequities in communities of color have constituted an area of academic and clinical interest for more than thirty years, with minimal popular appeal in my estimation. For months before the COVID pandemic, the VHEP had limited success working to redefine the ways clergy, faith, and clinical medicine intersected in communities of color. Then the COVID pandemic emerged, and attention spiked, especially when the federal government authorized vaccine distribution in December 2020. In addition to health equity, many organizations and groups including the United States government now focus on tangible ways clergy, faith, and clinical medicine can intersect to build healthier communities of color.

In my judgment, COVID made dysfunctional relationships between employment, healthcare, health insurance, and wealth in the United States more visible to people. Leaders from every walk of no longer could deny the healthcare system was not designed to take care of millions of people when they need care the most. Because of the largely privatized character of healthcare, scores of people lost access to medical services when they lost their jobs. Despite being a capitalist country, the federal government had to step in to provide assurances, forbearances, and related aid to unemployed or underemployed citizens, clinicians, and hospitals, among other people and entities, to keep the healthcare system afloat.[27] People in the United States spend more money on healthcare than people in any other country in the world; nevertheless, the federal government had to bail out the healthcare industry during the COVID pandemic.[28]

## Conclusion

The length and scope of the COVID pandemic has surpassed the estimates of many people in the United States and elsewhere in the world. Early in the pandemic, as it became more a partisan political issue than a public health issue, we at the VHEP made a wise choice to collaborate with faith-based organizations and institutions—Baylor University, the COVID-19 Prevention Network Faith Initiative Team, and the Drew Theological School—to follow the lead of Jesus and provide safe harbor for those whose health vessels did not sail smoothly. Though COVID waters have not calmed, attendant hardships have allowed the VHEP and its partners to highlight not only the benefits of universal healthcare but also consequences of the United States not having it. We now find more spiritual leaders requesting details about universal healthcare, Medicare for all citizens, and similar initiatives. That our work will embolden even more leaders, their congregants, and countless other people to demand government and healthcare officials reform the system is our hope.

As practicing Christians, we at the VHEP remain wary of policies and practices that overlook, ignore, blame, or demonize marginalized people. In Matthew 11, Jesus validated his messianic ministry on the basis of providing healthcare unbounded by cost when he told the disciples of John the Baptist "the blind receive their sight, and the lame walk, the lepers are cleansed, and the deaf hear."[29] Jesus did not respond with talk of spirituality, repentance, or piety; quite the opposite, he simply prioritized well-being. Aware of that act and countless similar others, we at the VHEP believe to intentionally maintain a system of healthcare that prioritizes profit or individuals who have the ability to pay for care is inconsistent with the practices of Jesus and his disciples. We therefore encourage spiritual leaders to emphasize that Jesus built his messianic ministry by freely providing healing and health-care to his community. In so doing, he provided a compass to guide people away from the rough waters of COVID toward safe shores.

## Notes

1  Maria Polyakova et al., "Racial Disparities in Excess All-Cause Mortality during the Early COVID-19 Pandemic Varied Substantially Across States," *Health Affairs* 40 (February 2021): 307–16; Thomas A. LaVeist, John M. Wallace, and Daniel L. Howard, "'The Color Line and The Health of African Americans," *Humboldt Journal of Social Relations* 21 (1995): 119–37.
2  Olajide Williams and Bruce Ovbiagele, "Stroking Out While Black—The Complex Role of Racism," *JAMA Neurology* 77 (November 2020): 1343–44.
3  Moti Gulersen, "Racial Disparities in the Administration of Antenatal Corticosteroids in Women with Preterm Birth," *American Journal of Obstetrics and Gynecology* 223 (December 2020): 933.
4  Boateng Kubi et al., "Theory-Based Development of an Implementation Intervention Using Community Health Workers to Increase Palliative Care Use," *Journal of Pain and Symptom Management* 60 (July 2020): 10–19.
5  For information about Myriad's *MyRisk* questionnaire, visit https://myriad-myrisk.com/genetics/.
6  Jordan Ciuro et al., "Health Care Disparities and Demand for Expanding Hereditary Breast Cancer Screening Guidelines in African Americans," *Clinical Breast Cancer* 21, (June 2021): e220–27, https://doi.org/10.1016/j.clbc.2020.08.010.
7  William D. Foulkes, "The Ten Genes for Breast (and Ovarian) Cancer Susceptibility," Nature Reviews Clinical Oncology, 18, (May 2021): 259–60, https://doi.org/10.1038/s41571-021-00491-3.
8  Information about the Drew Theological School Religion and Global Health Forum is available at https://www.drew.edu/theological-school/academics/centers-special-programs/religion-and-global-health-forum/.
9  Meghan L. Underhill, Tarsha Jones, and Karleen Habin, "Disparities in Cancer Genetic Risk Assessment and Testing," *Oncology Nursing Forum* 43 (July 2016): 519–23.
10  "WHO Director-General's Opening Remarks at the Media Briefing on COVID-19," *World Health Organization*, March 11, 2020, https://www.who.int/director-general/speeches/detail/who-director-general-s-opening-remarks-

at-the-media-briefing-on-covid-19. March 11, 2020. Although the COVID-19 pandemic has placed faith-based organizations in positions to offer valuable physical and mental healthcare services to their congregants and to communities at large, the pandemic also has provided unprecedented challenges to traditional church logistics. For example, not all churches are equipped to benefit from the type of webinars the VHEP has hosted with the New York Theological Seminary.

11 Jonathan M. Metzl and Helena Hansen, "Structural Competency: Theorizing a New Medical Engagement with Stigma and Inequality," *Social Science and Medicine* 103 (February 2014): 126–33; Jonathan M. Metzl, Aletha Maybank, and Fernando De Maio, "Responding to the COVID-19 Pandemic: The Need for a Structurally Competent Health Care System," *JAMA: Journal of the American Medical Association* 324 (July 1, 2020): 231–32.

12 As regards the type emergency room treatment African Americans receive I discuss in the main text, see Amrita Mukhopadhyay et al., "Racial and Insurance Disparities among Patients Presenting with Chest Pain in the US: 2009–2015," *American Journal of Emergency Medicine* 38 (July 2020): 1373–76.

13 United States Food and Drug Administration, "FDA Takes Key Action in Fight Against COVID-19 by Issuing Emergency Use Authorization for First COVID-19 Vaccine," December 11, 2020, https://www.fda.gov/news-events/press-announcements/fda-takes-key-action-fight-against-covid-19-issuing-emergency-use-authorization-first-covid-19.

14 Susan Milligan, "A Deadly Political Divide: Two Americas Are on Display as Political Conversations Turn to Vaccines and Election Results," *U.S. News and World Report*, July 23, 2021, https://www.usnews.com/news/the-report/articles/2021-07-23/coronavirus-vaccines-highlight-a-deadly-political-divide; Lydia Wheeler, "Religious Objections Stand in Path of Mask, Vaccine Mandates," *Bloomberg Law*, https://news.bloomberglaw.com/health-law-and-business/religious-objections-stand-in-path-of-mask-vaccine-mandates.

15 Simar Singh Bajaj and Fatima Cody Stanford, "Beyond Tuskegee—Vaccine Distrust and Everyday Racism," *New England Journal of Medicine* 384 (February 4, 2021): e12 (1–2), https://doi.org/10.1056/nejmpv2035827.

16 Victor Kiprop, "Countries with Universal Health Care," *WorldAtlas*, January 29, 2018), https://www.worldatlas.com/articles/countries-with-universal-health-care.html; Chris Slaybaugh, "International Healthcare Systems: The US Versus the World," *Axene Health Partners*, 2021, https://axenehp.com/international-healthcare-systems-us-versus-world/.

17 Pub. Law 111–148, 124 Stat. 119–124 Stat. 1025. (2010).

18 Cindy Ogolla Jean-Baptiste and Tyeastia Green, "Commentary on COVID-19 and African Americans. The Numbers Are Just a Tip of a Bigger Iceberg," *Social Sciences and Humanities Open* 2 (2020): 1–3.

19 Jean-Baptiste and Green, "Commentary on COVID-19 and African Americans."

20 Jean-Baptiste and Green, "Commentary on COVID-19 and African Americans."

21 Jean-Baptiste and Green, "Commentary on COVID-19 and African Americans."

22 For information about the "Let's Move" campaign, visit https://letsmove.obamawhitehouse.archives.gov/; and, among other sources, Jack Linshi discussed youth "This Chart Shows How Hard It Is to End Childhood Obesity," *Time*, February 9, 2015, https://time.com/3700930/childhood-obesity-michelle-obama-lets-move/.

23  Regarding the African Methodist Episcopal International Health Commission's general stances on obesity and COVID, see its *Guidelines for Reopening and Returning to Church Buildings* ([N.P.]: African Methodist Episcopal International Health Commission, 2021), 4.

24  James A. Greenberg, "Obesity and Early Mortality in the United States," *Obesity* 21 (February 2013): 405–12.

25  Andy Mead and Sutton Stokes, *How Should We Reduce Obesity in America?* (Dayton, OH: National Issues Forums Institute, 2016).

26  Farhad Islami et al., "Estimates of Lost Earnings from Cancer Deaths in US," *NewsRx Health and Science* (July 21, 2019): 195; Farhad Islami et al., "National and State Estimates of Lost Earnings from Cancer Deaths in the United States," *JAMA Oncology* 5 (2019): e191460, doi: 10.1001/jamaoncol.2019.1460; Sandy McDowell, "Study: Premature Deaths from Cancer in One Year Led to Loss of 8.7 Million Years of Life and $94 Billion of Future Earnings," *American Cancer Society*, July 3, 2019, https://www.cancer.org/latest-news/study-premature-deaths-from-cancer-in-one-year-led-to-loss-of-million-years-of-life.html.

27  David Blumenthal et al., "Covid-19 — Implications for the Health Care System," *New England Journal of Medicine* 383 (October 8, 2020): 1483–88.

28  Katherine Baicker and Amitabh Chandra, "Do We Spend Too Much on Health Care?," *New England Journal of Medicine* 383 (August 13, 2020): 605–8.

29  Matthew 11:5, King James Version.

# Part IV
# Spirituality and the Wellness of Black Minds, Bodies, and Souls

# 26 Nigerian Women, Mental and Physical Health, COVID-19, and Spirituality

*Samuel E. Oladipo, A. Christson Adedoyin, Jimoh W. Owoyele, and Hammed Adeoye*

## Introduction

During the nineteenth century, many European physicians other healthcare providers in Africa, particularly Nigeria, considered mental illness uncommon or inconsequential.[1] Since then, several epidemiologic studies have shown that mental illness is as frequent in Africa as it is elsewhere in the world.[2] Some studies explore mental issues by sex and gender,[3] while others investigate the prevalence of mental health in all people.[4] Yet other studies focus on mental health crises in specific countries, such as Nigeria, where in 2016 an estimated 20 percent to 30 percent of the total population of almost 200 million people suffered from mental disorders, according to one study.[5]

Although empirical data are not readily available for 2020 or 2021, the large number of published scholarly studies, daily news reports, and other reliable accounts of suicide and other self-inflicted tragedies in Nigeria attest to a rise in mental illness in the country since 2016.[6] Unfortunately, as of 2021, fewer than 10 percent of mentally ill Nigerians had access to adequate care.[7] Hence, there was an enormous unmet need for services.

A shortage of psychiatrists is partly responsible for the lack of sufficient mental healthcare in Nigeria.[8] Without them or other academics, clinicians, public officials, and similarly learned individuals who specialize in mental health devoting much attention the matter, public awareness of many disorders is poor, and misconceptions have been widespread for years. In 2006, the World Health Organization and the Nigerian Ministry of Health published a joint report on mental health policy that noted "no revision has taken place and no formal assessment of how much it has been implemented has been conducted…. No desk exists in the ministries at any level for mental health issues and only four per cent of government expenditures on health is earmarked for mental health."[9] The report also highlighted the unavailability of essential medicines at primary health centers, physicians to operate the centers, and shabby regulatory oversight on prescriptions for psychotropic medications.[10] Though Nigerians have made strides since 2006 to resolve such issues, this essay demonstrates that much work remains.

DOI: 10.4324/9781003214281-31

As regard Nigerian women, the primary focuses of the essay, organizations from across the globe have devoted much attention to their mental and physical health needs in the recent years, especially during the COVID-19 pandemic. For decades after Nigerians won independence from Great Britain on October 1, 1961, some organization recount, private and public entities in Nigeria struggled to provide adequate healthcare services to citizens. The pandemic worsened that ability. Since the Nigeria Centre for Disease Control confirmed the first incident of COVID on February 27, 2020, there has been daily increases in cases. With primary healthcare services insufficient to many Nigerians, people at the grassroots, especially women, have been hit particularly hard. This essay focuses on women—specifically, those in southwestern Nigeria—who have been affected disproportionately by mental and physical healthcare challenges resulting from the pandemic, but the essay does not ignore women in other parts of the world grappling with similar hardships.[11]

According to a United Nations policy brief published on April 9, 2020, as the pandemic spread around the world, COVID exacerbated difficulties that women had getting proper healthcare.[12] The report also cited age, disability, ethnicity, geographic location, race, and sexual orientation as factors influencing women's access to critical health services across the world.[13] In general, women were less likely than men to have such access, and urban women tended to have greater access to essential medicines and vaccines, to maternal and reproductive care, and to insurance coverage than rural women.[14]

Occupational sex and gender segregation also accounts for women being more vulnerable to exposure to COVID and other infectious diseases than men but having less access to adequate healthcare. Globally the 2020 United Nations policy brief noted, women made up 70 percent of the health workforce, and a considerable portion of that number performed frontline duties as physicians' assistants, midwives, and nurses, among other occupations.[15] Women also comprised the majority of health facility service staff, such as cleaners, laundry attendants, and caterers.[16] Those roles, too, made them vulnerable to COVID exposure and often not having personal protective equipment or equipment that fit properly worsened matters.[17] Finally, women were more likely than men to become unemployed when governments issued stay-at-home, lockdown, and shutdown orders.[18]

## Nigerian Women, COVID-19, and the Importance of Spirituality

While women in Nigeria typically live longer than men, women are more likely to become widowed, live in poverty, suffer from a chronic illness or disability, or lose informal support networks.[19] The probability of Nigerian women in one of those circumstances seeking help from formal secular sources is remote, given that doing so is antithetical to many local cultural norms; appealing to supernatural forces for assistance is more commonplace in many communities.[20] Indeed, many African communities are spiritually oriented; therefore, all members—and not simply women—look to other-worldly explanations for most things individuals encounter. Oftentimes, rather than visiting medical facilities, those seeking help turn to spiritual houses.[21]

While Africans in general value spirituality, it is of utmost importance to women, who give special attention to prayers, perceptions about God, and questions about the meaning of life when they experience difficult times.[22] In a 2020 research project, Samuel Oladipo and Jimoh Owoyele investigated why Nigerian women preferred spiritual help to orthodox medicine when faced with serious health challenges such as COVID-19.[23] Oladipo and Owoyele concluded that several factors influenced their general preference, and longstanding patriarchal culture that a male Nigerian to hold a bias against a female Nigerian was a principal factor.[24]

Culture is of enduring importance to Nigerian people. It encompasses their belief systems, traditions, and common practices. Indeed, culture is a potent force capable of impacting all aspects of life. Many Nigerian societies maintain beliefs and perpetuate practices that tend to relegate women to second-class status even though some belief and practices have serious mental and physical health implications.[25] For instance, the Yoruba view witchcraft in a positive manner for men but not for women. A male witch, or *oṣọ́*, is a powerful and respected person capable of using supernatural powers to influence a human behavior or experience.[26] An *oṣọ́* can proclaim in public his power and boast of the extraordinary power he alleges to have, causing some people to consider the appellation *oṣọ́* a mark of honor they use prefixally with their names (e.g., *Osonuga, Osolewa*).

*Àjẹ*, meaning female witch, is antipodean to *oṣọ́*.[27] *Àjẹ* suggests evil, devilish, abominable. Considering that many Yoruba believe *àjẹ*s are responsible for calamities and family deaths, among other terrible occurrences, no woman dares proclaim herself an *àjẹ* in public lest she risk being stoned to death.[28] Indeed, many women suffer deprivation, neglect, and oppressive treatment once others suspect them of being *àjẹ*s.

Nigerian women who face abuse because of local customs often experience serious psychological traumas leading to psychosis, depression, schizophrenia, and other mental health illnesses. Those who undergo extreme hardship might even confess to deaths with which they had nothing to do. Women who are fortunate enough to escape with their lives can end up in spiritual homes where they believe they can get compassion rather than neglect.[29]

Among the Igbos and the Ibibios in the southeastern Nigeria, there are similar cultural practices that put women at risk for mental health crises. For example, if a man dies before reaching old age, his wife or wives must prove having no part in the death by shaving hair, bathing the corpse, and drinking the dirty water she uses to bathe the corpse. Such practices, apart from posing direct threat to the general health and well-being of participating women, can lead to severe psychological traumas, mental illnesses, or psychosomatic disorders.[30]

In northern Nigeria, a man can divorce one wife or multiple wives by saying aloud he divorces her or them three times. Sometimes, divorces occur without a wife committing any offence, such as a breach of trust. Not unlike the Yoruba, Igbo, and Ibibio activities above, the acceptable traditions of men in northern Nigeria can induce severe mental challenges. Consequently, women in the region tend to resort to spiritual solutions to overcome various biases emanating from certain cultural practices.[31]

Stigmatizing is another cultural practice that affects women disproportionately in Nigeria. Such discrimination often prompts others to devalue or even hate targeted women, resulting in a broad range of negative consequences and painful experiences, especially for those who already suffer with mental illness.[32] Stigmatization routinely causes victims to be ashamed, embarrassed, or to lose hope. In relation to healthcare services, stigmatizing frequently occurs when people entrusted with patients' care instead isolate, avoid, or devalue the patients. During pandemics such as COVID-19, many people stigmatized as being infected become disturbed emotionally, mentally, psychologically, and even physically.[33]

In many Nigerian towns and villages, residents perceive outbreaks, epidemics, pandemics, and related catastrophes as abominations or reflections of evil; therefore, uninfected individuals often stigmatize, ostracize, or otherwise discriminate against infected individuals, with subsequent effects of such bias occasionally resulting in abuse more severe than infections themselves.[34] The magnitude of stigmatizing during the COVID pandemic has been so extensive that the National Centre for Disease Control in Nigeria has undertaken a massive campaign to slow the rate of stigmatization.[35]

Even some Nigerians who test negative for COVID have found it difficult to reintegrate into society because people, including their own relatives or close friends, avoid them like plague simply for being tested. To avoid stigmatization, we have found, women inflected with COVID or with mental illness often hide their condition. Many avoid licensed physicians, seeking assistance clandestinely by consulting traditional healers or spiritualists in worship centers.

Misinformation about illnesses is one reason many Nigerian women, as well as other people in the country, find themselves resorting to spirituality instead of seeking medical assistance. While the overall literacy rate in Nigerian is about 60 percent, countless inhabitants are ignorant about health issues, especially mental health issues, as well as professional services that might be able to help them.[36] Money is another factor. For many people in Nigeria, a country teeming with natural resources but whose masses are deprived financially, private medicine is too expensive to afford, and public medicine is lacking if not nonexistent. In their cases, turning to supernatural beings to overcome challenges such as COVID seems mandatory. Yet other

Nigerians think physicians and other formally trained medical workers are hexed. For example, in 2017, a full two years before the first diagnosed cases of COVID, a study conducted in southwest Nigeria revealed a prevalent belief in supernatural causation of schizophrenia among caregivers.[37] People associated the condition with Satanic influences (e.g., curses by the enemies of patients).[38] Because countless Nigerians believe spirits exist and are potentially evil instruments of envious or devilish people who wish to inflict insanity, depression, schizophrenia, paranoia, viral infections, and similarly troubling conditions on anyone they wish to punish or to oppress, it is feasible for the same Nigerians to believe good spirits can counterbalance the work of bad spirits.[39]

In Nigeria generally and in its southwestern quadrant specifically, people repose must trust in spiritual leaders. Essentially, traditional healers, pastors, imams, and comparably positioned individuals are second to God, or godly representatives on earth. Therefore, whatever they say or do is divinely ordained, including removing afflictions such as COVID. For those reasons, many people believe evil forces superimpose problems on humans, and God can help spiritual leaders solve humanly problems. Those ideas help explain why spiritual help-seeking remains a common practice in Nigeria during the COVID pandemic, especially among women in the Southwest. The same ideas constitute a major determinant to medical health-seeking in the same region and elsewhere in the country.[40]

## Nigerian Women and Agency in Response to COVID-19

Despite the many factors adversely impacting Nigerian women's mental and physical well-being during the COVID pandemic, they have responded well. In 2020, Samuel Oladipo and Jimoh Owoyele surveyed ninety-six women in the Southwest whose ages ranged from twenty-two to fifty-nine. Approximately, 69 percent of the women were married, 29 percent never wed, and less than 2 percent were widowed. Almost 57 percent were Christians, and 43 percent were Muslims. Educational levels ranged from first university degree holders to individuals with doctorates.[41]

All respondents believed the COVID was real, could be deadly if not properly treated, and recommended strict adherence to safety precautions. When confronted with questions about which types of treatments they should receive, medical or spiritual, 95 percent preferred spiritual. Every respondent said she would rather attend an organized prayer meeting or engage in an individualized prayer session to handle COVID than consult a physician or some other professional caregiver. That majority response, which applied to both Christians and Muslims, epitomized the general belief that God is supreme, knows everything, and can do everything. In fact, eight out of ten women whom Oladipo and Owoyele surveyed indicated they would attend healing services because they believed God could heal all diseases.[42]

As a further testament to the women's general faith in godly intervention, 86 percent supported prayer vigils and organized chain links to assist those inflected with COVID. Because governmental stay-at-home orders, lockdowns, and shutdowns restricted physical movement during the pandemic, many women organized vigils, using the internet and various technologies. Other women held hourly prayers online. One hundred percent of respondents confirmed they would use anointing oils, prayer tokens, and other items that spiritual leaders prescribed for healing, while 15 percent said they would combine scientific medicines with spiritual elixirs.[43]

## Conclusion

Mental health is as important as physical health to well-being, which in our judgment should be a primary societal goal. Unfortunately, for many Nigerian women, longstanding cultural obstacles and impaired access to available healthcare services make good mental health challenging. Consequently, Nigerian women often rely on spiritual resources that have been central parts of Nigerian society since antiquity to deal with phenomena such as the COVID pandemic. Their continued reliance on spirituality is significant, but in our opinion Nigerians should utilize every cultural, economic, political, or social resource at their disposal to improve not only women's health but also every sex or gender's health. In a bittersweet element of the pandemic, it has drawn attention to the need for comprehensive responses to mental and physical healthcare challenges.

## Notes

1 "Mental Health Care in Anglophone West Africa," *Psychiatric Services* 65 (September 2014): 1084–87, esp. 1084.
2 See, for example, *WHO-AIMS Report on Mental Health System in Nigeria* (Ibadan, Nigeria: World Health Organization and Nigerian Ministry of Health, 2006).
3 Mohammed Yaya, "Nigeria: Six Out of 10 Nigerian Women Have Mental Illness—Psychiatrist," *Daily Trust*, February 18, 2019, https://allafrica.com/stories/201902180060.html.
4 Socrates Mbamalu, "Nigeria Has a Mental Health Problem," *Al Jazeera*, October 2, 2019, https://www.aljazeera.com/economy/2019/10/2/nigeria-has-a-mental-health-problem.
5 Cheluchi Onyemelukwe, "Stigma and Mental Health in Nigeria: Some Suggestions for Law Reform," *Journal of Law, Policy and Globalization* 55 (2016): 63–68.
6 Tosin Philip Oyetunji et al., "Suicide in Nigeria: Observations from the Content Analysis of Newspapers," *General Psychiatry* 34 (January 13, 2021), 1–7, doi: 10.1136/ gpsych-2020-100347.
7 Modupeoluwa Omotunde Soroye, Obinna O. Oleribe, and Simon D Taylor-Robinson, "Community Psychiatry Care: An Urgent Need in Nigeria," *Journal of Multidisciplinary Healthcare* 14 (May 10, 2021): 1145–48; Elena Scappaticci, "Mental Health: Free Psychological Support in Nigeria in

Response to COVID-19," *iD4d Sustainable Development News*, September 21, 2020, https://ideas4development.org/en/mental-health-nigeria-free-covid-19-psychological-support/.

8 Socrates Mbamalu, "Nigeria Has a Mental Health Problem," *Aljazeera*, October 2, 2019, https://www.aljazeera.com/ajimpact/nigeria-mental-health-problem-191002210913630.html.

9 *WHO-AIMS Report on Mental Health System in Nigeria*, 5.

10 *WHO-AIMS Report on Mental Health System in Nigeria*.

11 Osagie Ehanire, "First Case of Coronavirus Disease Confirmed in Nigeria," *Nigeria Centre for Disease Control*, February 28, 2020, https://www.ncdc.gov.ng/news/227/first-case-of-corona-virus-disease-confirmed-in-nigeria.

12 "Policy Brief: The Impact of COVID-19 on Women" (policy brief, United Nations, April 9, 2020) (hereafter cited as UN, "Policy Brief").

13 UN, "Policy Brief," 10.

14 UN, "Policy Brief," 10.

15 UN, "Policy Brief," 10.

16 UN, "Policy Brief," 10.

17 UN, "Policy Brief," 9, 10.

18 UN, "Policy Brief," 2, 4, 9, 16, 18, 19.

19 Annamaria Milazzo and Dominique van de Walle, "Nutrition, Religion, and Widowhood in Nigeria," *Economic Development and Cultural Change* 69 (January 2021): 951–1001; Ayodeji Oginni, Babatunde Ahonsi, and Francis Ukwuije, "Are Female-Headed Households Typically Poorer than Male-Headed Households in Nigeria?," *Journal of Socio-Economics* 45 (2013): 132–37.

20 S. E. Oladipo and S. K. Balogun, "Age, Extraversion, Anxiety and Marital Status as Factors of Spiritual Help-Seeking Behaviour of Women in Ibadan Metropolis," *Educational Research* 1 (February 2010): 1–7.

21 Oladipo and Balogun, "Age, Extraversion, Anxiety and Marital Status," 2 (also employing the term *prayer houses*), 3, 6.

22 Mercy Amba Oduyoye, *Beads and Strands: Reflections of an African Woman on Christianity in Africa* (Maryknoll, NY: Orbis Books, 2004), 83–84.

23 Samuel E. Oladipo and Jimoh W. Owoyele, "Why Do Many Nigerian Women Seek Spiritual Help?" (unpublished paper, 2020).

24 Oladipo and Owoyele, "Nigerian Women."

25 Godiya Allanana Makama, "Patriarchy and Gender Inequality in Nigeria: The Way Forward," *European Scientific Journal* 9 (June 2013): 115–44, esp. 115.

26 Ilesanmi Akanmidu Paul, "The Survival of the Yorùbá Healing Systems in the Modern Age," *Yorùbá Studies Review* 2 (spring 2018): 103–9.

27 Paul, "Survival."

28 J. S. Eades, *The Yoruba Today* (New York, NY: Cambridge University Press, 1980), 125.

29 Olufunmilayo I. Fawole1, Omowumi O. Okedare, and Elizabeth Reed, "Home was not a Safe Haven: Women's Experiences of Intimate Partner Violence during the COVID-19 Lockdown in Nigeria," *BMC Women's Health* 21 (January 2021): 1–7, https://doi.org/10.1186/s12905-021-01177-9.

30 Immigration and Refugee Board of Canada, "Nigeria: A Ritual by the Name of 'Isiku' that a Widow is Subjected to Upon the Death of Her Husband," *Refworld*, May 4, 2000, https://www.refworld.org/docid/3ae6ad702c.html.

31 Tomike I. Olawande et al., "Gender Differentials in the Perception of Mental Illness among the Yoruba of Ogun State, Nigeria," *Ife PsychologIA* 26 (2018): 134–53.

32  Regarding stigmatization and mental health in general, see Patrick W Corrigan et al., "What Is the Impact of Self-Stigma? Loss of Self-Respect and the 'Why Try' Effect," *Journal of Mental Health* 25 (February 2016): 10–15; and Bernice A. Pescosolido, "The Public Stigma of Mental Illness: What Do We Think; What Do We Know; What Can We Prove?," *Journal of Health and Social Behavior* 54 (March 2013): 1–21.

33  Tiziana Ramaci et al., "Social Stigma during COVID-19 and Its Impact on HCWs Outcomes," *Sustainability* 12 (May 2020): 1–13, https://doi.org/10.3390/su12093834.

34  For general effects of people who internalize ostracism, physical abuse, and other discriminatory behavior across the globe, as opposed to Nigeria, see Corrigan et al., "What Is the Impact of Self-Stigma."

35  Timothy Obiezu, "Fear and Stigma Keep Nigerians from Helping Contact Tracers," *Voice of America*, July 30, 2020, https://www.voanews.com/africa/fear-stigma-keep-nigerians-helping-contact-tracers.

36  Oladipo and Balogun, "Age, Extraversion, Anxiety and Marital Status"; O.O. Latunji and O.O. Akinyemi, "Factors Influencing Health-Seeking Behaviour among Civil Servants in Ibadan, Nigeria," *Annals of Ibadan Postgraduate Medicine* 16 (June 2018): 52–60.

37  Osayi Igberase and Esther Okogbenin, "Beliefs About the Cause of Schizophrenia among Caregivers in Midwestern Nigeria," *Mental Illness* 9 (2017): 23–27.

38  Igberase and Okogbenin, "Beliefs."

39  Chikaodiri Nkereuwem Aghukwa, "Care Seeking and Beliefs about the Cause of Mental Illness among Nigerian Psychiatric Patients and Their Families," *Psychiatric Services* 63 (June 2012): 616–18; Oladipo and Balogun, "Age, Extraversion, Anxiety and Marital Status."

40  Increase Ibukun Adeosun et al., "The Pathways to the First Contact with Mental Health Services among Patients with Schizophrenia in Lagos, Nigeria," *Schizophrenia Research and Treatment* 2013 (January 2013): 1–8, http://dx.doi.org/10.1155/2013/769161; Victor O. Lasebikan, Eme T Owoaje, and Michael C Asuzu, "Social Network as a Determinant of Pathway to Mental Health Service Utilization among Psychotic Patients in a Nigerian Hospital," *Annals of African Medicine* 11 (January–March 2012): 12–20.

41  Oladipo and Owoyele, "Nigerian Women."

42  Oladipo and Owoyele, "Nigerian Women."

43  Oladipo and Owoyele, "Nigerian Women."

# 27 African American Palliative Care amid the COVID-19 Pandemic

*John C. Welch*

## Introduction

The novel coronavirus, or COVID-19, is a major health crisis across the globe. In the United States, and African Americans have been dispropor-tionately impacted in terms of infections and deaths.[1] Medical professionals have conducted numerous studies that identify underlying health factors that correlate with high risks of COVID infections among African Americans.[2] Obesity, cardiovascular disease, cerebrovascular disease, malignant neo-plasms, diabetes, high blood pressure, and asthma are foremost.[3] Because those conditions are prevalent among African Americans, they have greater risks of COVID infection and death than white people. The large numbers of African Americans employed as essential workers is an additional fac-tor.[4] Besides working conditions and fears of infection, which all ethnic groups have experienced, mental anguish attributable to psychological and emotional distress from generations of societal injustice in the United States has compounded physiological issues among African Americans. Scientists refer to that phenomenon as the allostatic load.[5]

The coupling of the physiological and the psycho-emotional components of health with terminal physiological issues, despite treatability, is what necessitates palliative care. I will demonstrate that a variety of accessibil-ity concerns exist for African Americans, leaving many to suffer unneces-sarily. While those concerns are hardly novel, I emphasize the COVID-19 pandemic illuminates an array of health disparities about which the medi-cal community has known but has not address properly for decades. In my judgment, old and new knowledge should spur a moral response from a broad coalition of members in the faith community.

If history serves as a guide, the longstanding epidemic of racism in the United States will cause professional healthcare and government institu-tions to do less to prevent COVID-19 from harming black people than white people. By offering palliative care, I submit, properly trained members of the faith community can join with other social service professionals in healthcare to reduce emotional and spiritual distress among patients with chronic and terminal illnesses the pandemic has exacerbated.

DOI: 10.4324/9781003214281-32

## Intersections of Palliative Care, Spirituality, and Healthcare Morality

Balfour Mount, a physician at the Royal Victoria Hospital in Montreal, introduced the *term palliative care* in 1974. There is no universal definition, but many authorities agree that it is designed to alleviate suffering for patients and their loved ones. Originally, palliative care was almost indistinguishable from end-of-life care, as both were melded with hospice care and focused on death.[6] In 1990, the World Health Organization (WHO) described palliative care as "the active total care of patients whose disease is not responsive to curative treatment. The control of pain, other symptoms, and of psychological, social, and spiritual concerns is paramount. The goal of palliative care is the achievement of the best possible quality of life for patients and their families."[7]

In 2002, the WHO redefined palliative care as "an approach which improves the quality of life of patients and their families facing life threatening illness, through the prevention and relief of suffering, by means of early identification and impeccable assessment and treatment of pain and other problems physical, psychosocial and spiritual."[8] The shift from "disease not responsive to curative treatment" to "life threatening illness" was the most crucial element of the revised definition (which definition did not assume that diseases could respond to treatment).[9] Organizations such as the European Association of Palliative Care and the International Association of Hospice and Palliative Care did not agree with every aspect of the new definition and therefore continued to advocate for a consensus description that expanded the care continuum beyond life-threatening conditions.[10]

Whatever the particulars, introducing "interdisciplinarity into the usual functioning of a multidisciplinary team" is key to effective palliative care, according to scholar Pierre Boitte.[11] Given continuous physiological and emotional distress within African American communities, which COVID-19 compounds, compassionate redress is needed in response to government policies that generate or that sustain socioeconomic inequities causing disproportionate levels of chronic and terminal disease among African Americans.

Palliative care attends to the physical, psychological, and spiritual needs of patients with chronic and terminal illnesses. Such care also supports their families. Nevertheless, African Americans tend to underutilize it for numerous reasons, including limited awareness of the availability of palliative care and doubts about its benefits. Such doubts often stem from a broader African American distrust toward the healthcare system, especially forms of care that unfamiliar or speculative. When asked, countless people offer the so-called Tuskegee Experiment as a significant reason for mistrust.[12] From 1932 to 1972, the US Public Health Service (along with Tuskegee Institute originally) used 600 African American men in Macon County, Alabama, in a syphilis research study under manipulative pretenses, including guarantees of medical insurance the service ultimately did not provide.[13]

Beyond unfair government experimentations, many African Americans are inclined to rely strongly on spiritual means when facing challenges and uncertainties. While numerous studies affirm the importance that many patients suffering from terminal and other advanced illnesses place on spirituality and religion as coping mechanisms, some practitioners have resisted incorporating spirituality in the delivery of care—despite evidence supporting its effectiveness in certain situations.[14] To integrate spirituality into palliative care, one should understand the roles that various medical professionals perform in such integration. Some professionals avoid asking patients about their spiritual beliefs because the questions seem to invade privacy. Even so, therapist Michael M. Olson and a group of his research colleagues suggested in 2006, "openness to discussions of spirituality contributes to both better health and better physician-patient relationships."[15]

Spirituality, in the context framed by Olson and company, can be beneficial not only to patients but also to caregivers, both professional and lay. Regarding African Americans, psychologist Ronald K. Barrett in 2002 proclaimed it was "almost unthinkable that you can have an honest, intelligent discussion about death and dying, unless you deal with the centrality of spirituality in the black experience."[16] Whereas Barrett believed spirituality was foundational to any honest and intelligent conversation about death and dying, I believe human dignity and other moral tenets are the foundations of conversations about palliative and hospice care. As disease decimates a patient's body, the patient's value system tends to become more pronounced. For example, in the midst of the suffering that can accompany a terminal malignancy, nearly every patient still wants others to recognize his or her worth. Such an expectation of respect often reflects a desire to suffer and ultimately die with dignity, though nurturing that dignity can be complex, especially in relation to African Americans due to the longstanding history of sociopolitical oppression and other forms of abuse.[17]

Insufficient access to healthcare has been a persistently insidious obstacle to black well-being. When COVID-19 began spreading rapidly across the United States in early 2020, hospital administrators throughout the country realized quickly their institutions had too few intensive care unit beds, ventilators, and other resources to meet the needs of actual or projected patients.[18] In March, the month the WHO declared COVID a pandemic,[19] New York Governor Andrew M. Cuomo predicted the state would need 30,000 such beds and 40,000 ventilators.[20] At the time the state possessed approximately 1,600 and 4,000, respectively.[21] Cuomo and others in his administration helped medical centers in the state double the number of ICU beds from 1,600 to 3,500 by utilizing beds on a naval medical ship called *Comfort* and by converting space inside the Jacob K. Javitz Convention Center of Manhattan.[22]

Of course not every American city had access to a seaport where a naval vessel could supplement a shortfall in medical beds. That being the case, the likelihood of every person with severe COVID-19 symptoms receiving adequate care was extremely low. That fact posed broad moral dilemmas to government officials, hospital administrators, and other individuals who had to decide who got potentially life-saving resources. In general, black, biethnic, and other people of color suffered disproportionately to white people.[23]

## The Need for Justice

Palliative care aims to alleviate the physical, psychosocial, and spiritual suffering of chronically ill people. Because a disproportionate number of people of color suffer with COVID-19, which induces psycho-spiritual distress, I believe healthcare administrators have moral and ethical obligations to allocate sufficient time and resources to address ethnic/racial disparities.

During the late twentieth century, as the palliative care movement matured in the United States, philosopher and physician Hugo T. Engelhardt Jr. helped popularize a now familiar inquiry regarding whether people were beneficiaries or victims of a natural lottery or a social lottery.[24] If one was disadvantaged because of a genetic predisposition, or was "born unhealthy," Engelhardt speculated, one had lost in the natural lottery, and other members of society had moral and ethical obligations to assist.[25] Engelhardt's contentions applied to efforts to raise awareness and, moreover, to support for birth defects such as Down Syndrome, Cerebral Palsy, and Spinal Bifida.

Engelhardt's social lottery constructs remain important to African Americans and their healthcare. While many Americans are born with serious health conditions, the natural lottery, many more African Americans are victims of the social lottery and its most persistent embodiment, racism. Distributive justice is a paradigm that seeks to address both lotteries. In 1976, medical ethicist Robert M. Veatch declared that gross social inequities in the United States were wrong and that, owing to power differentials between privileged and unprivileged Americans, the unprivileged were not situated well to represent themselves so the privileged often dismissed them.[26] For philosophers Tom Beauchamp and James Childress, justice is the "fair, equitable, and appropriate distribution determined by justified norms that structure the terms of social cooperation."[27]

In addressing distributive justice—especially health access disparities and the need for reform—ethicist Lisa Cahill's 2005 book, *Theological Bioethics*, builds on philosopher John Rawls's characterization of healthcare as an essential common good.[28] Cahill, however, qualified the issue of public responsibility for access to health by pointing out the need for spiritual responses from a variety of religious groups and respected theologians, who could undertake activism if necessary.[29] Her work is significant for my discussion of African Americans and healthcare. Among other things, she emphasized the importance of spirituality and religion to communal well-being.[30]

## Conclusion

If healthcare administrators improved board-certified hospital chaplains' capacities, their visibility, and integrated them into the treatment paradigm, the administrators would take an important step toward the healthcare reform I envision. Administrators also should review policies that create moral distress among healthcare practitioners, thereby affecting practitioners' well-being and their quality of care they delivery. The considerable amount of scholarship about such distress in multiple clinical disciplines can aid the administrators.[31]

Lawmakers also have important roles to perform to ensure the type of healthcare reform I propose. They should write and adopt legislation to expand access to care for those disadvantaged on account of racism and consequent socioeconomic inequities. Such legislation is crucial to promoting the dignity of human beings, a major part of making my health equity dream a reality.

## Notes

1　By late 2020, black and biethnic Americans were dying at 2.4 times the rate of whites Americans—ninety-two per 1,00,000 compared to thirty-nine per 1,00,000, respectively. "COVID-19 Is Affecting Black, Indigenous, Latinx, and Other People of Color the Most," *COVID Tracking Project*, September 15, 2020, https://covidtracking.com/race.

2　See for example, United States Centers for Disease Control and Prevention, "People with Certain Medical Conditions," May 13, 2021, https://www.cdc.gov/coronavirus/2019-ncov/need-extra-precautions/people-with-medical-conditions.html (hereafter cited as CDC).

3　CDC, "People with Certain Medical Conditions."

4　Ashley Imlay, "Why Utah Researchers Say Black Americans Face Higher Rates of COVID-19 Death Rates," *Deseret News*, September 8, 2020, https://www.deseret.com/utah/2020/9/8/21427384/utah-covid19-pandemic-326-new-cases-deaths-racial-disparities-university-of-utah.

5　Bruce S. McEwen, "Protective and Damaging Effects of Stress Mediators: Central Role of the Brain," *Dialogues in Clinical Neuroscience* 8 (December 2006): 367–81.

6　Ilora Finlay, "UK Strategies for Palliative Care," *Journal of the Royal Society of Medicine* 94 (September 2001): 437; Mary Pickett, Mary E. Cooley, and Debra B. Gordon, "Palliative Care: Past, Present, and Future Perspectives," *Seminars in Oncology Nursing* 14 (May 1998): 86.

7　World Health Organization, *Cancer Pain Relief and Palliative Care: Report of a WHO Expert Committee* (Geneva, Switzerland: World Health Organization, 1990), 11 (hereafter cited as WHO).

8　"WHO Defines Palliative Care," n.d., http://www.who.int/cancer/palliative/definition/en/.

9　Rien Janssens et al., "Moral Values in Palliative Care: A European Comparison," in Hank ten Have and David Clark, eds., *The Ethics of Palliative Care: European Perspectives* (Philadelphia, PA: Open University Press, 2020), 72–86 (first quotation on 75); "WHO Defines Palliative Care" (second quotation).

10　Lukas Radbruch et al., "Redefining Palliative Care—A New Consensus Based Definition," *Journal of Pain and Symptom Management* 60 (October 2020): 754–76.

11  Pierre Boitte, "Elderly Persons with Advanced Dementia," in Ruth B. Purtilo and Henk A.M.J. ten Have, eds., *Ethical Foundations of Palliative Care for Alzheimer Disease* (Baltimore, MD: Johns Hopkins University Press, 2004), 97–111, esp. 100.

12  Joel D. Howell, "Trust and the Tuskegee Experiments," in *Clio in the Clinic: History in Medical Practice*, ed. Jacalyn Duffin, 213–25 (New York, NY: Oxford University Press, 2005).

13  United States Centers for Disease Control and Prevention, "The Tuskegee Timeline," April 22, 2021, https://www.cdc.gov/tuskegee/timeline.htm.

14  Sian Cotton et al., "Spirituality and Religion in Patients with HIV/AIDS," *Journal of General Internal Medicine* 21, supplement 5 (December 2006): S10; "Palliative Care and Spiritual Care: The Crucial Role of Spiritual Care in the Care of Patients with Advanced Illness," *Current Opinion in Supportive and Palliative Care* 6 (June 2002): 273; Michael Stefanek, Paige Green McDonald, and Stephanie A. Hess, "Religion, Spirituality and Cancer: Current State and Methodological Challenges," *Psycho-Oncology* 14 (June 2005): 453; and George Handzo, "Spiritual Care for Palliative Patients," *Current Problems in Cancer* 35 (November–December 2011): 365.

15  Michael M. Olson et al., "Mind, Body, and Spirit: Family Physicians' Beliefs, Attitudes, and Practices Regarding the Integration of Patient Spirituality into Medical Care," *Journal of Religion and Health* 45 (summer 2006): 244.

16  Ronald K. Barrett and Karen S. Heller, "Death and Dying in the Black Experience," *Journal of Palliative Medicine* 5 (October 2002): 795.

17  Kathryn Proulx and Cynthia Jacelon, "Dying with Dignity: The Good Patient versus the Good Death," *American Journal of Hospice and Palliative Medicine* 21 (March/April 2004): 116.

18  Dante Chinni, "Tracking ICU Beds Reveals Potential Holes in Treatment," *NBCNews*, April 5, 2020, https://www.nbcnews.com/politics/meet-the-press/tracking-icu-beds-reveals-potential-holes-treatment-n1177046.

19  "WHO Director-General's Opening Remarks at the Media Briefing on COVID-19," *World Health Organization*, March 11, 2020, https://www.who.int/director-general/speeches/detail/who-director-general-s-opening-remarks-at-the-media-briefing-on-covid-19. March 11, 2020.

20  Lydia Ramsey Pflanzer and Jeremy Berke, "Converted Operating Rooms and Shuffled Patients: How NYC Scrambled to Turn 1,600 ICU Beds into 3,500 to Care for the Sickest Coronavirus Patients," *Business Insider*, April 9, 2020, https://www.businessinsider.com/coronavirus-nyc-more-than-doubled-its-icu-capacity-in-weeks-2020-4

21  David Jackson, "Trump Questions NY Request for 30,000 Ventilators: 'I Don't Believe You Need 40,000 or 30,000 Ventilators,'" *USA Today*, March 27, 2020, https://www.usatoday.com/story/news/politics/2020/03/27/coronavirus-trump-questions-new-yorks-request-30-000-ventilators/2924263001/; Pflanzer and Berke, "Converted Operating Rooms and Shuffled Patients."

22  "Converted Hospital Rooms and Shuffled Patients: How NYC scrambled to turn 1,600 ICU beds into 3,500 to care for the sickest coronavirus patients."

23  "Health Notes: People of Color Suffer Disproportionate Impact of COVID-19 Pandemic," September 3, 2020, *Yale School of Medicine*, https://medicine.yale.edu/news-article/health-notes-people-of-color-suffer-disproportionate-impact-of-covid-19-pandemic/; Pinar Karaca-Mandic, Archelle Georgiou, and Soumya Sen, "Assessment of COVID-19 Hospitalizations by Race/Ethnicity in 12 States," *JAMA Intern Medicine* 181 (January 2021): 131–34.

24  H. Tristram Engelhardt Jr., *Foundations of Bioethics*, 2nd ed. (New York, NY: Oxford University Press, 1996), 380.

25  Engelhardt, *Foundations of Bioethics*, 380.
26  Veatch and Branson, *Ethics and Health Policy*, 133–34.
27  Tom L. Beauchamp and James F. Childress, *Principles of Biomedical Ethics*, 6th ed. (New York, NY: Oxford University Press, 2009), 241.
28  Lisa Sowle Cahill, *Theological Bioethics: Participation, Justice, and Change* (Washington, DC: Georgetown University Press, 2005); John Rawls, *A Theory of Justice*, rev. ed. (Cambridge: Harvard University Press, 1999).
29  Cahill, *Theological Bioethics*, 132.
30  Cahill, *Theological Bioethics*.
31  Susan Houston et al., "The Intensity and Frequency of Moral Distress among Different Healthcare Disciplines," *Journal of Clinical Ethics* 24 (summer 2013): 98–112; Giulia Lamiani, Lidia Borghi, and Piergiorgio Argentero, "When Healthcare Professionals Cannot do the Right Thing: A Systematic Review of Moral Distress and Its Correlates," *Journal of Health Psychology* 22 (January 2017): 51–67.

# 28 Black Religion, Mental Health, and the Threat of Hopelessness during the COVID-19 Pandemic

*Danjuma G. Gibson*

> To be a Negro in this country and to be relatively conscious, is to be in a rage almost all the time.
>
> —James Baldwin (1961)

## Introduction: The Fatigue of Being Conscious

Catastrophic events in the United States often have affected black and brown communities disproportionately to other ethnic groups. Therefore, that healthcare inequity has revealed itself during the COVID-19 pandemic or that certain individuals have downplayed the significance of systemic racism, repeating hegemonic narratives that justify discrimination, does not surprise me. According to one belief, black and brown people have character flaws such as laziness that cause inequity.[1] Regarding COVID in particular, medical scholars Ibraheem M. Karaye and Jennifer A. Horney conducted research on social vulnerability, and their conclusions refute the biased ideas the aforementioned laziness belief epitomizes:

> In the U.S., 44 million adults are underinsured, including 48% of adults aged 19–64 years who face high copays and out-of-pocket costs. Nearly 2 million Americans lack running water in their homes, with Native Americans 19 times more likely and African Americans and Hispanics twice as likely to lack indoor plumbing than whites. This makes basic infection prevention practices, such as hand washing, less attainable for mitigating the spread of the disease. The lack of paid sick leave among low-wage earners, whose work often involves face-to-face interaction, also makes self-quarantining a less feasible option. In addition, because of low wages, many workers hold multiple jobs to support their families, which may further increase their risk of contracting or spreading COVID-19.[2]

Over the long run, the impact of COVID at the intersection of structural racism and inequity takes a severe toll on the mental health of communities, especially those forced to exist at the margin. In addition to ethnic minorities and poor people, those with mental disorders are particularly vulnerable.

DOI: 10.4324/9781003214281-33

In 2021, a team of scholars that included Benedetta Vai "found consistent evidence that patients with psychotic and mood disorders, and those taking antipsychotics or anxiolytics, represent susceptible subgroups."[3] Vai and her colleagues also concluded that "exposure to antipsychotic and anxiolytic drug treatments initiated before contracting COVID-19 was associated with severe COVID-19 outcomes."[4]

The findings of Ibraheem Karaye, Jennifer Horney, Benedetta Vai, and her associates remind me of a statement James Baldwin made in 1961 about conscious African Americans risking being enraged constantly.[5] As a theologian who also is a licensed psychotherapist, I believe the mental health field remains ill-equipped to address the intersection of structural racism, inequality, and the COVID pandemic. Those items have exacted serious psychological tolls on black and brown communities particularly, creating a breeding ground for hopelessness and nihilism. I propose mental health resources grounded in black religious experience are needed. As Audre Lorde declared in 1988, "caring for myself is not self-indulgence, it is self-preservation, and that is an act of political warfare."[6]

## Depoliticizing Hope

In this essay, I equate hope with the power of imagination. I define hope as the mental, spiritual, and emotional capacity and practice to imagine an improvement of circumstances in the future that does not yet exist in the present but that is grounded in the realities, truths, fears, joys, and concerns of the present. Psychic capacity, intentionality, creative imagination, and groundedness in reality, or truth telling, are key components of my definition; and courage, stamina, and tenacity of personal and communal intentionality are central to realizing it. In seasons of injustice, hope along with imagination tend to be the first human faculties to fail.

In a 1992 book titled *We Have Been Believers*, James Evans Jr. warned of hope that was disconnected from reality.[7] He stated the "hope of a people can never be separated from their history without dire consequences. A hope that does not come to terms with history can become unbridled optimism and idealism, or the cover for unchecked expansionism. History anchors hope," Evans continued.[8] But considering that "history and hope always belong to a specific community, they can mean different things to different people," he concluded.[9]

Hope, understood in the manner Evans described, represents the human faculty to creatively imagine a better future, thereby enabling individuals and communities to love deeply and fully in the present. They can live courageously for the next day despite the realities of evil and oppression of the current day. Hope is not static; it is dynamic. Hope is a practice of creative imagination. Depoliticizing and deconstructing hope as a virtue or proof of personal character, then, liberates individuals and communities to grieve and to mourn losses related to structures of injustice, such as oppression.

Grief and mourning are not antagonistic to hope; instead, grief and mourning are manifestations of hope. The capacity of hopeful imagination ebbs and flows with both the number and the complexity of challenges an individual or a community faces (and not as if circumstances do not impact the strength of hope or a community's capacity for hope).

## Black Religion, Transitional Therapeutic Spaces, and Cultivating Capacities of Hope

The idea that black churches can function as therapeutic spaces for black and brown communities is not a novel idea. In 1998, Cheryl Gilkes recognized that, "for black professionals who worked in overwhelmingly white settings, the cultural comfort of these black churches provided therapeutic relief from the micropolitics of being black in a white and unpredictably hostile world."[10] For black women in particular, Gilkes declared, the "church not only continues to function as a therapeutic community but it also reinforces women's sense of importance by thriving because of women's gifts and support in ways that are observable to the entire community in spite of institutional sexism."[11] In this essay, I develop Gilkes's idea of black religion as a therapeutic container by demonstrating how it accomplishes that mission.

Psychoanalytic theory long has observed the concept of play and transitional spaces, or objects, and their values to human growth and development. I conceptualize transitional spaces as areas between the inner worlds of individuals and the exterior worlds of realities. It is within those spaces, or with objects that represent the space, that significant psychic and emotional growth can occur for individuals and groups. Specifically, they can learn how to play in the space or, alternatively, to play with objects that represent the space.

By play I intimate the ability and the maturity to engage with abstraction, the subjective, and nonreality. According to Donald W. Winnicott, a man recognized internationally for his work on transitional space, it "is an intermediate area of experiencing, to which inner reality and external life both contribute ... an area that is not challenged, because no claim is made on its behalf except that it shall exist as a resting-place for the individual engaged in the perpetual human task of keeping inner and outer reality separate yet interrelated."[12]

I cannot understate the importance of the intermediary transitional space in terms of resisting hopelessness and the onset of nihilism. Both the interior world of a person or a group and the exterior world the person or the group contributes to transitional space, the area where the deep (and oftentimes unconscious or unrecognized) interior needs, desires, joys, concerns, and hopes of an individual or a group interact with the often uncontrollable, ruthless, and painful elements of the external world. In transitional space, similar to a child, one is able to play—that is, to exert omnipotent control over what is imagined and conceived in the space, or, quoting Winnicott, to exert "magical control."[13] A person or a group is able to realize in transitional space what he, she, or its members often are unable to accomplish in the exterior world. But it is by playing that personal emotional growth is achieved, that self-love, robust subjectivity, and agency are formed, that courage is cultivated, and thereby a constantly maturing engagement with the exterior world (i.e., reality) is achieved.

For black and brown people forced to exist at the margins in a Western social structure built on ideas that reflect the supremacy of whiteness, human capacities for play and imagination in transitional spaces represent final lines of defense between experiencing humanization and internalizing dehumanization. Winnicott expressed notions of play and imagination in terms of creativity:

> It is creative apperception more than anything else that makes the individual feel that life is worth living. Contrasted with this is a relationship to external reality which is one of compliance, the world and its details being recognized but only as something to be fitted in with or demanding adaptation. Compliance carries with it a sense of futility for the individual and is associated with the idea that nothing matters and that life is not work living. In a tantalizing way many individuals have experienced just enough of creative living to recognize that for most of their time they are living uncreatively, as if caught up in the creativity of someone else, or of a machine.[14]

Living *as if caught up in the creativity of someone else, or of a machine*, tends to be the experience of black and brown people who have come to the realization they are existing in spaces and institutions not designed with them in mind. Consequently, identifying transitional spaces in such institutions or spaces can be limited at best or at worse an exercise in futility where one's capacity for hope and sense of subjectivity wears away slowly. However, black and brown religious experiences and praxes have the potential to represent transitional spaces wherein they can strengthen their sense of hope and guard against the onset of hopelessness and nihilism.

## Conclusion: Strengthening Practices of Hope through Black Religious Experience

In addition to the depoliticizing of hope, this essay calls for a recognition and, moreover, an understanding of black religion as a possible transitional space for restoring and fortifying hope. The essay likewise advocates for a radical reclaiming of the multiplicity of worship modalities historically found in black religious heritage to increase the distribution channels of mental health resources available for black and brown people who are experiencing hopelessness and nihilism due to continual media images of black bodies being murdered with impunity in broad daylight by law enforcement agents or by white citizens, stories of private white citizens engaging in the deadly game of calling the police on black people engaged in mundane daily activities, legitimate accounts of slow justice or of no justice, and accurate reports of black people having greater percentages of COVID-19 infections and deaths collude to instigate hopelessness and eventually nihilism.

The intersection of the COVID pandemic with structural racism and injustice can instigate hopelessness and nihilism in marginalized communities. Black religion can serve as a transitional space where hope, understood as the capacity to imagine a better future, can be restored or reinvigorated. The internal praxis of the Black Church represents a transitional or liminal space in which individuals and groups can engage in play to exercise control over personal or communal visions for justice and equity. That act ultimately can contribute to the buildup of hope, which in turn can inform, underwrite, and eventually propel the external praxis of religion that is related to achieving liberation for black communities.

## Notes

1　Gregorio A. Millett et al., "Assessing Differential Impacts of COVID-19 on Black Communities," *Annals of Epidemiology* 47 (July 2020): 37–44; Eboni G. Price-Haywood et al., "Hospitalization and Mortality among Black Patients and White Patients with Covid-19," *New England Journal of Medicine* 382 (June 2020): 2534–43.

2　Ibraheem M. Karaye and Jennifer A. Horney, "The Impact of Social Vulnerability on COVID-19 in the U.S.: An Analysis of Spatially Varying Relationships," *American Journal of Preventative Medicine* 59 (June 2020): 321.

3　Benedetta Vai et al., "Mental Disorders and Risk of COVID-19-Related Mortality, Hospitalization, and Intensive Care Unit Admission," *Lancet Psychiatry* 8 (September 2021): 809.

4　Benedetta Vai et al., "Mental Disorders," 809.

5　James Baldwin et al., "The Negro in American Culture," *Cross Currents* 11 (summer 1961): 205–24, esp. 5 (containing the quotation that forms the epigraph, an excerpt from "The Negro Writer in America," a group discussion that Nathan Hentoff, erstwhile editor of *Downbeat*, moderated between Baldwin, Emile Capouya, Lorraine Hansberry, Langston Hughes, and Alfred Kazin in January 1961).

6　Audre Lorde, *A Burst of Light and Other Essays* (1988; repr., Mineola, NY: Dover, 2017), 130.

7　James H. Evans Jr., *We Have Been Believers: An African-American Systematic Theology* (Minneapolis, MN: Fortress Press, 1992).

8　Evans, *We Have Been Believers*, 141.

9　Evans, *We Have Been Believers*, 141.

10　Cheryl Townsend Gilkes, "Plenty Good Room: Adaptation in a Changing Black Church," *Annals of the American Academy of Political and Social Science* 558 (July 1998): 108.

11　Gilkes, "Plenty Good Room," 115.

12　D. W. Winnicott, *Playing and Reality* (1971; repr., New York, NY: Routledge, 2005), 3.

13　Winnicott, *Playing and Reality*, 12 (employing "[magical] omnipotent control"), 13, 15, 55, 63.

14　Winnicott, *Playing and Reality*, 87.

# Index

Note: Italicized page numbers refer to tables. Page numbers followed by "n" refer to notes.

access to care 21–22
Access to the COVID-19 Tools Accelerator 153
active listening 168–169
Adeboye, E.A. 126, 129
Africa: structural and systemic influences on COVID-19 impact 5–6; vaccination disparities 7
African Caribbean Evangelical Alliance 160
African Church of Philadelphia 19
African Diaspora 29
African Medicines Regulatory Harmonization Initiative 79
African Methodist Episcopal (AME) Church 19, 87–95; *Church Preparation and Response to Potential Pandemics* (International Health Commission) 94; Council of Bishops 94, 95; General Conference (1956) 94; General Conference (1976) 94; General Conference Commission 94; influenza, combating 90–93; International Health Commission 94; modern healthcare responses, ecclesial structuring of 93–95; responses to yellow fever outbreaks 87–90; Southwestern Georgia Conference 91
African Methodist Episcopal Zion Church 153
African Vaccines Regulatory Forum 79
Aina, A. 211
Akindayomi, J.O. 126
Allen, C.E. 91, 95

Allen, R. 19, 87, 91, 121–122, 142–146; *Narrative of the Proceedings of Black People, during the Late Awful a Calamity in Philadelphia, in the Year 1793: And Refutation of Some Censures, Thrown Upon Them in Some Publications, A* 88, 122, 145
AME *see* African Methodist Episcopal (AME) Church
American College of Obstetricians and Gynecologists 212
Amos, E. 138
Anderson, R. 115
Antigua: racial disparities in rates of COVID infections and mortalities 4
Argentina: racial disparities in rates of COVID infections and mortalities 4
Arnett, B.W. 89, 90
Ashmun Institute 100
"Ask the Docs: Preemptive Planning for Public Worship" 124
*Atlanta Constitution* 102
*Atlantic Monthly* 101

Baldwin, J. 217, 253
Barbuda: racial disparities in rates of COVID infections and mortalities 4
Barrett, R.K. 247
Batswana 67, 68, 73n1
Baylor University 231
BCSA *see* Black Church Supported Agriculture (BCSA)
Beauchamp, T. 248
beneficence 209
Berry, L.H. 94
Berry, L.L.: *Century of Missions of the African Methodist Episcopal Church, A* 93–94
Bethune, M.M. 122

Bianchi, D. 211
biopower 70
black aid workers 142–146
Black Church 36, 38–40, 227, 256;
    movement 19; role in mitigating
    food insecurity 62–63; solutions
    to historical healthcare problems
    178–181
Black Church Food Security Network
    62–63
*Black Church in the African American
    Experience, The* (Lincoln and
    Mamiya) 123
Black Church Supported Agriculture
    (BCSA) 63
black communities 39–40
black equality 146
black health 51–56; planetary
    perspective of 52–56
Black Lives Matter movement 35
black majority churches (BMCs):
    actual and potential responses to
    mental health challenges 186–188;
    backstories of 159–161; black mental
    health challenges and responses by
    185–189; mental health challenges,
    mapping dynamics of 186; resources
    of 159–161; responses to black health
    urgencies in UK 158–162, **159**;
    responses to COVID-19, 167–170,
    188–189
Black Mamas Maternal Association
    212
Black Maternal Health Association 212
Black Maternal Health Momnibus Act
    212
black mental health: challenges and
    responses by Britain's BMCs 185–189
black religion 253–254
Blake, C., Sr. 135–136, 140
BMCs *see* black majority churches
    (BMCs)
Boitte, P. 246
Boko-Haram 166
Bosque, J.A. 44
*Boston Globe* 31
Brazil: racial disparities in rates of
    COVID infections and mortalities 4
Britain *see* United Kingdom (UK)
*Brown* (1954) 113
Brown, M. 144
Brown, Pastor 63
Brown III, H. 62
Bruce, M. 39

Burnett, M.J. 94
Butchart, A. 70, 71
Butler, W.H.H. 92, 93
Byrd, W.M. 116n15
Byrd II, W. 19

Cahill, L.: *Theological Bioethics* 248
Canada: African-Canadian Civic
    Engagement Council 31; British
    North America Act of 1867, 29;
    and Haidi on infectious diseases,
    disputed linkages between 27–30;
    Innovative Research Group 31;
    racial disparities in rates of COVID
    infections and mortalities 3;
    structural and systemic influences
    on COVID-19 impact 5; vaccination
    disparities 6
Canadian Council of Churches 31
Carey, M.: *Short Account of the
    Malignant Fever … in Philadelphia,
    A* 145
Caribbean Conference of Churches
    (CCC) 150–151, 155
Caribbean Public Health Agency 7
Caribbean social vulnerabilities
    149–150
CARICOM 154
Carribean region 76; racial disparities
    in rates of COVID infections and
    mortalities 4; structural and systemic
    influences on COVID-19 impact 5, 6;
    vaccination disparities 7
Carter Metropolitan CME Church 115
Castro, F.R. 44
Catalyst Church, Philadelphia,
    Pennsylvania 21
categorical racism 190n16
Catherine, J. 99, 100
Catholic Doctors Association of Kenya
    78
CCC *see* Caribbean Conference of
    Churches (CCC)
CCCH *see* Collins Chapel
    Connectional Hospital (CCCH)
Centenary Biblical Institute (later
    Morgan State University) 122
Center on Budget and Policy Priorities
    58
*Century of Missions of the African
    Methodist Episcopal Church, A*
    (Berry) 93–94
chemical pollution 54
Childress, J. 248

Chile: vaccination disparities 7
Christian Church, in the Caribbean 150–152; responses to medical and economic challenges of the COVID-19 pandemic 153–154
Christianity 8–9, 18–19, 69
Christian Methodist Episcopal Church 113
*Christian Recorder* (formerly *Christian Herald*) 88–90
Church Agencies Network Disaster Operations (Can Do) 139
Churches Together in England 187
Church of God in Christ (COGIC) 134–140; approaches to healthcare infrastructure 137–138; ecclesial assessments 137–138; General Board 137; origin of 134–137; theological perspective on medical science 134–137
Church of the Nazarene 153
church responsiveness 8–9
civil society leaders 1
Civil War 91, 111
Clarkson, M. 143, 145
Clayton, L.A. 116n115
Cleage Jr., A.B. 62
CME *see* Collins Chapel Colored Methodist Episcopal (CME) Church
Coalition for Epidemic Preparedness Innovations 153
Coleman, M.H. 112
*Collection of Receits [Receipts] for the Use of the Poor, A* (Wesley) 111
Collins Chapel Colored Methodist Episcopal (CME) Church 110; responses to the COVID-19 pandemic 114–115; Women's Missionary Council 112
Collins Chapel Connectional Hospital (CCCH) 110, 113–116; as case study of Wesley's vision 112–114
Collins Chapel Old Folks' Home and Hospital (CCOFHH) 110, 111, 113, 118n24
Colombia: racial disparities in rates of COVID infections and mortalities 4
colonialism 148
colonial matrix of power 67; construction of African body within 70–71
colonial missionary healthcare paradigms 71–73

colonial racism 36–37
communalism 194
Conference of National Black Churches 115
"Convention on the Prevention and Punishment for the Crime of Genocide" 210
Cooper, L.A. 20, 22, 39
Cooper, R.S. 46
Cornerstone Faith Assembly 138
Council for International Organizations of Medical Sciences 80
Council of Black Led (later Majority) Churches 160
COVAX 153
COVID-19 pandemic: BMCs responses to 188–189; burden on health and wellness 203; in Caribbean Countries 149–150, **150**; CME Church responses to 114–115; in Cuba 48; extent of food security during 59–60; infections and mortalities, racially disproportionate 2–4; racializing religious institutions during 17–23; structural and systemic influences on 4–6
COVID-19 Prevention Network Faith Initiative Team 231
COVID Tracking Project 219
Crutchfield, C. 114
Cuba: COVID-19 in 48; Cuban Revolution (1959) 44; healthcare accomplishments 44–47, **45**; independence of 43–44; Latin American School of Medicine (ELAM) 45–46; *policlinicos* 46; War of Independence (1895–1898) 44
cultural competency 168
Cuomo, A.M. 247

*Daily Memphis Avalanche* 112
Dancy, B.L. 28
Daniels, J.K. 117n20
Daytona Literary 122
Del Pino, J.E. 121
deoxyribonucleic acid (DNA) 120, 121
Development Bank of Latin America 152
disciplinary power 70
Divine, J. 62
diviner-healers (*dingakas*) 67, 71
DNA *see* deoxyribonucleic acid (DNA)

Dominican Republic: racial disparities in rates of COVID infections and mortalities 4; vaccination disparities 7
Dortélus, D. 30
Drew Theological School 231
Drew Theological School Religion 227
Du Bois, W.E.B. 101; *Philadelphia Negro, The* 177

EAC *see* Evangelical Association of the Caribbean (EAC)
earth system 53
earth system science 53–55
Ebola ourbreaks 139, 166
ecologies 52–56
Edgell, P. 18
Eggers, R. 79
Egypt: International Conference on Population and Development 209
E.H. Crump Memorial Hospital 113
emotion regulation 212
empathy 169
employment, and food insecurity 60–61
Engelhardt, H.T., Jr. 248
enslavement, as slave healthcare deficit 116n15
environmental racism 52, 54, 57n10
Ethiopia 197
ethnic inequality 158
Etienne, C.F. 203
Europe 75, 76; medical science 36; vaccination disparities 7
European Association of Palliative Care 246
European Union 152
Evangelical Association of the Caribbean (EAC) 150–151, 153, 155
Evans, J., Jr.: *We Have Been Believers* 253

faith-sector leaders 1
faith-sector responses 7–9
FAS *see* Free African Society (FAS)
Feeding America 59–60
Fifteenth Street Presbyterian Church, Washington, DC 99, 101–104
film, as pedagogical tool for trauma- and resiliency-informed theology and liturgy 215–221; COVID-19 pandemic 218–220; *Open Wounds: A Story of Racial Tragedy, Trauma, and Redemption* 215, 217–218, 220, 221; storytelling 220–221

Flipper, J.S. 91
food insecurity 58–63; Black Churche, role of 62–63; employment and 60–61; housing instability and 61–62
food security: during COVID-19, extent of 59–60
Ford Foundation 113
Forten, C.L. 101
Foucault, M. 68, 70
Fowler, W. 103
France 148; racial disparities in rates of COVID infections and mortalities 3
Free African Society (FAS) 121
freedom 99–101
Friendship-West Baptist Church, Dallas, Texas 21

Gaede, B. 71
Gardner, L. 89
GDP *see* gross domestic product (GDP)
genomic literacy 194
genomics 193
Gere, R. 31
Ghana: racial health inequalities 37
Gilkes, C. 254
Glad Tidings International COGIC 138
Global Health Forum 227
Global North 28; racial disparities in rates of COVID infections and mortalities 3, 4; vaccination disparities 7
Global South 77; racial disparities in rates of COVID infections and mortalities 3, 4; vaccination disparities 7
Graves Drug 138
Great Depression 76, 113
Great Migration 62
Grimke, F.J. 99–105
Grimke, H 99
Grimke, S. 100
gross domestic product (GDP) 149, 150

Haiti: and Canada on infectious diseases, disputed linkages between 27–30
Haiti Teen Challenge 204
Hamer, F.L. 62
Hansen, H. 228
Harmony Presbytery of South Carolina 37
Harris, K. 182
Harris, T.A. 115
Harvard Law School 100

Haynes III,, F.D. 225
Healing Stripes Hospital 127
healthcare morality 246–248
health equity 225–232
health literacy 194
Heckler, M.M. 177
herd immunity 153
historical crisis mitigation, by black methodists 121–122
*History of the Colored Methodist Episcopal Church in America* (Phillips) 112
HIV/AIDS *see* human immunodeficiency virus/acquired immunodeficiency syndrome (HIV/AIDS)
hope: cultivating capacities of 254–255; depoliticizing 253–254; through black religious experience, strengthening practices of 255–256
Horney, J.A. 252, 253
House Energy and Commerce Committee 212
housing instability, and food insecurity 61–62
Hull (Boss) Jr., E. 113
human immunodeficiency virus/acquired immunodeficiency syndrome (HIV/AIDS) 27–32, 68, 75–77, 79, 114; in Nigeria 127–128; in the twenty-first century 30–31; in UK 158–161
Hunter, S.S. 28, 29

Ihekweazu, C. 166
image ontology 69, 70
IMF *see* International Monetary Fund (IMF)
imperialism 148
Independent Communications and Marketing 128
Indigenous healthcare paradigms 71–73
Industrial Training School for Negro Girls (later Bethune-Cookman University) 122
influenza 90–93, 104–105
intergenerational resiliency 217–218
intergenerational trauma 217
International Association of Hospice and Palliative Care 246
International Conference on Harmonization on Good Clinical Practice 80

International Geosphere-Biosphere Programme 55
International Monetary Fund (IMF) 130, 131n10
International Organization of the Francophonie 30
Irukwu, A. 187–189
Islam 193

Jacob K. Javitz Convention Center of Manhattan 247
Jamaica: racial disparities in rates of COVID infections and mortalities 4; vaccination disparities 7
Jean, M. 30
Jefferson Medical College 92
Jenkins, J.K., Sr. 21
Jim and Jane Crowism 102, 219
Jim-crow car legislation 102
job loss 5
Johns, V. 62
Johnson, W.B. 89, 96n14
Jones, Absalom 143, 144
Jones, Allen 19, 87, 91, 95, 121–122; *Narrative of the Proceedings of Black People, during the Late Awful a Calamity in Philadelphia, in the Year 1793: And Refutation of Some Censures, Thrown Upon Them in Some Publications, A* 88, 122, 145
Judeo-Christianity 193, 194
justice 209; need for 248; reproductive 209–210

Kamau, F. 138
Karaye, I.K. 252, 253
Kelly, R.L. 178, 182
Kennelly, J.F. 46
Kenya 75–81; Investigational Medicinal Products 80; Kenya Council of Catholic Bishops 77, 78; Kenya Medical Research Institute 79; medical experimentation on black bodies 76–77; Ministry of Health 77, 80; structural and systemic influences on COVID-19 impact 6; vaccine trials, race and ethical evaluations of 80–81; vaccine trials in 77–80
King, M.L., Jr. 20, 116, 177
Kloppers, P.J. 71
Ku Klux Klan 102

Lacks, H. 178–179
Landis, C. 150

262    *Index*

Latin America: racial disparities in rates of COVID infections and mortalities 4; structural and systemic influences on COVID-19 impact 5, 6; vaccination disparities 7
Leath, J.N. 95
Le Bonheur Children's Hospital 110
Lee, C.H. 117n20
Lee, J.C.H. 28, 144
"Let's Move" campaign 230
Lichtenstein, A. 77
Lincoln, C.E. 104; *Black Church in the African American Experience, The* 123
Lincoln University 100
Lioyd, V. 18
LMS *see* London Missionary Society (LMS)
Locht, C. 75
London Missionary Society (LMS) 57, 68, 69
low-wage jobs 5
Lucini, B.A. 152

Mackenzie, J. 73n2
Madison, J.H. 89
*Mahoko a Becwana* 67–68
Malloy, P. 77
Mamiya, L.H.: *Black Church in the African American Experience, The* 123
Marsh, V.M. 194
Martin, J.C. 113
Martin, W.S. 113
Mason, C.H. 134
Mbembe, A. 69
McBride, D. 112
McNeill, L.H. 180
Medicaid 212
medical science 36
Meharry Medical Department (formerly the Meharry Medical Department of Central Tennessee College) 111
Meharry Medical Department, Central Tennessee College 112
meningitis 76
mental health 237–242, 252–256
Methodism 110–111, 120
Methodist Episcopal Church 121
Methodist Episcopal International Health Commission 230
Metzl, J.M. 228

Mexico: racial disparities in rates of COVID infections and mortalities 4
Mignolo, W.D. 67
Miller, K. 101
Mira, J.-P. 75
Moeti, M. 78
Moffat, R. 69, 73n3
Moltmann, J. 51
Montague, E. 99, 100
Moroka, M.T. 68
Moshabela, M. 71
Mother Bethel African Methodist Episcopal (AME) Church 144, 145
Mother Bethel Church, Philadelphia 92
Mottley, M.A. 149–150
Mwiti, G.K. 216
Myriad's *MyRisk* questionnaire 227

NAACP *see* National Association for the Advancement of Colored People (NAACP)
Namaste, V.K. 31
Namibia: racial disparities in rates of COVID infections and mortalities 3; structural and systemic influences on COVID-19 impact 6
*Narrative of the Proceedings of Black People, during the Late Awful a Calamity in Philadelphia, in the Year 1793: And Refutation of Some Censures, Thrown Upon Them in Some Publications, A* (Allen and Jones) 88, 122, 145
National AIDS Trust 161
National Association for the Advancement for Colored People 113
National Association for the Advancement of Colored People (NAACP) 101
National Church Leaders Forum 161, 188
Netherlands 148
New St. Paul COGIC 138
New Testament 37
New York Theological Seminary 228
Niagara movement 101
Nigeria: Centre for Disease Control 238; Federal Ministry of Health 166; government response to COVID-19, 166–167; in historical perspective 165–166; HIV/AIDS 127–128; Ministry of Health 237; National Bureau of Statistics 166; National Centre for Disease Control

240; Public Health Institute 166; Redeemed Christian Church of God (RCCG) 126–130; spirituality 238–241; structural and systemic influences on COVID-19 impact 5; women and agency in response to COVID-19, 241–242
nonmaleficence 208–209
North America: medical science 36; vaccination disparities 7
Northern-based Methodist Episcopal Church, Meharry 112
North Georgia AME Church 91

Obama, B. 181, 230
Obama, M.: "Let's Move" campaign 230
Oladipo, S. 239, 241
Old Folks' Home and Hospital 113
Old Testament 37, 104–105
Olson, M.M. 247
*Open Wounds: A Story of Racial Tragedy, Trauma, and Redemption* 215, 217–218, 220, 221
Operation Higher Ground 62–63
oppression 18, 36, 37, 102, 204–206, 212, 239, 241, 253; reproductive 210; sociopolitical 247; systemic 206
Organisation for Economic Co-operation and Development Centre 5, 152
Orguñez-Garcia, P. 46
*Ottawa Citizen* 31
Owoyele, J. 239, 241
Oxfam International 4

palliative care 245–249
Pan American Health Organization 153, 154
Parks, R.M. 144
pastoral care 202–206
Pentecostal Assemblies of the West Indies 153
Peru: racial disparities in rates of COVID infections and mortalities 4
Pew Research Center 120, 165
Pfizer 76
*Philadelphia Negro, The* (Du Bois) 177
Phillips, C.H.: *History of the Colored Methodist Episcopal Church in America* 112
physical health 237–242
Pittsburgh Annual Conference 90, 92
planetary boundaries 55

Pleasant Hope Baptist Church 62
*Primitive Physic* (Wesley) 111
Project CHURCH (Creating a Higher Understanding of Cancer Research and Community Health) 180–181
Prostate Health Education Network 181
Protestant Episcopal Church of North America 19
Protestantism 18
psychoanalytic theory 254
public health 204–205
Puerto Rico: racial disparities in rates of COVID infections and mortalities 4

Quijano, A. 67
Quirot, A. 45

race and religion, intersecting 18–19
racial equality 142
racial inequality 158
racial injustice 145
racialized discourse, in the twenty-first century 30–31
racialized healthcare inequities 35–40; history of 36–39
racialized religion and COVID-19 pandemic: access to care 21–22; exposure risks 19–21
Rah, S.-C. 223n29
Randolph, A.P. 144
Rawls, J. 248
RCCG *see* Redeemed Christian Church of God (RCCG)
Red Cross 102
Reddick III, L.L. 114
Redeemed Christian Church of God (RCCG): approaches to prevent HIV/AIDS 127–128; Healing Stripes Hospital 127; Redeemers *Aids Initiative for People and Community* (formerly the Redeemed Aids Programme Action Committee) 128; responses to contemporary health urgencies in Nigeria 126–130
redemptive potentiality 218
Regional One Health 110
religion: and race, intersecting 18–19
Religious Society of Friendz 100
Rendez-Vous Church 202, 204, 205
reproductive health 208–213
reproductive justice 209–210
respect for autonomy 208

Rhone, T. 138
Ridley, J.H. 112, 117n20
Rivers, S. 117n20
Roberts, B.W. 89
Room In The Inn Homeless Ministry 115
Ross, L. 210
Ross, W.P. 89, 90
Rowley, K. 154
Rush, B. 87–88, 143
Ryan White HIV/AIDS program 181

salvation 68
Sampson, W.W. 89
Santana, M.-A. 28
SARS-CoV-2 (severe acute respiratory syndrome coronavirus 2) 128, 178, 192, 195, 202
*Scribner* 101
Seawright, H.L. 94
Senagal: structural and systemic influences on COVID-19 impact 6
Setswana: colonial missionary healthcare paradigms 71–73; contested power over black bodies 68–69; Indigenous healthcare paradigms 71–73; medical practices 67–73; missionary mindset 68–69
Shaffer, C.T. 92, 93
Sharma, A. 152
Sharp Street Memorial UMC 122
Shi, J. 216
*Short Account of the Malignant Fever ... in Philadelphia, A* (Carey) 145
SIDS *see* small island developing states (SIDS)
Sister Song (or SisterSong) 210, 212–213
slavery 99–101, 145, 148
small island developing states (SIDS) 150, 154
Smith, B. 117n20
Smith, W.M. 148
social depravation 190n16
Soil to Sanctuary Market 63
Solinger, R. 210
SOS Racisme 75
South Africa 144; arrival of missionaries in 70; green (nature conservation) and brown (social justice) agendas, tension between 56n2; racial disparities in rates of COVID infections and mortalities 3–4; structural and systemic influences on COVID-19 impact 5

sovereign power 70
Spanish-American War 91
spirituality 39, 238–241, 246–248
SSA *see* sub-Saharan Africa (SSA)
Steffen, W. 55
Stevenson, B. 101
St. George's Methodist Church 19, 144
stigmatization 194
St. James Church 138
St. Jude Children's Research Hospital 110
storytelling 220–221
St. Paul's AME Church, Washington 93
Structural Adjustment Program 127, 131n10
sub-Saharan Africa (SSA): Africa Centres for Disease Control and Prevention 196; Africa Taskforce for Novel Coronavirus 196; cultural and religious influences on genetic interventions in 192–197; racial disparities in rates of COVID infections and mortalities 3; structural and systemic influences on COVID-19 impact 5
*Sun* 113
supportive close relationships 212
Sutter Health 179
systemic racism 63

*Télémaque* 144
tetanus vaccine 77
Thairu, Y. 129
*Theological Bioethics* (Cahill) 248
thingification of black bodies 71
Traditional Health Practitioners Act (22 of 2007) 72
transitional therapeutic spaces 254–255
Trinidad and Tobago: racial disparities in rates of COVID infections and mortalities 4; vaccination disparities 7
Trump, D.J. 115, 137, 182
Turner, H.M. 89
Tuskegee Experiment 246
Tuskegee Study of Untreated Syphilis in the Negro Male 178

Uganda: structural and systemic influences on COVID-19 impact 5
UMC *see* United Methodist Church (UMC)
Underwood, L. 212

United Kingdom (UK) 148; Adult
Psychiatric Morbidity Survey (2014)
185; black majority churches 185–189;
Department of Health 185; *Guide to
Healthy Living: Mosques* (PHE) 161;
HIV/AIDS 158–161; Housing Act
of 1996, 186; Mental Health Act of
1983, 185; National Health Service
(NHS) 160; National Health Services
Information Centre for Health and
Social Care 186; Office of National
Statistics 158; *Positive Faith* (PHE)
161; Public Health England (PHE)
158, 160, 161, 188; racial disparities
in rates of COVID infections and
mortalities 3; vaccination disparities
6–7
United Methodist Church (UMC):
dialectical model of COVID-19
response 123–124; Multi-Ethnic
Center for Ministry of the
Northeastern Jurisdiction 124;
responses to COVID-19, 120–124
United Nations 173n34, 238
United Nations Economic Commission
for Latin America and the Caribbean
152
United Nations Educational, Scientific,
and Cultural Organization 152
United Nations Nigeria Isolation
Center 129
United States (US) 17, 75, 148, 151;
Bureau of Justice Statistics 216;
Bureau of Labor Statistics 20;
Centers for Disease Control and
Prevention (CDC) 17, 35, 76–77,
94, 120, 134–137, 166; Constitution
19; Coronavirus Aid, Relief, and
Economic Security Act 21; Dental
Health Act 182; Department
of Health and Human Services
212; disease, disaster, and racial
reckoning in 1790s Philadelphia
142–144; First Amendment of
the Constitution 20; healthcare
inequities in 35–40; Health Equity
and Accountability Act of 2020,
182; Healthy Start Initiative 181;
Maternal Care Access and Reducing
Emergencies Act 182; Mothers and
Offspring Mortality and Morbidity
Awareness Act of 2019 (MOMMA)
182, 184n28; National Institute of
Allergy and Infectious Diseases

137; National Institutes of Health
181; National Institutes of Health
(NIH) 76; National Prison Statistics
program 216; Patient Protection and
Affordable Care Act 181, 230; Public
Health Service 246; reckoning with
racial illness 144–146; structural and
systemic influences on COVID-19
impact 5; Thirteenth Amendment
to the US Constitution 220; *Unequal
Treatment: Confronting Racial and
Ethnic Disparities in Health Care*
(Congress) 177, 178; United States
Department of Agriculture (USDA)
59
University of Abuja Teaching Hospital
129
University of California-Merced
study of COVID health impact on
California workers 5
University of the Western Cape 51
Unthank, T.C. 93
Urban Institute: Health Reform
Monitoring Survey 59
US *see* United tates (US)

vaccination disparities 6–7
Vai, B. 253
Vanbert Health Equity Project (VHEP)
225–232, 233n10
Veatch, R.M. 248
Venezuela: vaccination disparities 7
Vesey, D. 144
VHEP *see* Vanbert Health Equity
Project (VHEP)
Volcy, J. 202–205

Waters, J.C. 88–89
*We Have Been Believers* (Evans) 253
Wemos Foundation 78, 81
#WENEED2SURVIVE 123
Wesley, C. 121
Wesley, J. 110, 121; *Collection of Receits
[Receipts] for the Use of the Poor,
A* 111; holistic vision and mission
110–112; *Primitive Physic* 111
West Angeles Cathedral 138
Weston, N. 99
Wild, W. 72
Williams, D.R. 20, 22, 39, 211, 220
Williams, H. 70
Williamson, H., Sr. 115
Wilson, W. 102
Winnicott, D.W. 254, 255

Winters, L. 78
Witchcraft Suppression Act (3 of 1957) 71
Wolff, N.. 216
Women of African Descent for Reproductive Justice 209–210
women of color, impacts of COVID-19 on 211–213
Women's Parent Mite Missionary Society 90
Womeodu, R.J. 124
Woodson, C.G. 101
World Bank 131n10; 2019 Human Capital Index 203
World Council of Churches 151
World Health Organization (WHO) 17, 45, 77–79, 94, 105, 114, 149, 166, 202, 219, 227, 237, 246; Commission on Social Determinants of Health 1
World Medical Association 80

World War I 90, 102, 103, 230
World War II 186
Wright, R.R., Jr. 93

yellow fever outbreaks, AME responses to 87–90
Young, Q. 182n3
Yukich, G. 18

Zdanowicz, C. 48
Zethar Al-Umma Foundation 170
Zion World Prayer and Missions (ZWPM) 165, 167–170; active listening 168–169; cultural competency 168; effective engagement 169–170; empathy 169
Zuma, T. 71
ZWPM see Zion World Prayer and Missions (ZWPM)

3 20